GENDER AND SEXUALITY
IN CHINESE MEDICINE

Extraordinary Chinese Medicine
The Extraordinary Vessels, Extraordinary Organs,
and the Art of Being Human
Thomas Richardson with William Morris
ISBN 978 1 84819 419 9
eISBN 978 0 85701 371 2

Heart Shock
Diagnosis and Treatment of Trauma with Shen-Hammer
and Classical Chinese Medicine
Ross Rosen
Foreword by Dr. Leon Hammer
ISBN 978 1 84819 373 4
eISBN 978 0 85701 330 9

Treating Emotional Trauma with Chinese Medicine
Integrated Diagnostic and Treatment Strategies
CT Holman, MS, LAc
ISBN 978 1 84819 318 5
eISBN 978 0 85701 271 5

The Art and Practice of Diagnosis in Chinese Medicine
Nigel Ching
ISBN 978 1 84819 314 7
eISBN 978 0 85701 267 8

Psycho-Emotional Pain and the Eight Extraordinary Vessels
Yvonne R. Farrell, DAOM, LAc
ISBN 978 1 84819 292 8
eISBN 978 0 85701 239 5

Counselling Skills for Working with Gender Diversity and Identity
Michael Beattie and Penny Lenihan with Robin Dundas
ISBN 978 1 78592 741 6
eISBN 978 1 78450 481 6

GENDER AND SEXUALITY IN CHINESE MEDICINE

CATHERINE LUMENELLO

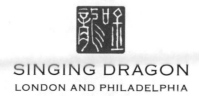

SINGING DRAGON

LONDON AND PHILADELPHIA

First published in 2020
by Singing Dragon
an imprint of Jessica Kingsley Publishers
73 Collier Street
London N1 9BE, UK
and
400 Market Street, Suite 400
Philadelphia, PA 19106, USA

www.singingdragon.com

Library of Congress Cataloging in Publication Data
A CIP catalog record for this book is available from the Library of Congress

British Library Cataloguing in Publication Data
A CIP catalogue record for this book is available from the British Library

ISBN 978 1 84819 379 6
eISBN 978 0 85701 335 4

Printed and bound in the United States

Certified Chain of Custody
Promoting Sustainable Forestry
www.sfiprogram.org
SFI-01268

SUSTAINABLE FORESTRY INITIATIVE

SFI label applies to the text stock

For Clara,
and all our children,
that they may live free.

Contents

SECTION III: THE SEXUAL JOURNEY

SECTION IV: THE EMOTIONAL LANDSCAPE

Acknowledgments

The writing of any book is simply not possible without the contributions of many participants in the initial conceptualizations, the refinement of thought and word, and the actual publication and presentation of the work itself. Without Claire Wilson, Emily Badger, Hannah Snetsinger, and the entire Singing Dragon team, this book would simply not exist. I am grateful they offered me the opportunity to flex my wings and see what happened. My colleagues and peer reviewers, Leslie Romero, Angela Rosen, and Nigel Ching, deserve a hefty nod of credit for agreeing to support the efforts of a first-time author. I am also truly indebted to my colleague and assistant on this project, Alex Andrew, who gifted me with mad editing skills, laughter, and budding friendship as we navigated quick sands of theory and language.

Over the years there have been many patient people that supported and witnessed me processing my journey as practitioner, healer, and writer – which is not always a pretty process. There were violent scribbles on wine-stained hotel bar napkins, interrupted family meals, long periods of silent contemplation, and a few critically timed motorcycle rides. I remain grateful to so many people – students, clients, teachers, lovers, acquaintances, kinksters, and poly-folk – that have contributed their wisdom in untold ways, as well as challenging me time and again to communicate better in both word and action.

Specifically I must recognize Janet K. Bardwell for fifteen years of connection, support, and mutual love for Art, Qigong, and Chinese Medicine. My Buddhist and Yoga-loving therapists Peg Kaufman and Lara Darrow for facilitating humor and child-like curiosity on the journey of spiritual self-discovery. Folk musician Namoli Brennet for poetry and sound that reflects the desolate places where beauty comes rough and raw. And I am honored to acknowledge Carolyn L.H. Fort, EJ Millstone, and Michelle W. Bower for the most amazing friendships, deep and challenging conversations, and snorting laughter that has lifted me off the floor multiple times.

Finally, there are those closest to my heart and home, whose loving commitment I both treasure and surrender to each day. Matthew L. Gould arrived exactly on time during the writing of this book, heralding profound lessons in trust, compassion, and unabashed joy-seeking. For a full decade Benjamin D. Heckman has offered me unconditional adoration and agape, both calling out my craziness and meeting me exactly where I am with contemplative, raucous meep-ing. Ben is also an amazing co-parent to our own little light, Clara T. Lumenello, who keeps me grounded with snuggles, giggles, play, and singing her to sleep every night with our song. You three are my anchor, the breeze, and the stars.

Disclaimer

The information in this book is designed for healthcare professionals well versed in Chinese Medicine and the tradition of Acupuncture. There is no one Chinese Medicine methodology preferred over any other for concerns related to gender and sexuality. In fact, this book blends Classical, Five Element (Five Phases, *Wu Xing*), Japanese, Medical Qigong, and TCM diagnosis concepts with both well-known (Acupuncture, Herbs, Tuina) and the more esoteric (Essential Oils, Gemstone Therapy) modalities of Chinese Medicine. It is assumed that the reader:

- is proficient in the differential diagnosis techniques particular to their tradition

- will prioritize individual evaluation of any client, including overall health and Constitution, over printed theory to determine the most appropriate treatment principles and modalities

- will thoroughly research any modalities with which they are unfamiliar before recommending or practicing them (see Bibliography)

- will consider the treatment options provided throughout this book as examples rather than a 'prescription' for any given condition.

CONDITIONS OF THE SPIRIT

Regardless of the presence of physical symptoms, many issues related to gender and sexuality are considered Spirit conditions. When developing a comprehensive treatment plan, the importance of psycho-spiritual etiology affects choice of modality, point selection, needle insertion technique, length of treatment session time, and intention-setting. For example, treating Blood Deficiency caused by emotional stress with nourishing Herbal Formulae and Diet is important, but inviting the client to recognize just how much stress their psyche is subject to (the true cause for 'depletion' of the Blood) is the real key to full recovery.

OVERTREATMENT

Throughout this book is a note to avoid 'excessive' or 'over' treatment of the Extraordinary Vessels. Practitioners are reminded that any acu-point and its associated channel can be damaged by either aggressive technique or frequent use, so reverence for the power of *any* point is appropriate.

Extraordinary Vessels are special, as they serve as the reservoirs for Yin, Yang, Qi, and Blood. Damage to these structures can come from the aggressive or frequent needling already mentioned, or it may arise from asking them to 'mobilize' when they are too deficient to offer assistance. An example of this is to needle the Ren Mai when there is already a system-wide Yin Deficiency. A better initial approach would be a combination of Essential Oils, Gemstones, Herbal Formulae, Diet, and Qigong to nourish and stabilize the overall Yin substances before stimulating the Vessel with Acupuncture.

Notes on the Text

TERMINOLOGY

Choosing a simplified term that refers to multiple communities with various needs was not easy. Diverse Gender and Sexuality (DGS) was selected to represent the many facets of gender, sexuality, and relationship choices as a method of inclusion, but it is not meant to imply that the unique concerns of each individual are the same as any other.

ABBREVIATIONS

Throughout the text, abbreviations are used to refer to various channels, including:

- Extraordinary Vessel – EV
- Lung – LU
- Large Intestine – LI
- Stomach – ST
- Spleen – SP
- Heart – HT
- Small Intestine – SI
- Urinary Bladder – UB
- Kidney – KI
- Pericardium – PC
- San Jiao – SJ
- Gallbladder – GB
- Liver – LV

Preface

I come to this project after 15 years specializing in severe emotional stress and Trauma recovery, with extensive experience working in the LGBTQ+, BDSM, and polyamorous communities. I have also taught at two Chinese Medicine schools in the United States, and independently taught Qigong for self-cultivation and external healing. In each of these settings I've witnessed deep yearning for unbiased, frank, and empowering information about gender, sex, sexuality, and relationship. After fielding hundreds of questions from clients, colleagues, and students of all gender and sexual identities, this text covers many of the questions I was asked, as well as some that no one dared speak out loud.

As a child growing up in the 1970s and 1980s, there were no popular books, television shows, advertisements, or movies with two mommies, consensual triads, or gender-diverse individuals. Raised in New England (which remains steeped in the anti-sexual morality of Puritanism), there simply were no informed discussions or language debates around sexuality. I first heard the term 'bisexual' in my late teens, and only with extensive searching discovered 'queer' in my mid-20s. It wasn't until my mid-30s that I met an openly polyamorous person, and shortly thereafter attended my first event at a BDSM club. With lack of language and exposure to these concepts in my youth, realizing my own identities has not been an easy process and the ability to discuss sex openly is a skill I've slowly achieved. Unburdened contemplation of gender and sexuality issues was simply not part of my formative years, just as it had not been for generations before me.

But this has changed.

We are in the midst of an unprecedented era of human history. A large portion of humanity now has the opportunity to consider life beyond their daily survival needs, along with access to an international community of opinion. The open-mindedness of American, European, and certain indigenous cultures has spread across the globe, penetrating even the most remote and conservative populations. From the comfort and privacy of their living rooms, millions can dip their toes in the palace of Travel and Adventure to help broaden their perspective, and many are using this window to delve into the most important of spiritual questions: 'Who am I?'

The quest for self-actualization is not unique to individuals from the Diverse Gender and Sexuality (DGS) communities, but the opportunity for *every person* to express their thoughts and desires is a very recent phenomenon. The increasing visibility of DGS perspectives obviously brings more possibility to explore, but it has also stirred intense backlash and unfortunate reminders that prejudice has not been eliminated from our own communities. As issues of gender, sex, sexuality, and relationship continue to expand within the global consciousness, Chinese Medical professionals must compassionately embrace each person's journey into these fundamental aspects of existence. Open-hearted acceptance will not only allow all our clients to express their truest selves, but will also keep the profession at the forefront of holistic medicine worldwide.

To best serve the wide spectrum of human experience, the first section of this text identifies changes that are necessary within the practice of Chinese Medicine. Each of us has likely been raised with cultural bias, so we must simultaneously learn to be better allies *and* agree to eliminate professional practices that can easily cause physical or emotional harm. The second section examines binary thinking and gender constructs through Yin–Yang theory, the Three Treasures, and the spiritual journey of the Nine Palaces, with a chapter dedicated to gender transitioning concerns. In the third section, sex, sexuality, and relationship come to the forefront, with a thorough overview of sexual energetics and the basics of sexual and emotional attraction, as well as individual chapters dedicated to sex-based health concerns and relationship power dynamics.

The most important section may be the last, which examines emotional etiology. As Chinese Medicine practitioners, we know that *all chronic disease involves emotion*, so as international violence and persecution remains on-going, it is critical to consider emotional etiology (including Secrecy, Repression, etc.) for every individual *regardless of their current or assumed identity*. Although this book does not specifically address issues of intersectionality among minority populations (such as women, people of color, and those adversely impacted by classism), the concepts presented regarding the role of cultural oppression in the creation of emotional etiology certainly apply.

The global conversation around gender and sexuality will certainly not end soon. The visible presence of LGBTQ+ actors, politicians, and sports icons, as well as drag queen competition, polyamorous relationship, and BDSM-themed entertainment have brought these issues to the forefront of consciousness for both the general public and the next generation. Children growing up in the age of increasing possibility will only continue to raise their voices, and Chinese Medicine must be ready to meet all of humanity with open-hearted healing.

May we each choose the path of Love.

Vermont, USA
June 2019

Section I

A PRACTICE OF LOVE

Whenever a Great Physician treats disease…[he] should first of all develop a marked attitude of compassion. He should commit himself firmly to the willingness to make every effort to save every living being.

– Sun Si-Mao[1]

1   As quoted in Hicks, Hicks, and Mole 2011, p.40.

TERMINOLOGY: BASIC DEFINITIONS

(an incomplete list)[1]

- **BDSM** (abbreviation for Bondage, Discipline/Domination, Sadism/Submission, Masochism) a wide variety of erotically charged behaviors engaged in by consenting adults, which may or may not involve emotional or sexual intimacy – *see also Kink*

- **Cisgender** a person whose anatomical sex and gender identity align (i.e., assigned male at birth, identifies as male)

- **Closeted** in a state of secrecy in regard to one's sexuality, especially used in regard to homosexuality (i.e., 'in the closet')

- **Gender** a combination of one's internal self-perception of their own gender (i.e., Gender Identity), and the external display of dress, demeanor, and social behavior (i.e., Gender Expression)

- **Heteronormative** a world view that promotes heterosexuality as the norm in regard to sexual orientation, often with prescribed gender roles

- **Homophobia** a form of dislike or prejudice toward homosexual people

- **Kink** a sexual practice or desire often highly specific to the individual that is considered outside cultural norms – *see also BDSM*

- **Monogamy** the practice of being sexually and/or intimately involved with only one person at a time

- **Polyamory** the practice of being sexually and/or intimately involved with more than one person at a time, with the knowledge and consent of all parties

- **Sex** the act of physical, sexual intimacy between consenting adults

- **Sexuality** a person's preference for specific styles of sexual contact, and their capacity for sexual feelings, desire, and activity

---

1   More definitions are found at the beginnings of Sections II and III.

- **Straight** a heterosexual person; someone attracted to the 'opposite' sex based on anatomical differences or gender identity (i.e., a female attracted to a male, and vice versa)

- **Transgender** (also called Transsexual) a person whose anatomical sex and gender identity do not align (i.e., assigned female at birth, identifies as male)

- **Queer** a person whose gender, sexual identity, and/or orientation does not correlate with heteronormative or binary gender expectations; also used as an umbrella term for the entire LGBTQ+ community

Chapter 1

HEALING FROM WITHIN

- Identifying Blocks
- Five Element Treatments
- Addressing Root Emotions
- Physical Obstructions: Qi and Phlegm

Classism, homophobia, racism, sexism, and xenophobia have left a mark on each of us, typically at such an early age that most people cannot remember another way of being. Although exposure to prejudice is no individual's fault, it is the responsibility of every adult to address the consequences head-on. In order to do that, each person must first realize that they – just like everyone else – has been raised with cultural bias.

None of us was born with prejudice. These unhealthy beliefs are taught and enforced by multiple cultural structures including educational institutions, religious traditions, community or family members, and consumer marketing. Though not always based in personal experience, these opinions may be strongly defended by the individual that clings to them. Whether one's bias is openly evidenced by word or action, or covertly lying deep in the subconscious, unhealthy belief will form obstructions that can impact the physical, emotional, or spiritual health of the individual.

As Hicks, Hicks, and Mole wrote, 'Practitioners who strive to accept themselves are likely to also accept whatever arises from their patients' (2011, p.39). Only by accepting the possibility that each person – including ourselves – has been exposed to prejudice is it possible to 1) do something about it, and 2) help others. In order to do this, we must also recognize that unhealthy belief can come from inside any group or culture, including the Diverse Gender and Sexuality (DGS) communities. Over the years I have heard unsettling comments from individuals with various identities and backgrounds:

- Bi- or pansexuality doesn't exist – that person is *just closeted*, or needs to *pick a side*.

- Homosexuality, queer-ness, and/or LGB-identity is *only a 'white people thing'.*

- Polyamory is *more evolved* than monogamy.

- *Everyone* is kinky, no matter what they say.

- *All* pornography and those that view it are disgusting.

Each of these statements reflects the presence of unhealthy belief and cultural bias.

As practitioners and healers of Chinese Medicine, our own biases can interrupt the ability to fully accept, have compassion for, and truly love our clients. However large or small, conscious or subconscious our beliefs may be, if we choose to ignore the possibility of prejudice toward others, our capacity to heal is reduced. Without addressing our own internal obstructions and the underlying beliefs that created them, then, as Sun Si-Mao instructed, our commitment to 'save every living being' will falter. This chapter includes methods to help recognize the presence of prejudice, as well as methods to transform these opinions through Five Element theory, by addressing root emotions, and by treating the physical substances – Qi and Phlegm – that can directly prevent proper movement and evolution of thought.

IDENTIFYING BLOCKS

Each person has been exposed to prejudice. Whether conscious or subconscious, the presence of unhealthy belief forms obstruction at the physical, emotional, or spiritual level. Fortunately, it is possible to discern one's own internal blocks to self-knowledge, emotional growth, and spiritual potential. One method available to all practitioners is quiet, introspective meditation on topics related to gender, sexuality, or relationship.

The goal of this practice is to identify any emotions or physical sensations that can pinpoint the location of an obstruction. Fortunately, getting started is relatively easy! One only needs a short period of time to sit or rest – even ten minutes will sometimes do – and a comfortable place to do so. Once you've settled in, breathe deeply, allowing the mind to settle and the day's events to pass. In the space of silence, ask yourself simple, open-ended questions related to DGS topics, such as:

- When did I first hear this belief?

- How did I learn this idea?

- How does this make me feel?

- Where do I feel something?

When asking introspective questions, it is important to remain open-hearted and forgiving, free of self-blame, with simultaneous loving attention to emotions and physical sensations. The purpose of the practice is to dive as deeply as possible into the roots of belief. It will likely take more than one session for superficial emotions to step aside and allow deep-rooted opinions to surface, so patience is key to this process.

Over time, one might notice clear memories that surface, or clouded visions of memory that are difficult to recall. There may be strong emotions that rise up with specific words or images. Perhaps a chronic tension spot flares up, or just an overwhelming sense of fatigue, hunger, or other physical sensation. Any emotional or physical symptoms experienced in this process can indicate areas of concern or suggest methods of self-treatment, so take note of these experiences. After a few sessions, there should be clear evidence of consistent memory, emotion, or physical sensation that is triggered; these are the areas to target through self-treatment. If no consistencies are found, there are three options to consider: more frequent (and potentially longer) sessions that allow for more introspection in order to get to the root; pursuing another method of introspection such as through Qigong practice; or the possibility that Fluid Stasis (Phlegm or Blood) has obfuscated the root.

Once the root of prejudice is uncovered, self-treatment can begin. It takes consistent intention and time to retrain one's thoughts, so expect it to take weeks or months to unwind at each level. Plan to repeat the process of introspective questioning at regular intervals (i.e., monthly, semi-annually) to see what new information may have come forth, ready to be released.

FIVE ELEMENT TREATMENTS

One method of releasing prejudice is based in Five Element theory. Imagery, emotions, or physical symptoms one discovers through the introspective meditation discussed above may easily fall into elemental correspondences. For example, one might see flashes of green, while feeling angry or frustrated and physically bound, unable to move; these are all indicative of Wood Element issues.

For those that practice Qigong, both Five Healing Sound and Five Healing Color forms (see Appendix III) can help confirm the presence of a Five Element block. These forms can also be used to diagnose obstructions if the introspective questioning method did not resonate. For example, while doing these exercises in the traditional generating sequence order, one or two exercises may prove more difficult, in the physical movement, sound tone, or color visualization; this can be indicative of a blocked area.

The complete list of Five Element correspondences (i.e., organs, tissues, sounds, emotions, etc. – see Appendix I) may be helpful in identifying areas of concern, but the following is a list of common complaints that correspond to Five Element blocks:

- Water: Terror, strong temperature changes (both hot and cold), libido or pelvic area stimulation, arthritic pain aggravation, lumbar or sacroiliac pain, urgent need to urinate, difficulty visualizing a 'gemstone quality' black-blue, overall movements are too slow.

- Wood: Anger, headaches, shoulder tension, blurry vision, hard to stretch the right side of the body, sounds are too loud, sense of overall impatience.

- Fire: Anxiety, palpitations, hot flashes or heat sensations (especially in the Upper Jiao: hands, chest, face), overall movements are too fast.

- Earth: Queasy stomach, clenched abdomen, weak legs and arms, difficulty visualizing a golden/honey yellow (often a dark mustard-green or -brown), sound is consistently high-pitch or off-tone.

- Metal: Chest tightness, shortness of breath/shallow breath, cough with/without Phlegm, difficulty visualizing a silvery white color (often dark grey).

Five Element obstructions are treated through the generating and control sequences, along with clearing Qi Stagnation and/or Phlegm as needed. Treatment is focused on righting the elemental issue(s) so that the entire system has proper flow; this will likely take some time to unwind. Primary self-treatment modalities are Acupuncture/Acupressure, Qigong exercises, and Essential Oils.

- Acupuncture/Acupressure: Use various Mother–Child combinations to nourish or disperse (such as LU 5 and KI 7, for Metal–Water), or Control cycle combinations to disperse (such as Heart 3 and 8, for Water–Fire); use gold beads for tonification, silver for dispersal, and stainless steel for neutrality (seeds in general are neutral, and preferred by some clients).

- Qigong: Five Healing Sound and/or Five Healing Color Qigong can be used for diagnosis as well as treatment. To re-align thinking patterns and overall health, treat the dysfunctional Element by doing a greater number of that particular movement/meditation.

- Essential Oils – *Note: Rotate oils or use blends for greater efficacy*:

  – Water: Basil, Cedarwood, Clove, Geranium, Frankincense, Spruce

- Wood: Chamomile, Jasmine, Lavender, Lemon, Sweet Marjoram, Peppermint, Rose, Rosemary, Vetiver

- Fire: Cinnamon, Frankincense, Jasmine, Sweet Marjoram, Neroli/Orange Blossom, Rose, Sage, Sandalwood, Valerian, Ylang Ylang

- Earth: Bergamot, Cardamom, Coriander, Lemongrass, Neroli/Orange Blossom, Orange, Patchouli

- Metal: Eucalyptus, Fir, Myrtle, Sweet Marjoram, Peppermint, Pine, Rosemary, Spruce, Thyme.

ADDRESSING ROOT EMOTIONS

If a Five Element approach doesn't resonate, working with underlying emotions may prove helpful. There are two emotional groups that are often found at the root of prejudice toward DGS communities: Shame – Guilt – Repression, and Anxiety – Worry – Fear. Again according to Hicks *et al.*, 'It is often hard for practitioners…to have the same level of compassion if the patient has feelings such as jealousy, resentment, insecurity, and self-loathing. These are regarded as less acceptable emotions and may incur disapproval from practitioners, especially if practitioners have repressed these feelings in themselves' (2011, p.40). When left untreated, any buried emotions can become triggered during client interactions, leading to lack of empathy or the potential for muddled diagnosis. Outside the office, interpersonal communication and connection may be impacted at every level, thwarting the ability to confidently represent one's practice or attract appropriate clientele.

Shame, Guilt, or Repression typically result from a combination of intuitive knowledge that a specific belief or behavior is wrong, frustration of being unable to escape the bias, and the suppression of natural curiosity or desire to change as 'bad.' These heavy and binding emotions typically affect the Middle and Lower Jiao organs, and can be difficult to self-diagnose. Treatment is focused on 'lightening the load' through elevating the Spirit, coursing bound Qi, and harmonizing the Middle and Lower Jiaos (as appropriate). Clearing areas of Qi Stagnation or Phlegm may also be needed, and is addressed below.

The primary self-treatment modalities for Shame, Guilt, and Repression are Qigong, Essential Oils, and Lifestyle, specifically regular walks in nature. Acupuncture and Herbal Formulae are also appropriate, and talk therapy or mental health counseling is highly recommended to navigate this particular terrain. The following are just a few suggestions; these methods are more fully covered in Section IV.

- Qigong: Flying and open arm movements which lift the body: Five Animal Frolics–Crane; Sheng Zhen Qigong: Heaven Nature/Kuan Yin Standing–Boat Rowing in the Stream of Air, Traveling Eastward Across the Ocean; Butterfly Form.

- Essential Oils: Chamomile, Frankincense, Lavender, Mimosa, Narcissus, Sandalwood, Violet, Ylang Ylang.

- Lifestyle: Walking in nature with good-quality air to increase the movement of *Zong*/Chest Qi and the overall Qi Mechanism; eating smaller meals to encourage smooth digestion and easy passing in the Middle and Lower Jiaos; living one's authentic life without apology.

Anxiety, Worry, and Fear result from the desire to 'fit in' properly to avoid personal harassment: 'Am I doing it right?' 'Will they think I'm one too?' These emotions can affect any Jiao, but they each have a general tendency: Anxiety in the Upper Jiao, Worry in the Middle and Upper Jiao, and Fear in the Lower and Upper Jiao. Each of them can obstruct the proper functioning of the Chong Mai, so the basic treatment principles are to calm and nourish the Shen-Spirit (i.e., nourishing the Blood/Yin to anchor the Shen) and to harmonize the Chong Vessel. Opening the San Jiao pathways and clearing Qi Stagnation and Phlegm (see below) may also be needed.

The primary self-treatment modalities for Anxiety, Worry, and Fear are Acupressure/Acupuncture, Qigong, and Gemstones; Essential Oils are also applicable. *Note: Although Acupressure/Acupuncture is appropriate for occasional regulation of the Chong Mai, Qigong, Gemstones, and Essential Oils are more appropriate for daily self-treatment to avoid damage to the EV.*

- Acupressure/Acupuncture:

  – To regulate Chong Mai: SP 4, LV 3, PC 6 (used individually, or in combination), applicable Ren and Kidney Channel points on the torso, ST 30

  – To calm and nourish the Shen: SP 6, LV 8, HT 6, Ren 17, Yintang.

- Qigong:

  – To align the Ren, Du, and Chong: Hun Yuan Gong–Opening and Closing Heaven and Earth; Microcosmic Orbit

  – Sitting and Lying postures to calm and nourish the Shen-Spirit: Buddhist Greeting, Qi Circulation/Tai Yang Circulation, Daoist Napping/Shao Yin Circulation.

- Gemstones: Amethyst, Amazonite, Bloodstone, Coral, Garnet, Jasper (Red), Jade (Lavender), Lapis Lazuli, Obsidian, Meteorite, Moonstone, Pearl, Opal, Ruby, Sapphire, Smoky Quartz, Sunstone, Unakite.

- Essential Oils: Frankincense, Lavender, Mimosa, Narcissus, Sandalwood, Vanilla, Vetiver, Violet, Ylang Ylang.

PHYSICAL OBSTRUCTIONS: QI AND PHLEGM

When prejudice and unhealthy belief are encountered from a very young age, the development of Qi Stagnation and Phlegm is extremely likely. The first response to a blatantly intolerant and unjust message is almost always confusion: 'Why is this happening?' or 'Why did they say that?' Whereas an adult mind may quickly move through this phase to outrage, an immature mind will not understand how to categorize such an incident, leading to 'churning' of thought, where the system attempts to process the incident over and over again. This repetitive processing initially creates Qi Stagnation, as the confusion is unable to flow properly through the system. If these thoughts are not properly dealt with or are frequently re-triggered, the body fluids will eventually stagnate as well. Thought is insubstantial in nature, but is related to the Yi-Intellect aspect of the *Wu Shen* and through Five Element correspondences to the Dampness pathogen, so chronic churning of body fluids from confusion leads directly to the creation of insubstantial Phlegm.

Signs of Phlegm may be minimal or fluctuate dramatically. One might see a come-and-go tongue coat or wiry-slippery pulse. There could be mild confusion or outrage that arises only when the triggering topic is debated. Symptoms of 'clouding the orifices' (blurry vision, nasal or ear congestion, sleepiness or poor concentration) may appear only sporadically as the insubstantial Phlegm gets stirred up by triggers, but then resettles back to the subconscious once more. The biggest problem with Phlegm is that by clouding the orifices it prevents the individual from experiencing the truth, thereby thwarting the process of change. One great description of the evidence of Phlegm comes from Caroline Myss (n.d.), an internationally renowned medical intuitive: 'I always try to observe when people turn off their attention span, because allowing yourself to be distracted, or falling asleep, often indicates an unconscious effort to avoid hearing content that holds the potential of personal empowerment.'

Clearing Qi Stagnation and Phlegm starts with increasing free flow through-out the body. The basic principles are to course Qi and clear Phlegm; the primary self-treatment modalities are Diet and Lifestyle, specifically regular, frequent physical movement (which may include Qigong). Adjunct modalities include

Acupressure/Acupuncture, Herbal Formulae, and Gemstones to break up Qi and Phlegm accumulations. Phlegm makes it difficult to remember any initial incident where unhealthy beliefs were set in, and can make it seem impossible to think clearly or find appropriate resolution methods. If you think Phlegm is obstructing the healing process, get another professional on board – preferably a Chinese Medicine practitioner and/or mental health specialist (e.g., talk therapist, counselor, etc.) – to help your eyes, ears, and mind perceive more clearly.

- Diet: Avoid high-fat foods, processed foods, dairy, wheat, beer, and other Dampness/Phlegm-producing foods; incorporate Phlegm-clearing foods (i.e., almonds, celery, garlic, mustard greens, jasmine green tea, onion, parsley, pear, scallions, thyme, walnuts, etc.); eating smaller meals may also help clear and prevent further accumulation.

- Lifestyle: Walking, biking, or any form of smooth, self-paced movement to promote freedom of internal movement; for those that primarily work at a desk, frequent stretching, standing, or walking around the office.

- Qigong: Silk-Reeling Qigong; Hun Yuan Gong–Grinding the Corn; Sinking the Turbid and Washing the Organs; Gathering the Rice.

- Acupressure/Acupuncture: Liver and Gallbladder Channels (especially LV 3, 8, GB 20, 21, 30–34, 40, 41), Dai Mai (GB 41–SJ 5), ST 8, 40, SP 3, 6, 9, SJ 17, Du 20.

- Herbal Formulae: Xiao Yao Wan, Jia Wei Xiao Yao Wan, Er Chen Wan, Liu Jun Zi Wan, Bi Xie Sheng Shi Wan, Bu Nao Wan.

- Gemstones: Amethyst, Agate, Agate-Jasper, Amazonite, Amber, Azurite-Malachite, Garnet, Hematite, Jasper, Lapis Lazuli, Malachite, Nephrite Jade, Obsidian, Pyrite, Peridot, Ruby, Sapphire, Tourmaline, Unakite.

SUMMARY

» Everyone has been exposed to prejudice and needs to address the internal physical, emotional, and spiritual consequences of unhealthy belief.

» Unhealthy belief, even when subconscious and hidden, causes obstructions which can be self-treated using Chinese Medicine theories.

» Meditation and Qigong are two ways to identify unhealthy beliefs and any blocks to spiritual growth.

» Physical and energetic blocks may correspond to the Five Elements, and can be treated with Five Element generating and control sequence theories.

» Shame, Guilt, and Repression are heavy and binding in nature. They are treated by 'lightening the load' and elevating the Spirit, coursing the Qi (systematically), and harmonizing the Middle and Lower Jiaos. The best modalities to elevate the Spirit are 'flying' Qigong movements, Essential Oils, and walks in nature.

» Anxiety, Fear, and Worry can affect any chamber of the San Jiao as well as obstruct the proper functioning of the Chong Mai. They should be treated by calming the Spirit and harmonizing the San Jiao and the Chong. Consider Qigong, Gemstones, and Essential Oils to treat the Chong in order to avoid damage.

» Qi Stagnation and Phlegm is characterized by poor memory, confusion, or excessive rumination without the ability to find resolution. It is treated by coursing the Qi and clearing Phlegm. Diet adjustments and regular exercise are critical components to an effective treatment plan.

» Talk therapy or mental health counseling may be needed to unwind deeply ingrained beliefs, especially when Phlegm is involved.

Chapter 2

A WELCOMING PRACTICE

- Outside the Office

- Paperwork Guidelines

- Treatment Considerations

If I speak in the tongues of men and of angels, but have not love, I am only a resounding gong or a clanging cymbal. If I have the gift of prophecy and can fathom all mysteries and all knowledge, and if I have a faith that can move mountains, but have not love, I am nothing.

– 1 Corinthians 13.1–2[1]

Without question, all health professionals seek to improve their clients' overall physical and emotional well-being. Even when practitioners have the best intentions, minority individuals – including the Diverse Gender and Sexuality (DGS) communities – may still experience a wide range of reception. Within an environment that clearly embraces gender and sexuality concerns, every client is able to be open and honest about pertinent medical information, sharing those specific details that a good diagnosis and treatment plan may hinge upon. In an environment where acceptance is uncertain, a client might choose to conceal bits of information in order to get unbiased treatment, but in doing so may inadvertently obscure the root of their condition and thwart excellent care.

This chapter covers a variety of ways that practitioners and business owners can ensure each of their clients receives the best, and most respectful, care possible – *no matter how a specific client identifies*. Given that the majority of DGS individuals have likely experienced intolerant behaviors first-hand, it is important for any

---

1 *New Revised Standard Version Bible: Anglicized Edition, copyright © 1989, 1995 National Council of the Churches of Christ in the United States of America.*

medical professional to gain trust by 1) doing the personal work to unwind internal bias (see Chapter 1), and 2) becoming a genuine ally to the DGS communities.

Becoming an authentic, outspoken, and open-hearted ally happens *well before* a potential client ever enters the clinic. Each practitioner must therefore take the time to educate themselves about gender, sex, sexuality, and relationship structures, and re-analyze business or healing practices that can easily ostracize prospective clients. It is critical that highest priority is placed on each client's perception of safety and sense of 'belonging,' which impacts all decisions regarding clinic set-up, paperwork, interpersonal interactions, treatment intention, choice of modality, and lifestyle suggestions.

OUTSIDE THE OFFICE

As Mark Twain said, 'Travel is fatal to prejudice, bigotry and narrow-mindedness, and many of our people need it sorely on these accounts. Broad, wholesome, charitable views…cannot be acquired by vegetating in one little corner of the earth all of one's life' (1984, p.521). In Chinese Medicine, Travel and Adventure is considered one of the Nine Palaces of 'life's curriculum,' the challenges that each person must face on their pre-destined path (see Chapters 4, 7). The Travel and Adventure Palace emphasizes the need to learn about and move away from cultural bias by immersing oneself in a new perspective.

Fortunately, Travel does not always necessitate getting far away from home – it can happen almost anywhere. Attending DGS events (such as Pride Parades, HIV+/AIDS fundraisers, and informational events at BDSM clubs or 'adult toy' stores) and reading books or listening to podcasts about these topics is a conscious choice to engage the challenge of Travel and Adventure, while stimulating the Yi-Intellect and expanding Shen-Spirit awareness. Of course, exposure to new vocabulary, candid dialogue, and other perspectives may trigger areas of subconscious belief that require further healing (see Chapter 1), but when allowed to flow properly, they will also precipitate healthy changes in one's personal and professional life. With just a little bit of time and effort, practitioner-allies will be more easily able to perceive the business or healing practices that could alienate would-be clients.

Prospective DGS clients typically look for images and verbal clues that they will be emotionally and physically safe prior to entering a practice. The way a business presents itself in advertising and marketing materials is the first impression a potential client, DGS or otherwise, will consider. Business cards, brochures, websites, and other materials have always used non-verbal clues to indicate business focus or target specific clientele. Consider what images represent a sports medicine or orthopedic acupuncture practice, versus a cosmetic acupuncture practice or a focus on infertility and women's health. Visual indicators of imagery and font selection indicate the style of practice, and whether it might be a 'good fit' for any potential client.

At an international level, the rainbow flag is probably the most recognized symbol of LGBTQ+ rights. Use of this image automatically denotes acceptance of diverse sexual orientation and gender identity, with potential openness to mixed relationship styles. Using a rainbow flag or written 'LGBTQ-friendly' notation on advertising materials, hanging an actual rainbow flag or window decal at the office entrance, and posting a non-discrimination policy addressing sexual orientation, gender expression, and relationship structure are simple acts of recognition that go a long way toward creating a sense of safety for DGS clients.

> Having a practice that clearly welcomes DGS individuals grants freedom of expression to everyone that walks in the door. You may be pleasantly surprised how open *all* your clients become!

PAPERWORK GUIDELINES

Once a DGS client enters an office, even a small act denoting lack of acceptance can turn them away. The forms clients fill out offer them more clues about the inclusivity of the practice; this is where various check boxes may become an affront. In order to communicate respect and encourage information sharing, categories related to gender, sex, and relationship require re-examination from a DGS perspective.

Gender

Assumptions about gender are made early in the client–practitioner relationship. Labeling a person's gender starts right at the top of an intake form, where it asks a client to select a title: Mr., Mrs., Ms., or Miss. These options reflect the binary gender system; i.e., two options only, female or male. As this field is not always required, individuals wishing to avoid unnecessary categorization may simply leave this option blank, but another option already exists.

In 2015, the Oxford English Dictionary inducted a new title to be used by genderqueer, agender, or gender non-binary individuals that prefer to identify as neither male nor female. Although not yet widely used, 'Mx.' is helping fill the need for new language to reflect the expanding cultural understanding of gender. Using this, and/or a fill-in-the-blank option, is one way to indicate an open-minded environment.

Incorrect pronoun use is another obstacle during the initial stages of connection and trust-building. Starting any conversation with gendered language use, even if addressing someone with a traditional term of respect such as Sir, Mister, Miss, Ma'am, or Lady, can derail the entire process. This is especially true for transgender and genderqueer clients, where each person may have different preferences. One step in the right direction is to ask each person their 'pronoun preference'; if preferred, this could be done with another series of check-boxes:

'How would you like to be addressed?'

☐ He, Him

☐ She, Her

☐ They, Their

☐ Other – please describe: _____

Sex

Gender describes one's self-perception and/or visual presentation to the world, and the issues discussed above are about how to address clients in line with their self-perceptions. Gender actually has nothing to do with a person's physical anatomy, but intake forms frequently mis-use this term. When asking about anatomy, the correct term is 'sex' (for more on the distinctions between gender and sex, see Section II).

The majority of intake forms only have two check boxes for sex: female or male. These options are driven in part by insurance companies, but when considering the contemporary understanding of human anatomy, there are actually *at least four* options to include: female, male, intersex, and transgender. Practitioners that specialize in treating transgender or LGBTQ+ clientele may offer even more options in this category, or create a formal distinction between sex and gender identity, such as:

Sex

☐ Female

☐ Male

☐ Intersex

☐ Transgender – please describe: _____

■ Gender

☐ Female

☐ Male

☐ Queer or Non-binary

☐ Agender

☐ Other – please describe: _____

Another option is to *not have any check boxes* in relation to title, gender, sex, or pronouns,[2] instead just allowing clients to fill out the health information sections that pertain to them as applicable (i.e., gynecological and genito-urinary health), and then *asking them directly* during the interview process about pronoun use or other concerns as applicable.

Relationship

The typical selection in regard to relationship status is 'single, married, divorced, widowed.' Although this terminology is sometimes required by insurance companies, these insufficient options do not reflect the real and complex relationship structures of many people's lives: those that have divorced and are remarried; those that are partnered in long-term relationships but choose not to be married; and those that are polyamorous with multiple partners, whether or not they are married.

Further, the automatic assumption that a married individual is sexually monogamous eliminates potentially pertinent questions and/or medical testing in regard to sexually transmitted infections (STIs). This is critical information, as STI symptoms can mimic other complaints, such as yeast infections, urinary tract infections (UTIs), or cysts. Any space for 'Spouse's Name' (specifying the non-plural) also reflects the cultural bias toward monogamy. Putting aside the assumption that 'married = monogamous' is critical to being a sex-positive healthcare professional. Consider the following alternative to better reflect the diversity of sexual relationships:

---

2   This may not be possible if your office accepts insurance!

▓ Check as many as apply:

☐ Single

☐ Dating

☐ Married/Partnered – how long: _____

☐ Divorced – how long: _____

☐ Monogamous

☐ Polyamorous

☐ Other – please describe: _____

Married ≠ Monogamous

As a healthcare professional, it is important to respectfully inquire how many sex partners a client currently has and how often they get STI tested.

Other Health

When looking at a client's overall health, surgical history provides another way to demonstrate openness to information sharing. Instead of saying 'List surgical history here,' try any of the following:

- List any surgeries, including cosmetic or gender-transforming.

- List any surgical, physical, or emotional trauma.

- List any surgeries, large scars, or history of abuse (physical, emotional, sexual).

Another option is a separate area that invites a client to 'List any other life experiences (surgery, trauma, injury, etc.) that might be pertinent.'

Although especially helpful for assessing transgender health and abuse history, asking these questions also provides a venue for any client to tell their unique story. By allowing an individual to tell their story, trust is built, etiology may be clarified, and clients can even stimulate their own spirit-healing process.

TREATMENT CONSIDERATIONS

In every aspect of treatment space interaction, there is the very real possibility of 'wrong treatment' – that which goes against the nature of the individual. Within Chinese Medicine there are multiple gender- or sex-based practices that can throw off diagnostic certainty, lessen treatment efficacy, or even cause adverse effects. The first area of concern is that of intention – the mindset with which a practitioner enters a treatment space. The attitude of a practitioner will translate across every aspect of the client–practitioner relationship, including diagnosis, treatment, and follow-up, so it is important to be compassionate and energetically clear, without judgment, criticism, or agenda.

Beyond one's intention, there are multiple pitfalls to avoid in order to prevent harm to DGS clients. Unfortunately, these incorrect practices are ingrained in the global practice of Chinese Medicine and continue to be taught. Therefore, all aspects of treatment, *especially intention setting, pulse diagnosis, needling techniques, herb formula selections, and Qigong practices*, must be re-evaluated to ensure correct treatment for all clients, no matter how they identify.

Intention Setting

Misaligned intention is something to be acutely aware of when treating DGS individuals. When a client agrees to receive, they 'let their guard down' and relax, allowing the Wei Qi boundary to soften so an energetic exchange between client and practitioner may form. A practitioner will enter and exit this space of exchange multiple times during treatment, bringing with them any personal feelings about asexuality, gender-play, homosexuality, kink practices, polyamory, etc. When negative judgments or inappropriate treatment goals enter the energetic space, they can do harm to a client at any level – physical, psychological, and/or spiritual – and potentially exacerbate the root etiology as well.

For example, any false belief that a client's gender or sexuality is a mistake or divergence – as in 'they have diverted from their path' – is an incorrect assessment based in cultural bias. Treating any person with the intention that they can switch their identity or orientation to a more culturally appropriate presentation is based in homophobia, gender oppression, and/or sex-shaming. Chinese Medicine is a powerful healing modality where the practitioner's emotions, beliefs, and treatment goals must be free of judgment in order to prevent an array of adverse effects for DGS clients. Doing the personal work to eliminate unhealthy belief, such as outlined in Chapter 1, is therefore *critical for every practitioner*.

Pulse Reading

In many forms of Chinese Medicine, pulse diagnosis is heralded as *the major palpatory finding* under the Four Examinations of Observation, Hearing/Smelling, Interrogation/Asking, and Palpation, and is generally considered one of the top three for diagnosis of a condition (along with tongue and interview).

Most pulse systems teach that healthy male pulses will be stronger on the left and weaker on the right, and conversely that healthy female pulses will be stronger on the right and weaker on the left. When working with self-identified LGBTQ+ clients, these generalities are not consistently valid within a range of healthy individuals. Specifically with queer, transgender, and bi/pansexual identified persons, the pulse strength is often in opposition to these guidelines, or switches strength at various times (such as with menstrual cycle phases).

The ability for the strength of the pulse to switch sides is due to the operation of two organ systems: the Heart and the Spleen. The Heart is responsible for 'making' the Blood, and for 'governing' its circulation through the blood vessels. The Spleen not only contributes the Gu Qi that enriches the quality of the Blood, but it also 'controls' the Blood by keeping it in the blood vessels that circulate it. The Heart, as the seat of the Emperor, reflects the mood of the entire Kingdom (i.e., the Body). The Spleen, as the seat of Post-Natal Qi, reflects the day-to-day energy of the body. The influence of the Heart and Spleen's functions to make, govern, and control the Blood mean that the pulse is primarily a reflection of *current* emotions and energy. In other words, the pulse is the answer to 'Who am I *today*?' This explains the ease with which the pulse sides can switch strengths, especially among individuals that have more fluid identity.

Unfortunately, the pulse strength guidelines do not always apply to those *outside* the DGS communities either. Repressed identity or sexuality is a potential cause for someone that isn't already DGS identified, but a strength-switch does not consistently correlate with deeper signs of Repression. A better conclusion to draw from the overall pulse strength is simply the reflection of the state of Qi/Yang (right side) and Blood/Yin (left side), *without any attachment to the client's gender or sex*.

Needle Insertion

Acupuncture is also taught using sex-based rules, specifically with Extraordinary Vessel (EV) treatments. EVs are typically needled based on sex, using opening points for women on the right, opening points for men on the left, and couple points on the opposite side. An example of this with a female client is using the opening point for the Ren vessel (Lung 7) on the right side, and the couple point (Kidney 6) on the left. The mnemonic 'women are always right' is sometimes used to help students remember these rules.

In Japanese Acupuncture styles, pulse and hara diagnosis have 'women are right' rules as well. Many practitioners believe the pulse must be taken first on the right side for women, first on the left side for men. For proper Hara/abdominal palpation, the practitioner must stand on the right of a female client, the left side for a male client. There is also a rule to always needle women on the right side first, men on the left, especially for Back Shu points.

Again, these rules do not generally apply to DGS individuals. When one takes the time to palpate the EV points for stickiness, tenderness, or vacuity, the findings for those who self-identify as homosexual (i.e., gay or lesbian) are consistently opposite the sex-based rules. Among those who identify as sex- or gender-fluid (i.e., queer, transgender, and bi/pansexual), there is an even wider variety of results, with palpatory findings frequently switching sides back and forth, just as the pulses do.

Relying on sex-based acupuncture techniques can actually cause damage to an individual by going against the natural flow of their Qi Mechanism. Within the field there are a few accounts of 'old guard' acupuncturists trying to change a client's sexual orientation 'back' to heterosexuality. Though these tales are generally unreliable, the symptoms described have a degree of truth to them. One wrong treatment creates generally minor symptoms, including slight dizziness, mild headaches, vague digestive upset (bloating, nausea/queasiness), or just feeling 'off' in a variety of ways. In my own office one client described feeling as if they were standing next to their body; another described feeling uncomfortably bent to the side like a boomerang. Ongoing wrong treatment will create more severe symptoms, such as vertigo, migraines, vomiting, and mental unrest. Many of these complaints, along with anxiety, depression, insomnia, and mild bipolar states, have all presented in clients that appeared to have consistently received *unintentionally wrong treatment* before entering my practice.

Side effects of inappropriate treatment may be reported while needles are still in place, immediately upon rising from the treatment table, or within a few hours post-treatment. If it was only one wrong treatment and the client's Constitution is generally strong, it is possible for mild symptoms to fade away on their own. With consistently wrong treatment that goes against the client's nature however, only a short series of *right* treatments with Acupuncture or Medical Qigong can reverse the condition. In order to avoid this situation, needle insertion decisions must no longer be based on outdated assumptions relating to gender, sex, or sexuality. For the benefit of all our clients, *the rules of Acupuncture related to sex and gender must be discarded immediately.*

Herbal Formulae

In clinical practice, accurate initial pattern diagnosis is often baffled by various lifestyle factors, such as Dampness from diet. When a client presents with a great mixture of patterns, any sex-biased training may lead to wrong treatment. Sex-based notions such as 'men only get Kidney Yang/Qi Deficiency' (i.e., not Kidney Yin Deficiency) or 'only women get Blood Deficiency' can get in the way of developing an accurate diagnosis. In reality, client Constitution and lifestyle factors dictate pattern development far more than their gender or sex.

When examining the categorization of any formula as 'women's' herbs, there are a few formulae that specifically target the menses (such as Tong Jing Wan), but there are plenty of more generalized remedies as well. Due to sex-based educational training, practitioners may not consider using one of these for a male-identified client even when the symptoms and treatment principles are in alignment. For example, both Nu Ke Ba Zhen Wan and Liu Wei Di Huang Wan are considered 'women's formulas,' but the patterns addressed – Blood and Spleen Qi Deficiency or Liver–Kidney Yin and Blood Deficiency respectively – are incredibly commonplace among both men and women due to the extreme physical and mental stress that working people experience.

These sex-based biases frequently interrupt proper treatment for clients that present as male, but they are also problematic for those with fluid identity or for those undergoing gender transitioning (hormones, surgery, etc.). The process of herbal selection therefore, must also be *free of assumption related to gender, sex, or sexuality*.

Qigong Practice

Qigong is not immune to gender- and sex-bias, with both hand positions and directional movements taught differently for men and women. For example, in a simple standing pose to store Qi in the Lower *Dan Tian*, the palms being connected right-over-left or left-over-right is taught based on perceived gender. Or, when regulating the bowels, starting with circulating the abdominal Qi clockwise or counterclockwise is another gender-based teaching.

For those that are not energetically sensitive or have limited intention, these methods can be practiced incorrectly for years without significant harm. But for individuals with increased sensitivity, 'wrong practice' is another form of wrong treatment – that which goes against the nature of the individual. The symptoms of wrong practice are incredibly similar to those of wrong treatment with Acupuncture: dizziness, headaches, digestion, and emotional upset while performing the practice are commonplace, and should be watched for. Deeper symptoms such as extreme temperature fluctuations, hot flashes, vertigo, and vomiting reflect the involvement of EVs; *these practices must be stopped immediately* and evaluated by a professional Qigong teacher or Master-level practitioner to confirm correct practice for the individual.

I have abandoned all of the sex-based rules in my own Qigong practice and teaching. Instead, I inform students that this way is how I was taught this information, but *personal comfort while practicing is always more important than following the rules*.

Symptoms of 'wrong treatment' – i.e., going against the nature of the individual – with Acupuncture, Herbs, or Qigong will impact the physical body with dizziness, headaches, digestive upsets, or just feeling physically 'off.' Ongoing wrong treatment can affect the emotional and spiritual levels with anxiety, depression, insomnia, and even acute episodes of manic-depression.

CLIENT EXAMPLE

A genderqueer female client in their 40s was in a motor vehicle accident one week ago, with only mild soft tissue injury (bruising and swelling). They describe feeling 'off-kilter' since the accident, with mild dizziness, fatigue, various aches and pains, and visual cloudiness that comes and goes. The accident was from the side at relatively low speed, but the car was fully spun around. The client is also overweight, with a history of whiplash injuries from horseback riding years prior. The acute signs of whiplash are confirmed with Manaka-style Hara diagnosis. Because the client could not lie face down comfortably, this was addressed using the Du and Dai Vessels with general points to promote healing and reduce swelling (Stomach 36–Large Intestine 10 in combination, Spleen 6, 9, Kidney 3, Gallbladder 34, etc.).

The client felt better immediately after the treatment, but called the next day feeling much worse. Now they are nauseous with a strong headache and increased dizziness; *this is the evidence of wrong treatment*. Treatment of the Du and Dai is repeated, but the opening-couple points are located opposite the initial treatment. Teishin (non-puncturing needle) stimulation is also used at the Four Doors (Ren 12, 6, Stomach 25 in combination) to re-anchor the system at 'Home' (Ren 8), along with gentle pole Moxa stimulation at Kidney 1 for grounding and Taiji pole rectification. All symptoms completely cleared during treatment, and a follow-up was scheduled for five days later to ensure the original symptoms did not return. *Note: In my own practice, this client would not be charged for the second treatment, as it repaired the unintentionally 'wrong' treatment originally provided.*

CLIENT EXAMPLE

A heterosexual male in his early 30s presents with acute insomnia, teeth grinding, and stress levels that are related to graduate school. He is also a chronic sleepwalker (since childhood), which runs in his family from both maternal and paternal sides. He is currently single and is feeling lonely so far from home. His tongue and pulse both suggest Liver and Kidney Blood-Yin Deficiency with mixed Heat, so the primary modalities are Herbal Formulae and Diet – physical substances to nourish the Yin and Blood – along with Acupuncture treatment to help clear Heat, calm the Spirit, and course the Channels to prevent tooth grinding.

Diet recommendations focused on cooking methods (soups, stews, and steamed foods to nourish fluids) as well as ocean foods and leafy greens to nourish Water and Wood elements. Herbal Formulae started with a combination of Liu Wei Di Huang Wan and Chai Hu Long Gu Mu Li Wan to repair the fluids and clear excess Heat, then to Liu Wei Di Huang Wan with Xiao Yao Wan (Jia Wei Xiao Yao Wan during the hot months) for long-term management of stress and Constitution. Acupuncture included Ren, Chong, and Du vessels to address the major patterns of Yin, Blood, and Heat, along the Gallbladder Channel to reduce present-day stress, and ashi points around the jaw and teeth. *Note: His sleepwalking is clearly an inherited trait, so the Blood and Yin Deficiency is likely Constitutional. Long-term Blood and Yin nourishment for symptom management will typically be needed, regardless of lifestyle factors.*

SUMMARY

» Office paperwork and intake forms offer clues about the inclusivity of the practice.

» Being an ally requires reflection on office policies and treatment practices – ensuring that DGS clients feel accepted is the priority.

» Be careful to avoid assumptions regarding pronoun use, relationship status, sexuality, and/or gender.

» Exposure to new cultures and experiences precipitates healthy growth for practitioner-allies and helps build empathy for DGS clients.

» One's intention will affect diagnosis, treatment, and any follow-up plan, so it is important to be energetically clear, without judgment, criticism, or agenda about DGS clients or their struggles.

» Gender-based pulses are not consistent among LGBTQ+ individuals. The pulse can be opposite or switch back and forth, especially among queer, transgender, bi/pansexuals, or anyone with more fluid identity.

» Sex-based Acupuncture needling can cause damage to a DGS individual by going against the natural flow of their Qi Mechanism.

» The patterns addressed by 'women's' Herbal Formulae are incredibly commonplace across the lines of gender and sex, typically due to the extreme physical and mental stress in the modern workplace.

» Symptoms of wrong treatment with Acupuncture, Herbs, or Qigong practices include dizziness, headaches, digestive upset, hot flashes, and emotional distress (anxiety, depression, insomnia, etc.).

THE YIN–YANG OF GENDER

Breaking down that us-and-them binary is part of the work of love.

– bell hooks 2017

TERMINOLOGY: GENDER IDENTITY AND GENDER EXPRESSION

(an incomplete list)[1]

- **Agender** (also called Genderless) a person that sees themselves existing without gender

- **Androgynous** a person that presents with both masculine and feminine elements

- **Butch** a person that presents as physically, mentally, or emotionally masculine

- **Cisgender** a person whose anatomical sex and gender identity align (i.e., assigned male at birth, identifies as male)

- **Drag king** a person who performs masculinity in a theatrical setting

- **Drag queen** a person who performs femininity in a theatrical setting

- **Femme** a person that presents as physically, mentally, or emotionally feminine

- **FTM or F2M** (abbreviation) a Female-to-Male transgender person, at any stage of transition

- **Gender fluid** (also called Bigender) a person that does not feel their gender is fixed, or whose presentation does not consistently correlate with cultural binary gender expectations

- **Genderqueer** a person that does not identify with either binary gender; also used as an umbrella term for all gender non-conforming identities

- **Gender non-conforming (GNC)** a person that does not identify with either binary gender, or that presents outside of cultural binary gender expectations (i.e., a masculine woman or a feminine man); also used as an umbrella term for all gender non-conforming identities

---

1   More definitions are found at the beginnings of Sections I and III.

- **Gender normative or gender straight** a person whose gender identity or presentation aligns with cultural binary gender expectations (i.e., a feminine woman or a masculine man)

- **Intersex** a person whose anatomical sex organs and/or DNA does not align with cultural binary gender expectations

- **MTF or M2F** (abbreviation) a Male-to-Female transgender person, at any stage of transition

- **Transgender** (also called Transsexual) a person whose anatomical sex and gender identity are not aligned (i.e., assigned female at birth, identifies as male)

- **Transvestite** (also called Crossdresser) a person that wears clothing in opposition to cultural binary gender expectations for purposes of relaxation, fun, or sexual gratification. *Note: This is often classified as a kink, and is not to be confused with transgenderism/transsexuality, or with Drag king/queen performance*

- **Two-spirit** an Indigenous Native American person whose gender identity or presentation does not consistently correlate with cultural binary gender expectations, often seen as fulfilling the expectations of both binary genders; Indigenous communities developed this term in 1990, and it is not considered culturally appropriate for use by non-Natives

- **Queer** (similar to Genderqueer) a person whose gender, sexual identity, and/or orientation does not correlate with heteronormative or binary gender expectations; also used as an umbrella term for the entire LGBTQ+ community

Chapter 3

NEGATING THE BINARY

- Two Give Birth to Three
- Trans(cending)Gender
- Gender Play

There's a real simple way to look at gender: Once upon a time, someone drew a line in the sands of a culture and proclaimed with great self-importance, 'On this side, you are a man; on the other side, you are a woman.' It's time for the winds of change to blow that line away.

– Kate Bornstein 1994, p.21

The concept of gender as a social construct – a concept or practice that is *not innate, but created* – has been explored through academia and the sciences for well over 50 years. Historical evidence clearly demonstrates that labeling dress and other mannerisms as 'masculine/male' or 'feminine/female' differs greatly from one culture to another, as well as within the same community over time. In conservative heteronormative cultures, it is assumed that gender is unchangeable, binary, and always consistent with anatomical sex. In other words, males are expected to feel masculine, and act, dress, and behave in masculine ways; females are expected to feel feminine, and adopt feminine dress and behavior. In the reality however, there is a wide variety of both sex and gender. Various fish, amphibians, reptiles, birds, and even a few mammals have the capacity to display characteristics of either or both sexes, and some have the ability to change sex during the course of their lifetime. Although not able to change their anatomy without surgical intervention, human beings also remain subject to the infinite variety of biology.

According to the United Nations (n.d.), intersex is the term for individuals 'born with sex characteristics (including genitals, gonads and chromosome patterns) that do not fit typical binary notions of male or female bodies.'[1] This includes the physical absence of gonads and/or sex organs (i.e., ovaries, testes, uterus, vagina, penis), as well as differences in chromosomal patterns from the standard XY (male) or XX (female). It can also include the shaping and size of an individual's genitalia, although this classification lacks both uniform and science-based definitions. A 2000 study published in the *American Journal of Human Biology* (Blackless *et al.* 2000) estimates that one in 1666 individuals (just over 0.06%) have something other than XY or XX chromosomes, and that a full 1 percent of the population are born with visible physical differences. One percent may seem small, but with a current global population hovering near eight billion, that is an estimated 70–80 million intersex individuals.

The regular occurrence of intersex within the human population demonstrates a wider variety of anatomical possibilities than is culturally expected in a binary system. This can be viewed as an inverse bell curve of 'culturally acceptable' genital appearance (see Figure 3.1), where examples of 'perfect' genitalia (again, a highly subjective, non-scientific classification) exist at the endpoints, with the majority in the large zones toward either side of the minority midpoint. And at that exact midpoint is intersex, where either the anatomical appearance and/or the genetic code no longer matches binary expectation.

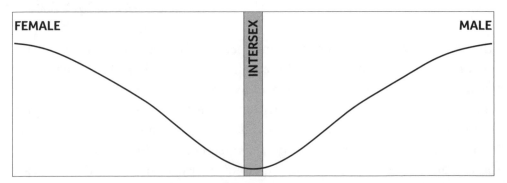

Figure 3.1: Genital Appearance

---

1   'It is important to note that "Intersex" has replaced "hermaphrodite" as the appropriate term for human beings' (United Nations n.d.).

Intersex traits may be apparent at birth, but for many these traits emerge at puberty or are genetically determined during fertility testing. Children identified in infancy may undergo surgical procedures to make their genital structures conform to cultural expectation; in some cases this involves gender reassignment surgery. These procedures are often done before the individual is old enough to participate in informed consent and can cause unfortunate and life-long suffering, including infertility, pain, incontinence, numbness, loss of sexual sensation, and mental health issues. Due to cultural oppression, extreme levels of Shame and Secrecy are common among intersex individuals (see Section IV for treatment of these emotions).

Anatomical sex is often conflated with gender. But gender itself is an umbrella term incorporating internal and external characteristics which may or may not correlate with each other or to one's anatomy. Sam Killermann[2] created *The Genderbread Person* (Figure 3.2) to help demonstrate this point.[3] *The Genderbread Person* has three variables that are of importance to this chapter: Gender Identity, Gender Expression, and Biological Sex (see Chapter 8 for issues of attraction). This text defines Gender as 'a combination of one's internal self-perception of their own gender (i.e., Gender Identity), and the external display of dress, demeanor, and social behavior (i.e., Gender Expression).' Therefore, gender identity is an internal knowing of the self; a generally un-changing characteristic which reflects the Shen-Spirit. Gender Expression is an external presentation that can easily change to reflect personal preferences or adapt to cultural norms; in this way it reflects the emotions as they are the 'spirit of the moment.'

In Daoist philosophy and foundational Chinese Medical theory, anatomy, emotions, and spirit are all considered forms of Qi. Qi is the basis from which all life is created, coming directly from the Wuji. And the Wuji is the origin of endless possibilities, including the great spectrums of gender and sex.

---

2   See www.itspronouncedmetrosexual.com
3   www.genderbread.org

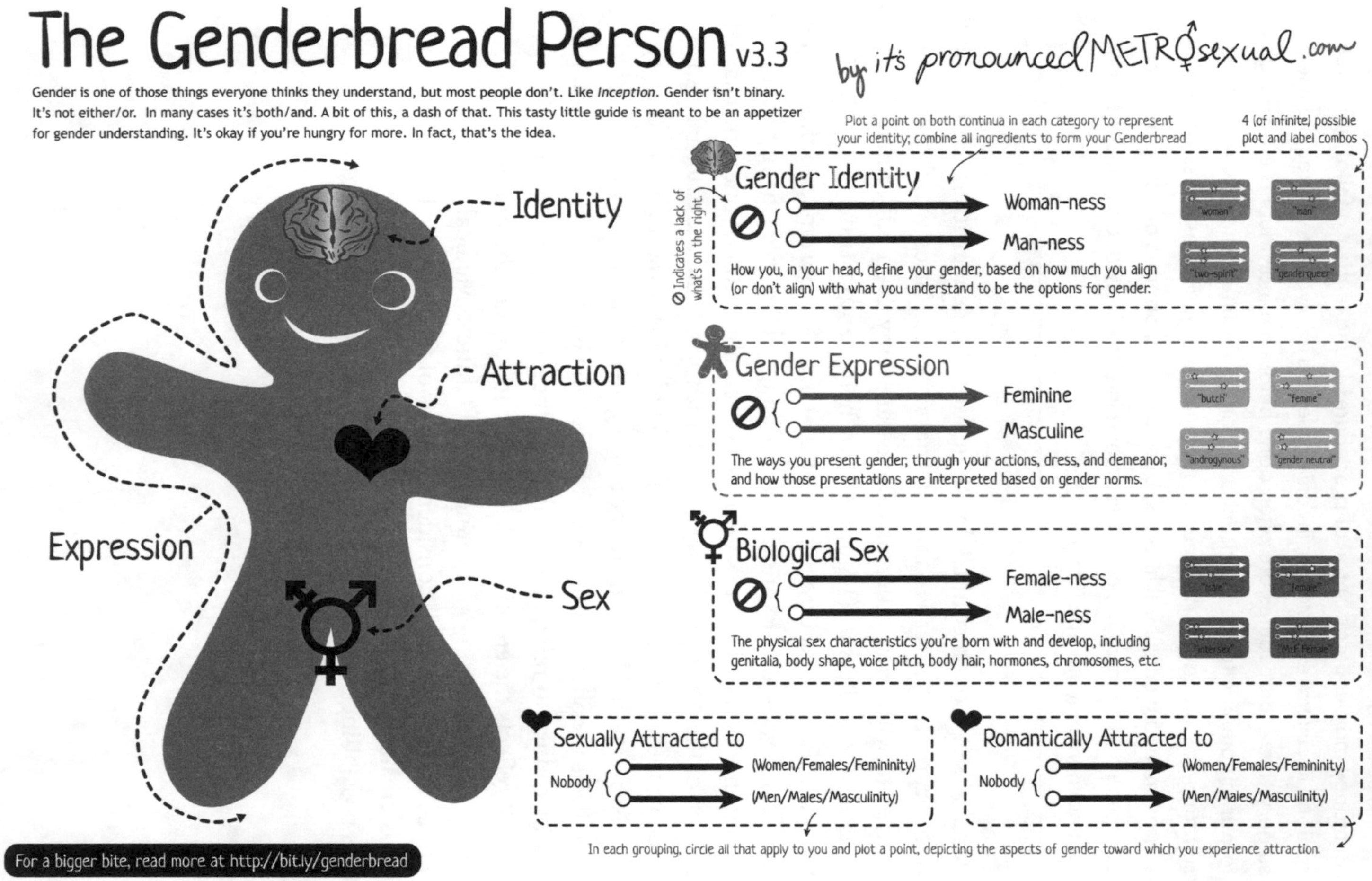
The Genderbread Person v3.3
by it's pronouncedMETROsexual.com
Gender is one of those things everyone thinks they understand, but most people don't. Like Inception. Gender isn't binary. It's not either/or. In many cases it's both/and. A bit of this, a dash of that. This tasty little guide is meant to be an appetizer for gender understanding. It's okay if you're hungry for more. In fact, that's the idea.
Identity
Attraction
Expression
Sex
For a bigger bite, read more at http://bit.ly/genderbread
Plot a point on both continua in each category to represent your identity; combine all ingredients to form your Genderbread
4 (of infinite) possible plot and label combos
⊘ Indicates a lack of what's on the right.
Gender Identity
Woman-ness
Man-ness
How you, in your head, define your gender, based on how much you align (or don't align) with what you understand to be the options for gender.
"woman"
"man"
"two-spirit"
"genderqueer"
Gender Expression
Feminine
Masculine
The ways you present gender, through your actions, dress, and demeanor, and how those presentations are interpreted based on gender norms.
"butch"
"femme"
"androgynous"
"gender neutral"
Biological Sex
Female-ness
Male-ness
The physical sex characteristics you're born with and develop, including genitalia, body shape, voice pitch, body hair, hormones, chromosomes, etc.
"male"
"female"
"intersex"
"MtF female"
Sexually Attracted to
Nobody
(Women/Females/Femininity)
(Men/Males/Masculinity)
Romantically Attracted to
Nobody
(Women/Females/Femininity)
(Men/Males/Masculinity)
In each grouping, circle all that apply to you and plot a point, depicting the aspects of gender toward which you experience attraction.

Figure 3.2: The Genderbread Person

TWO GIVE BIRTH TO THREE

Dao gives birth to One
One gives birth to Two
Two give birth to Three
Three give birth to ten-thousand things
The ten-thousand things carry yin and embrace yang
They mix these energies to enact harmony

– Lao Tsu[4]

Zhang Zai (1020–1077 CE) is credited with being the first person to propose that the Wuji state is entirely composed of Qi. He expanded on the previous notion that Qi could concentrate and scatter, stating that it is Qi which gathers to create material substances (i.e., the creation of life), and that it is this same Qi that disintegrates back to the Wuji state upon death. This implies that the Wuji state is a form of scattered Qi, and the duality represented by the Taiji is born from this scattered – yet interconnected – Qi.

Wuji is commonly translated as 'the great void,' but this implies that the Wuji state is completely empty, that nothing is contained within. I prefer the translation offered by contemporary Qigong Master Li Jun Feng, who refers to Wuji as a state of 'one-ness' where all things are interconnected and inseparable. Li also states that Qi – pure Qi such as that existing in the Wuji – is a form of unconditional love.

> … love is the Source of All – love that is unconditional, selfless and totally free. It is from this that qi came into being, flowing out of unconditional love. From timelessness, from wuji, qi created the universe of non-definable reality. From this non-dual reality, yin and yang came into being and blended together giving rise to the world of duality. Wuji became taiji. So it is qi that created the universe and it is unconditional love that gave birth to qi. (Li 2004, p.viii)

One-ness and unconditional love offer a new understanding of the state where all is blended beyond the measure of individuality or duality; a place from which the Taiji, the ten-thousand things, and a myriad of anatomical sex and genders can be formed (see Figure 3.3).

The Taiji symbol is a simplified, two-dimensional representation of a constant, multi-dimensional movement. It is not just cyclical in nature, but spherical. As practitioners, we know that the phases of Yin–Yang are constantly in flux, never static. The spherical movements of the Taiji contain the same movements as the Qi Mechanism within the human body: up, down, in, and out. This constant churning is life itself, for Yin and Yang only stop their cycling (or at least slow

4   As translated from Chapter 42 of the *Tao De Jing*, quoted in Newell 2011.

down dramatically) upon death. The implication contained within the Taiji is that life and all living beings are constantly transforming themselves through the various cycles of Yin and Yang, be they diurnal, seasonal, annual, lifetime, or unknown to the human realm.

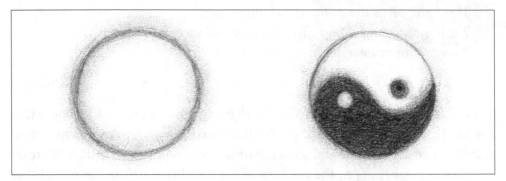

Figure 3.3: From Wuji – One-ness, comes Taiji – Duality

Anatomy, emotions, and spirit are all forms of Qi, the same Qi that came from the Wuji. Physical anatomy, including biological sex, is a very dense and slow-moving form of Qi that changes over a long period of time, such as with aging. Emotional states are a more quick-moving Qi, able to shift with thought and action. Gender expression is an aspect of emotion as it also changes day to day or moment to moment, such as with more masculine or feminine clothing choices and mannerisms.

Spirit is the fastest-moving form of Qi, able to sense and adapt to the immediate environment, yet it is also deeply anchored to the Jing-Essence of our Constitution and our ancestral culture. Gender identity, which is not as mutable as gender expression, comes from this blend of Shen-Spirit and Jing-Essence – it is *who we know ourselves to be*. Anatomy, emotions, and spirit – like all things in this universe – derive directly from the Qi of the Wuji, the place of unconditional love and infinite possibility. The labeling of possibility into different categories is the purview of the Taiji; it is where the duality of Yin–Yang comes into play.

Binary gender theory posits that masculine and feminine qualities do not change, they are constant and unwavering. Yin–Yang principles demonstrate exactly the opposite: all aspects of existence – including sex and gender – come in a variety of presentations and are in constant flux:

- Relative Opposition – no one aspect or thing is inherently Yin or Yang by itself, all is examined in comparison to another.

- Interdependence – no aspect can exist without the other; there can be no Yang without Yin and vice versa.

- Infinite Divisibility – no aspect is only Yin or Yang, they are infinitely divisible into further comparisons of Yin and Yang.

- Inter-transformation – both Yin and Yang give rise to one another at specific stages of development based on two factors: internal conditions (i.e., inherent nature) and the passing of time.

- Mutual Consumption – Yin and Yang are constantly re-balancing to prevent (and/or self-treat) pathological states.

Relative Opposition dictates the comparative existence of both *Ultimate Yin* and *Ultimate Yang* states, but Infinite Divisibility dictates that there must also be *Yin within Yang, Yang within Yin*, and every permutation between. Interdependence dictates that no one thing, or aspect of existence, is inherently Yin or Yang by itself; all is interconnected and must be viewed in comparison. All of these states are, of course, in constant flux, with Inter-transformation and Mutual Consumption constantly re-balancing the equation.

In other words, there is no masculine without the feminine, just as there is no day without night, or sunshine without shadow. Each person must therefore have both Yin and Yang aspects, and the ability to transform into, or express, either or both. This is a perfect description for the great variety of gender presentations – including gender-fluid, queer, and transgender – as well as the need for expansive and inclusive language.

Figure 3.4 demonstrates Yin–Yang theory at play with issues of gender identity and expression. The North and South poles of Water and Fire are the 'Ultimate' positions of Yin and Yang. They are shown here by hyper-gendered states, i.e., hyperfemininity or hypermasculinity. These poles could be represented by a female beauty pageant contestant in full regalia, and an over-developed, muscular male boxer about to enter the ring. The East and West poles are where Yin and Yang are transforming into each other; where the feminine is transforming into the masculine, and vice versa. There are dozens of gender identities and expressions that could hold the East–West positions: drag kings and drag queens, femme bois and butch dykes, and MTF and FTM transgendered individuals are just a few possibilities. At the central position, where there is a blending of the four poles, everything stabilizes as neutral. Here again, there are multiple options to represent neutrality, including androgynous, gender non-conforming, or genderqueer persons. It is important to emphasize again that the Taiji is not static: on a day-to-day basis any individual can choose how to express themselves.

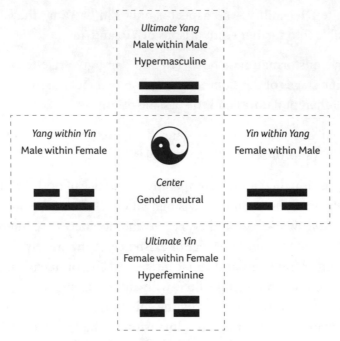

Figure 3.4: The Yin–Yang of Gender

TRANS(CENDING)GENDER

As healers trained in a philosophy of dualities, we have the ability to understand the fluidity of nature at a profound level. By translating this level of understanding to all aspects of our treatment, we can offer all patients including the transgendered, the type of sensitivity and high level of care they deserve.

– Elizabeth Sommers and Kristen Porter 2003a, p.5

Transgender and transsexual are two commonly used terms to describe a person whose anatomical sex and gender identity differ. Transsexual is a more outdated term, but is still commonly used to denote individuals that wish to change their anatomical sex (through hormones, surgery, etc.). Transgender is a newer term, which applies to individuals that do not conform to gender norms, but may or may not wish to change their sex. Transgender is commonly used in opposition to cisgender, with the implication that those who feel comfortable in their alignment of sex and gender are cis, and those that do not feel in alignment are trans. In other words, there are cis-males, cis-females, trans-male-to-female, and trans-female-to-male. These options can also translate into the four poles of Yin–Yang theory, as shown in Figure 3.5.

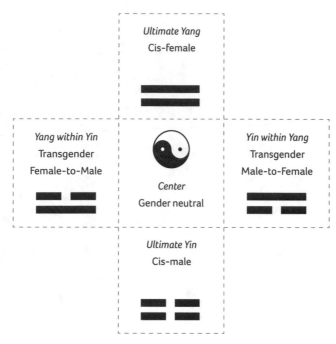

Figure 3.5: Transgender Yin–Yang I

Unfortunately, Figure 3.5 starts to resemble dipolar 'this versus that' thinking, such as is found in a binary gender system. Fortunately, Western culture has greatly expanded in the last two decades, offering newer language that rejects the concepts of binary genderism: gender-fluid, genderqueer, gender non-conforming, and gender-variant are just a few of these options. As fluid itself is a solution that is flexible, ever-shifting, and lacking a fixed physical shape, gender-fluid is perhaps the best term to represent the ever-changing *Yin within Yang*, *Yang within Yin*, and the churning center of the Taiji. Figure 3.6 attempts to correct binary concepts by showing gender-fluid as both the 'between states' of *Yin within Yang* and *Yang within Yin*, as well as the center point of infinite possibility. Transgender and cisgender take position as the opposing Ultimates, with cis represented by the more Yin-physical aspect, and trans represented by the more Yang-energetic aspect.

The roots of a person's gender identity are based in a combination of Shen-Spirit and Jing-Essence (see Chapter 4). These are deeply ingrained in a person's Constitution and therefore not likely to dramatically change over the course of a lifetime. The two exceptions that can push one's identity to change over time are 1) oppression and repression, where an individual has been denied the possibility of self-awareness due to cultural pressures, and 2) the lack of accessibility to language that accurately describes one's experience. Although there are some aspects of gender that are difficult to change, one's gender expression – the external display – can always change day to day.

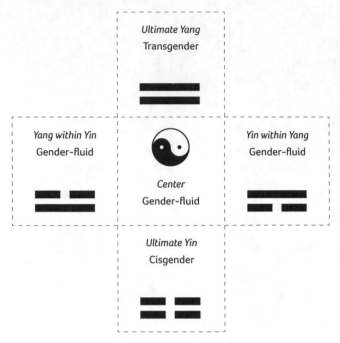

Figure 3.6: Transgender Yin–Yang II

Never Judge a Book by its Cover

At first glance, someone might appear gender-normative or gender-straight, easily fitting binary gender categories through their dress and mannerisms; it is important to realize that this is often done because of cultural pressure to conform. Those who specialize in treating transgender, gender-fluid, or gender non-conforming clients will emphasize again and again that asking people their identity and choice of pronouns (and consistently honoring those choices) goes a long way toward trust-building in every relationship.

GENDER PLAY

It is widely accepted that children develop a sense of their gender identity early, by the age of three. If there is cultural support, most children, including transgender individuals, are able to verbalize this knowledge by the age of five. Refinement of concepts and full comprehension of gender identity and its implications within one's culture would clearly take more time than this, but it is clear that children know exactly who they are from a very early age.

Gender expression is the outward presentation of this identity, shown to the world primarily through clothing, hairstyle, mannerisms, and roles. Another way that people can physically and energetically transform their gender is through the use of prosthetics. Drag queens and transgendered MTFs might use gluteal enhancers and breast forms to reshape their bodies. Drag kings and FTMs may 'pack' their genitalia, using bound socks, small dildos, or commercially produced items to visually flesh out the area. Prosthetics not only help portray the appearance of one's gender identity, but can also help people 'feel' more like the chosen gender by altering the shape of the energetic field.

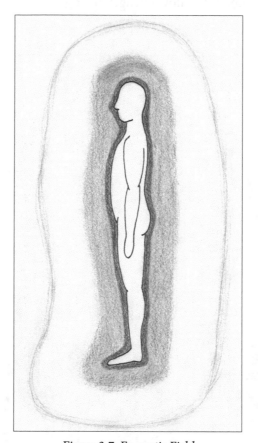

Figure 3.7: Energetic Field

Figure 3.7 demonstrates the energetic field which extends from the body, consisting of three levels that correspond to the physical, emotional, and spiritual aspects. These fields are commonly used in Medical Qigong, Qigong for self-cultivation, and Taiji practices. Taiji sword practice is actually the perfect example of prosthetic use, as one aims to feel the inanimate object – in this case a sword – as an extension of the arm and body. By allowing their Qi to flow into and around the sword extension, it is incorporated into the practitioner's energetic field, which not only enhances their sword technique but also transforms their overall energetic field shape.

'Packing,' breast forms, and other gendered prosthetics can alter the shape of the person's external energetic fields in this very same way, creating a better sense of comfort – of physical 'right-ness' – for the wearer. Figure 3.8 shows the changing shape of the energetic field for individuals wearing breast and genital prosthetics. For transgender individuals suffering from gender dysphoria, a form of emotional distress related to the 'mismatch' of gender identity and anatomical sex, the energetic flow changes from prosthetic forms can provide welcome respite.

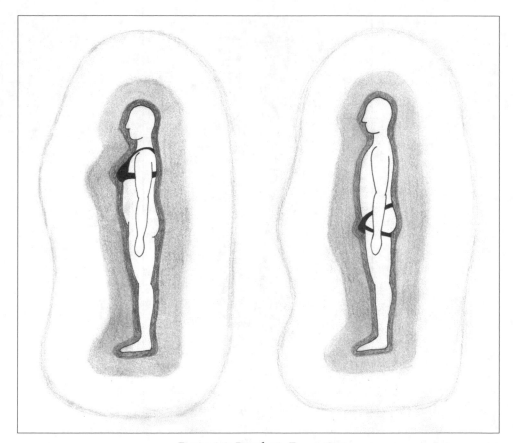

Figure 3.8: Prosthetic Energetics

Gender expression and gender identity do not have to be in perfect alignment at all times. Experimentation with gender expression is extremely healthy and not to be considered pathological or kinky.

Clearly the majority of obstacles to more gender-fluid or transgender expression are created by cultural norms, so each person must choose for themselves how to best address these issues for their own emotional and physical safety. The emotional impact of gender repression is discussed later in this book (see Section IV), but the acute impact on the Earth organs is worth noting here.

The Earth organs are located at the seat of the Middle *Dan Tian,* where they nurture the Post-Natal Qi through the creation of Gu Qi. In order to do this, these organs take in the food and drink, deciding which aspects (nutrients, etc.) to physically accept, and which to reject: i.e., the Clear versus the Turbid. Psycho-spiritually, the process of Earth acceptance relates to the self: *Am I accepted in this world? Am I able to accept myself?* Damage to the Earth organs is common in individuals that have a good grasp of their gender identity – i.e., who they know themselves to be – but who are not allowed to express that openly and uninhibitedly.

The Earth organs are vulnerable to damage anytime an individual does not feel personally accepted by their culture, with some specific symptoms that commonly correlate:

- Digestive complaints related to Phlegm, Stagnation, or Yang Deficiency – especially food stagnation, abdominal bloating and pain, diarrhea/constipation/IBS, gallstones.

- Menstrual issues from Qi or Blood Stagnation – especially *pain* (dysmennorhea, endometriosis, fibroids), but also clots, irregular cycles, and amenorrhea.

- Auto-immune conditions associated with Qi Stagnation and stress – especially allergies.

- Mental health issues related to Qi or Blood Stagnation, Phlegm, or Yang Deficiency – especially depression and anxiety.

My own daughter (born female sex) verbalized her gender identity as 'girl' around the age of four. At this time she also told stories about her infancy and childhood (up to age three) as the time 'when I [was] a boy.' In a heteronormative culture where 'male' is the assumed linguistic neutral, her preschool-age word choice regarding self-knowledge of gender identity aligns well with current research. As she becomes exposed to more terminology and her level of gender comprehension refines, she may choose different verbal descriptors to reflect her experience.

SUMMARY

» Neither anatomical sex nor gender are binary. All of life must follow the principles of Yin–Yang theory: relative opposition, interdependence, infinite divisibility, inter-transformation, and mutual consumption.

» Gender is a social construct, and an umbrella term for identity and expression.

» Gender identity is one's internal self-perception of their own gender. It is deeply ingrained, not likely to change, and related to the Shen-Spirit.

» Gender expression is the external display of dress, demeanor, and social behavior. It can change from day to day and is related to the Emotions, the Earth Organs, and the Post-Natal Qi.

» Cultural oppression and limited access to language/terminology are the biggest obstructions to an accurate self-assessment of gender identity.

» Never assume an individual is cisgender; it is best to ask clients about their preferred identity and choice of pronouns.

» Prosthetics can help a person to alter their Qi flow and energetic fields, enabling them to feel more comfortable in their chosen gender presentation.

» Earth organ symptoms related to acceptance include various digestive and menstrual complaints, allergies, depression, and anxiety.

Chapter 4

A SPIRITUAL JOURNEY

- Nine Palaces and the Extraordinary Vessels

- Three Treasures and the *Wu Shen*

- Treatment Options

How an individual's Constitution is formed remains an issue of debate within Chinese Medicine. This is due in large part to the different spiritual perspectives of the founding philosophies, Buddhism, Confucianism, and Daoism. For example, a Confucian might state that an individual's Constitution is driven by family: that children take on the elemental nature that complements and blends well into the birth-family dynamic. Conversely, a Daoist might argue that the elemental nature is not determined by the family at all: one is born into the circumstances and Constitutional alignment that is necessary to uphold the individual's Heavenly Contract.

Those that affirm the concept of a Heavenly Contract generally agree that this is formed in the Wuji, from which all things are possible. It is an agreement between a pre-incarnate Spirit and the Heavenly Emperor that dictates the challenges that must be faced in a given lifetime *before* the Spirit is granted a human form in which to manifest and learn these lessons. The Heavenly Contract then is part of the Pre-Heaven or Pre-Natal Qi that comes into the new life. These lessons can play out via family, culture, geographic area, Constitution, and, of course, anatomical sex, gender identity, and sexual identity.

Obviously the concerns of Diverse Gender and Sexuality (DGS) individuals can be a life-long journey of self-discovery. In Nigel Ching's 2016 talk at TCM Kongress – Rothenburg, Ching spoke about the gender journey in relation to the Dao:

My own gender idenity and presentation, and transgenderism in general, relates to *De* – how the *Dao* is manifesting. I am manifesting my true self. My *Dao* is that there is a discrepancy between my physical gender and my gender identity. A female heart in a male body. My *Dao* is to be different from other people, but this is in reality exactly the same for each and everyone of us. None of us are normal. Normality is a common prison, that we are each of us both prisoners and prison guards in, at the same time. If we step outside of the prison bars and manifest our true selves, then we follow the *Dao* in its manifesting. This is *De*.

De is translated as original nature or virtue, referring to an individual's innate capacity for following their truth, their path, their way. As Lonny Jarrett states, *De* is, then, 'that aspect of heaven, as it exists within each of us, that the vicissitudes of life may never harm. *De*, as the primordial influence of heaven, remains pure and untouched in each person's depths' (2001, p.46). Ching understands that the journey of gender identity and transgenderism is a journey of Destiny; it is how the challenges of the *Dao* are manifesting, offering an opportunity to cultivate and remember the true *De*.

Of course, each person still has the privilege of choice. No matter what the Heavenly Contract dictates, individuals may choose to acknowledge and follow their nature, or they can turn away from it. As Jarrett also states, 'Heaven may will us a unique nature, but it cannot force us to manifest that destiny… Just as an emperor cannot command people to be upright, so heaven cannot mandate each of us to treasure the gift of *de*' (2001, p.46).

The Nine Palaces

1. Health	4. Relationship	7. Career
2. Wealth	5. Creativity and Children	8. Wisdom
3. Prosperity	6. Travel and Adventure	9. Home

NINE PALACES AND THE EXTRAORDINARY VESSELS

The spiritual challenges of the Heavenly Contract are brought into one's life via the challenges of the Nine Palaces. The Nine Palaces are a series of inter-related, repeating lessons that must be undertaken and resolved by each individual in order to avoid reincarnation. This can be viewed as a college program where everyone has the same prerequisites, but each person chooses a particular course to fulfill the requirements in their own way. Each person's major field of study was also chosen for them before the program even began: this is the *Dao*, the way of Destiny.

The first eight palaces correspond to the *Ba Gua* commonly used in both Feng Shui and martial arts practices, each with their corresponding trigrams and elemental associations. These palaces are Health, Wealth, Prosperity, Relationship, Creativity and Children, Travel and Adventure, Career, and Wisdom. The ninth and ultimate position is located at the center of the *Ba Gua*: this is 'Home.' In regard to the challenges of gender and sex, four palaces are of greatest interest: Health, Relationship, Travel and Adventure, and Home.

Health is the first and most important palace for any individual; it is the foundation upon which all others are built and must be addressed in order to fulfill the remaining palaces. Perfect health is not the goal here. Instead, Health focuses on how we take care of ourselves as a reflection of self-worth and the inherent value in identifying and caring for our true needs. When an individual is taught negative self-image (such as 'I'm a freak' or 'No one will ever love me' or 'I am evil') then their perception of self and ability to maintain Health – emotional, physical, and spiritual – will be impacted. For example, a transgender person with crippling gender dysphoria may experience difficulty in adequately caring for the physical body that is the cause of emotional distress, preferring to dissociate from physical care (including preventative medical care such as PAP smears, breast exams, STD testing, etc.).

Health reflects the Yang-Wood Element in terms of the ability to grow and navigate the challenges of life with courage. As part of this palace, each individual must recognize their own inappropriate beliefs or habits that are contributing to poor health, and instead cultivate a positive relationship with the self through both physical and mental self-care.

> When culture teaches people to feel bad about or to hide their true selves – pretending to be heteronormative, monogamous, 'straight,' etc. – the impact on self-esteem in undeniable. As belief in one's self is the foundation for spiritual growth in the Health Palace, none of the other Nine Palaces can be properly fulfilled until this challenge is overcome.

Although Wealth and Prosperity lie between, the fourth palace of Relationship builds directly on the challenges to self-worth and self-care that were faced in Health. This palace addresses relationship to self and to others, in that the cultivation of healthy internal abundance (through self-love/self-worth) is critical for the development of healthy external relationships of any kind. If a person is able to identify and address their needs without self-criticism (the lesson of Health), then they can develop healthy, authentic interaction with others. Without feelings of internal abundance, a person might choose abusive relationships that negate self-worth, or attract co-dependent relationships that reflect an internal landscape of insecurity, vulnerability, and desperation to feel needed or desirable.

Travel and Adventure is the sixth palace, also called the palace of Opportunity. This palace represents one's engagement with the external world, learning new ways of doing, seeing, and thinking outside of the 'comfort zone.' The spiritual journey of gender and sex involves being open-minded, pushing against cultural and personal boundaries, and granting one's self the latitude to engage without judgment. Associated with Yang-Metal, this palace also involves release of one's attachment to the known: once we set out to travel to a new place or learn something new, there is no guarantee of returning the same person as when we left. Curiosity, adaptability, and resilience are all required for Travel and Adventure, especially when we might encounter the unexpected. Cultural messages of homophobia, misogyny, and slut-shaming are especially problematic to this palace in relation to DGS issues. They are also the cause for many emotional states in Section IV that would prevent someone from reaching the ultimate palace: Home.

Home is the final palace, a place of sanctuary and comfort at the center of the *Ba Gua*. It is the experience of contentment where nothing is lacking. Any pain or suffering is met not with overwhelming Fear or Sadness, but with curiosity and willingness to adapt. It takes belief in self-worth, construction of a wellness-promoting lifestyle, the ability to maintain empowering relationships, and flexible engagement with new experiences and beliefs (as well as facing the other five challenges) to arrive here. It is possible to glimpse this palace without having fully realized the other eight, but life will continue to dole out the other challenges until all Nine Palaces are truly fulfilled. For DGS individuals going against conservative cultural traditions, this journey toward Home may require extraordinary effort.

Oppressive cultural messages can create impediments to self-worth (impacting Health and Relationship), or limit one's ability to explore and grow (impacting Travel and Adventure). As practitioners of Chinese Medicine, we can serve all of our clients by being an excellent ally (see Section I) and demonstrating a firm belief in their spiritual journey – no matter where it takes them. We can also help them to face the Nine Palace challenges through the influence of the corresponding Extraordinary Vessels (EV).

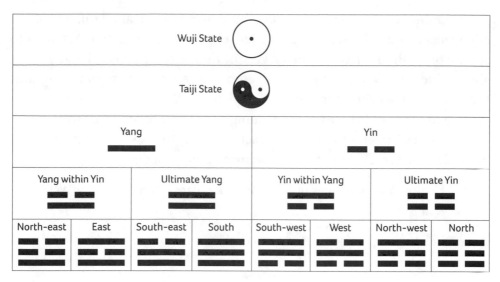

Wuji State	
Taiji State	
Yang	Yin
Yang within Yin	Ultimate Yang	Yin within Yang	Ultimate Yin
North-east	East	South-east	South	South-west	West	North-west	North

Figure 4.1: Development of the Ba Gua

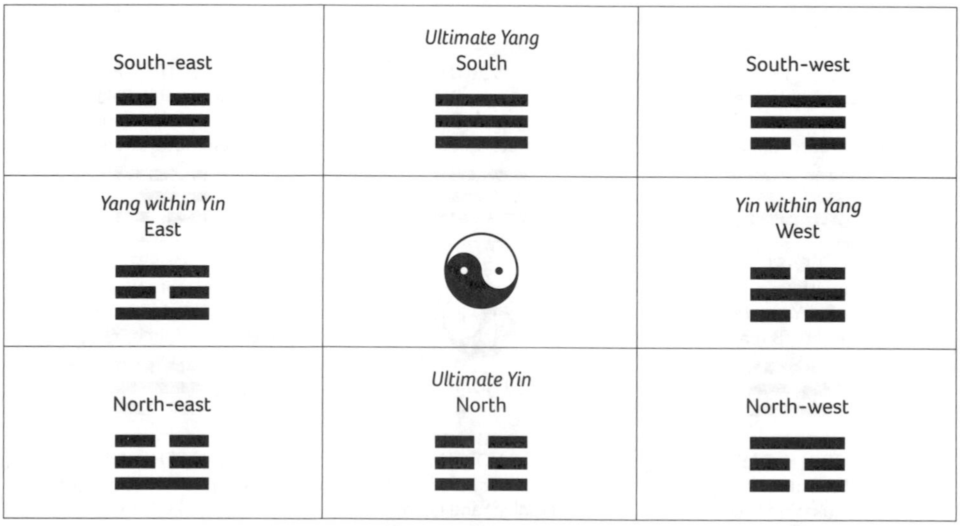

South-east	Ultimate Yang South	South-west
Yang within Yin East		*Yin within Yang* West
North-east	Ultimate Yin North	North-west

Figure 4.2: The Ba Gua

Figure 4.1 shows the formation of the eight trigrams of the *Ba Gua*. The diagram starts with an open – but not empty – circle: the Wuji. Originating from the Wuji came the Taiji: the blending of Yin and Yang. The duality of Yin and Yang is represented by a solid line (Yang) and a broken line (Yin). Building on Yin and Yang are the Four Directions (*Ultimate Yin, Ultimate Yang, Yin within Yang, and Yang within Yin*), which are represented by two lines. These are further differentiated into the full set of eight trigrams. Figure 4.2 shows the trigrams arranged according to the *Ba Gua*, placed at the Four Directions (East, South, West, and North) and their four midway points.

In Leslie Franks' *Stone Medicine*, she shows a classical alignment of the Nine Palaces with the eight trigrams (2016, pp.34–38). In Keiko Matsumoto and Stephen Birch's *Extraordinary Vessels*, they show a classical system that aligns different EV master point correspondences with these same trigrams (1986, pp.6–7). As shown in Figure 4.3, by putting these systems together, each of the Nine Palaces has two corresponding EVs. Logic follows that treating the Extraordinary Vessels can directly impact the ability to respond to the lessons of particular palaces. Of particular importance in this chapter are:

- Health Palace – issues of self-worth, self-care – treat the Yang Wei or the Ren Mai.

- Relationship Palace – issues of relating to others – treat the Yin Qiao or the Dai Mai.

- Travel and Adventure – issues of vulnerability, flexibility, new experiences – treat the Chong or Yin Wei Mai.

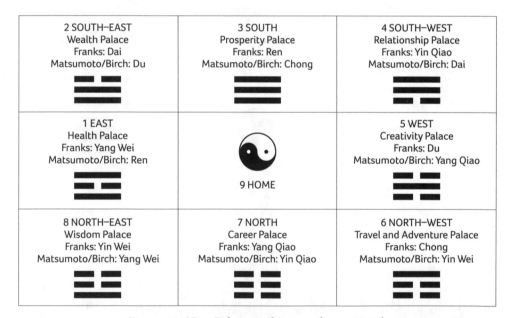

Figure 4.3: Nine Palaces and Extraordinary Vessels

Spiritual journey treatments are best done with gentle and consistent technique. Because EVs are easily damaged with over-treatment, Acupuncture and Herbal Medicine are not always the best modalities. An alternative approach uses Gemstones, which have a particular affinity for facing the challenges of life. Gemstones work best with direct skin contact, and can only reach full potential when they are able to interact as a grouping. Select an appropriate few from the following:

- Health: Carnelian (Red Chalcedony), Chrysoprase, Aventurine Green, Green Jade, Septarian Nodules (Dragon's Egg), Sodalite, Turquoise.

- Relationship: Beryl (Pink or Golden Yellow), Blue Lace Agate, Charoite, Chrysocolla, Green Garnet (Tsavorite, Uvarovite, Demantoid), Kunzite (Pink Spodumene), Red or Pink Tourmaline/Rubellite, Rhodonite, Rose Quartz, Seraphinite, Zincite.

- Travel and Adventure: Blue Beryl/Aquamarine, Hematite, Kyanite, Labradorite, Moonstone, Smoky Quartz, Turquoise.

When considering the EV correspondences, one could also add:

- Health: Beryl (Pink Morganite), Diamond, Moonstone, Peridot, Snow-flake Obsidian, Sugilite.

- Relationship: Hemimorphite, Pearl, Stalactite, Zircon.

- Travel and Adventure: Chong – Amethyst, Azurite, Coral, Epidote, Lepidolite, Obsidian (Black, Gold Sheen, Rainbow, Snowflake) Spinel, Topaz, Unakite.

Unfortunately, the palace of Home cannot be treated using the EV correspondence system. Home is only attained by accomplishing the challenges of the other eight.

When working with clients, it is important to remember that courage is required to face any life challenge, but especially those challenges that go against cultural norms. As the Nine Palaces are transmitted into human life upon creation, the Jing-Essence and *Yuan*/Source Qi of Kidney Yang are intimately related to these challenges. Of course, one of the most common obstructions to following one's *De* is Fear, which will deplete both Water and Wood Elements, inhibiting courage. It is only the strength and stability of Water and the Lower *Dan Tian* that can enable an individual to ignore Fear in order to manifest and integrate their gender and sexuality through the Three Treasures.

THREE TREASURES AND THE *WU SHEN*

The challenges of the *Dao* come into the human form via the Three Treasures of Jing–Qi–Shen, which are associated with the three forces of Earth–Humanity–Heaven. Although the three forces are not heavily emphasized in Chinese Medical theory, these terms are used extensively in cultivation practices (i.e., Qigong and other internal alchemy traditions). In this system, there are Three Treasures associated with each force: Heaven has the sun, moon, and stars, Earth has soil, wind, and water, and Humanity has Jing-Essence, Qi, and Shen-Spirit.

Jing, the Essence associated with the Water Element, is the Treasure with the most physical substance of Humanity's Three Treasures. It sits in the Lower *Dan Tian* – 'heavenly elixir' or 'red cinnabar field' – and is associated with the force of Earth. Shen-Spirit is the most insubstantial Treasure. It is intimately related to the Fire Element of the Upper Jiao and associated with the force of Heaven. Qi is a blend of Jing-Essence and Shen-Spirit, so it is found in the Middle Jiao associated with the forces of Humanity.

The Three Treasures are in constant interaction, interconnected via the Taiji pole. Their relationship is perhaps best illustrated by steam rising from a cooking pot, heated by the flames of Jing-Essence and the *Ming Men* Fire. This pot contains the food and fluids of culture, which form the foundation of Post-Heaven Qi. As the Qi is warmed by Jing, steam rises up from the pot, manifesting the Shen-Spirit. Without the flames of Jing underneath the pot of Qi, there would be no steam rising up from the Qi, and no Shen-Spirit to follow the mandate of Heaven (see Figure 4.4).

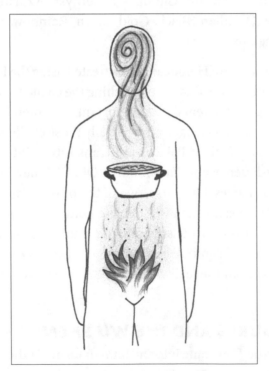

Figure 4.4: The Three Treasures

Anatomical sex, gender expression, and gender identity are easily viewed in relation to these Three Treasures. In the *Dan Tian* of the Lower Jiao resides the Jing-Essence, which is related to the Water Element, the *Yuan*/Source Qi that is spread by the San Jiao, and the ability of the physical form to grow and reproduce. Just as steam cannot rise if there is no flame, the Shen-Spirit cannot remain in the Earthly realm if there is no physical form. Therefore, the Earth, Jing-Essence, and 'flame' of the Three Treasures are associated with the physical human body and one's anatomical sex.

Gender identity is one's internal self-perception of their gender. Although identity is a generally unchanging characteristic deeply anchored to the Jing-Essence, it can only properly manifest when the emotions of self-awareness and self-acceptance are allowed to flow uninhibited. In this way, gender identity is the steam on top of the cooking pot. Although the verbalization of one's identity is related to the perspective and language of one's culture, the *truth* of one's identity is related to the influence of Heaven and the Shen-Spirit.

Whereas gender identity is deeply personal and does not easily shift, gender expression is highly influenced by culture. It is a painful reality that many people do not feel comfortable displaying identity because of social expectations. Gender expression is responsible for navigating this terrain, choosing how and when to present one's authentic self to the world. Choice of gender expression can shift day to day or moment to moment, just as Qi is able to follow thought. In these ways, gender expression is associated with the Middle *Dan Tian* and the forces of Humanity. Table 4.1 shows the alignment of sex, gender expression, and gender identity in relation to the Three Treasures of Humanity.

Table 4.1: The Three Treasures of Gender and Sexuality

Force	Location	Treasure	Influence	Aspect
Heaven	Upper *Dan Tian*	(Wu) Shen Spirit	Self-perception, awareness and acceptance	Gender identity
Humanity	Middle *Dan Tian*	Qi Post-Natal Qi and Emotions	Cultural expectations and day-to-day decisions	Gender expression
Earth	Lower *Dan Tian*	Jing Essence	Physical form	Anatomical sex

When considering issues of gender as a spiritual journey, it is important to remember that there are actually five forms of Shen-Spirit. The *Wu Shen* includes the Hun, Shen (the 'little' Shen related to the Heart), Yi, Po, and Zhi, each with their own attributes and elemental correspondences. Three are of primary importance to how an individual interprets their gender and sex: the Hun, the Shen, and the Po.

Table 4.2 re-examines the Treasures based on these three aspects of the *Wu Shen*. The Po, 'corporeal soul' of the Lungs and Metal Element, is activated when a newborn takes their first breath. It is intimately connected to the physical body, and remains with it through death. Therefore, the Spirit of the Po best corresponds to the most physical aspect of the Three Treasures, the force of Earth as manifesting through anatomical sex.

The Shen is associated with the Heart and the Fire Element. It manages the flow of emotions by using the Blood to circulate experiences throughout the body for comprehension and integration. Shen is directly connected to the Post-Natal experience of the individual's culture and the Qi of Emotions, so it is associated with the force of Humanity and one's gender expression.

The Hun is the 'ethereal soul' associated with the Liver and the Wood Element. The Hun is said to 'travel outside the body' during sleep, receiving dream messages from the Wuji that Wood can transform into action. Destiny comes from the Wuji as well, so by bringing forth messages from the dream world the Hun uses Wood's courage and direction to help manifest the truth of gender identity – who we intuitively know ourselves to be – at the conscious level.

Table 4.2: *Wu Shen* and the Three Treasures

Force	Location	Wu Shen	Aspect
Heaven	Upper *Dan Tian*	Hun	Gender identity
Humanity	Middle *Dan Tian*	Shen	Gender expression
Earth	Lower *Dan Tian*	Po	Anatomical sex

Three Treasures and *Wu Shen* Review

- Anatomical sex – related to physical form, the forces of Earth, Jing-Essence, the flames of the Water Element, and the spirit of the Po (Metal Element). The Lower *Dan Tian* is located in the lower abdomen incorporating the Uterus/*Zi Bao* in females and the Essence Palace/*Jing Gong* in males.

- Gender expression – related to emotions and the movements of Qi, Post-Natal Qi (Earth Element), the forces of Humanity (culture), and the Shen-Spirit (Fire Element). It is supported by the Middle *Dan Tian* located at the center of the chest (Ren 17).

- Gender identity – related to *Wu Shen*, the forces of Heaven, and the Hun. It is supported by the Upper *Dan Tian* located at the center of the head (Min Tang).

TREATMENT OPTIONS

When treating the spiritual journey of gender and sex through the Three Treasures and Five Spirits, the primary area of focus is the Lower *Dan Tian* and the force of Earth. The interaction of the physical body, Jing-Essence, and the Po are the flame that ignite and inspire the other Treasures, and there are three potential treatments to consider:

1. Warming the Lower *Dan Tian* to 'build up' the Jing-Essence.

2. Aligning the three *Dan Tian* to better integrate the Jing–Qi–Shen.

3. Harmonizing the Lower *Dan Tian* through the Ren, Du, and Chong Vessels.

1. Warming the Lower *Dan Tian*: Building the Flame

Here the Jing is not able to connect with Qi and Shen, due to improper activation from either Deficiency or obstruction in the Lower Jiao. Symptoms of Middle and Upper Jiao organs are deficient in presentation because the Qi and Shen are unsupported by Jing. Due to the lack of warmth, Qi impact is likely digestive system, Yang and/or Qi Deficiency, and Earth organ focused. Shen impact is likely of a depressive nature affecting the Hun or the Shen, but anxiety is also possible when lack of warmth has allowed Yin excess to accumulate. The client may deny the opportunities for growth that life presents to them: 'Oh, but I can't do *that*!' Or they may complain of lack of self-awareness, a sense of belonging, or the courage to face that which is already intuitively known.

- Treatment Principles: Warm the Kidneys, *Ming Men* Fire, Nourish Jing-Essence, Harmonize the San Jiao (clear obstructions as needed – see option 3 below, or Section IV).

Primary Modalities

- Acupuncture and Moxabustion: Du 3, 4, UB 22, 23, 25, 31–35, Ren 4–6, 8, 12, Zigong, ST 25–27; consider Acupuncture only for Ren 13–17, Du 6–11, Yintang–Taiyang–Du 20 (in combination) and other points of the *Mu Xi/ eye system*. *Note: Always pair points in the Lower Jiao with Middle and Upper Jiao points to harmonize the San Jiao and connect the Three Treasures.*

- Herbal Formulae: Wu Zi Yan Zong Wan, Huan Shao Wan, Jin Gui Shen Qi Wan, You Gui Wan, Ba Ji Yin Yang Wan, Er Xian Wan, Zuo Gui Wan.

- Qigong: Five Animal Frolics–Bear; Hun Yuan Gong–Opening and Closing Heaven and Earth.

Secondary Modalities

- Diet: Warming foods such as cinnamon, garlic, ginger, lamb, rosemary, shrimp, venison, walnut; small meals are appropriate for those with food stagnation concerns.

- Lifestyle: Small amounts of daily cardiovascular exercise (10–20 minutes) to raise the body temperature, preferably during the hours of 3–5 pm to activate Kidney Yang.

Location of the Three *Dan Tian*

There are two different locations of the three *Dan Tian*. In most theoretical systems, they are located in the lower abdomen near Ren 4–6, in the center of the chest (Ren 17), and in the ventricular space at the center of the head. Some Qigong theories place the Middle and Upper *Dan Tian* in slightly different locations: at the solar plexus area (Stomach/Ren 12), and the center of the chest (Ren 17). This second set is thought to better align with the Three Treasures, placing the Jing-Essence in the *Zi Bao*/Uterus in women or Room of Essence in men, the Post-Natal Qi in the Stomach (as the source of food and fluids that create Gu Qi), and the Spirit at the center of the Chest where the Zong Qi and Blood are formed.

---

2. *Dan Tian* Alignment: Integrating the Treasures

The Three Treasures are connected via the Taiji pole of energy that extends from the perineal floor (Ren 1) along the anterior aspect of the spine to the crown chakra (Du 20/Bai Hui). To align the three *Dan Tian*, one focuses on the connection between the Lower and Middle – the flames and the cooking pot – to ensure that the steam of the Spirit is able to rise naturally on its own. Clients will likely present with flip-flopping or conflicting ideas and goals, unable to move forward in their lives because of constant switching of direction or focus. Depression and postural concerns are likely to present, including mild kyphosis and scoliosis.

- Treatment Principles: Stimulate and Harmonize the *Dan Tian* and the Taiji pole (*Note: In Medical Qigong the Chong Vessel is thought to align with the Taiji pole and they are often considered the same structure*).

Primary Modalities

- Acupuncture: KI 1–KI 16–Du 20 in combination to stimulate the Taiji pole (can substitute KI 16 with Moxa on Ren 8); Chong Vessel (LV 3–SP 4–PC 6 in combination); points around Ren 3–6 (Lower), Ren 12–17

(Middle), Yintang–Taiyang–Du 20 and other points of the *Mu Xi*/eye system (Upper).

- Medical Qigong: Harmonize the three *Dan Tian* (*Note: To avoid the potential for Shen-disturbance, always focus in the Lower and Middle* Dan Tian *with more repetition, more time, and finishing with the Lower* Dan Tian):

    - Circling (clockwise) over the three *Dan Tian*: in the order of Lower–Middle–Upper–Middle–Lower

    - Holding the three *Dan Tian*: In the order of Lower–Middle, Middle–Upper, Upper–Lower, and end with the Lower only

    - Taiji pole activation: Gentle stimulation at Du 20, visualizing the connection to Kidney 1; then gentle stimulation at Kidney 1, visualizing the connection to Du 20; end by closing both portals from Kidney 1.

- Qigong: Hun Yuan Gong–Opening and Closing Heaven and Earth.

- Lifestyle: If postural issues are present, bodywork may be appropriate to treat chronic, improper musculoskeletal or structural alignment (Massage, Tuina, Rolfing, Myofascial Release/MFR, etc.).

The Ancestral Vessels: Ren, Du, and Chong Mai

Ren is most often translated as the vessel of 'conception,' but Ren also means 'to accept' and 'to hold something in front of the abdomen' (Matsumoto and Birch 1986, p.3). Jeffrey Yuen (2017) says the Ren Mai is the vessel of bonding, helping establish a sense of stability and support in order to counterbalance the emotion of Fear.

Du Mai is translated as the 'governing' vessel. It represents the archetype of the general, someone that exerts control over a certain domain. It is intimately related to the para-spinal muscles that develop in infancy, allowing a child to sit upright, crawl, and eventually stand, coming face to face with cultural expectations. The Du helps maintain individuality and the ability to 'stand up for one's self' amidst pressure to conform.

The Chong Mai is considered the 'thoroughfare' or 'penetrating' vessel, but Matsumoto and Birch offer another view: 'Chong means a street. It is used to express the idea of passing or transformation. In some contexts chong refers to alchemical transformation, two entities "crashing together" to produce something different' (Matsumoto and Birch 1986, p.3). Jeffrey Yuen (2017a) describes the Chong as a vessel of 'rectification' that reconciles the differences between cultural expectation and who we know ourselves to be. The Chong is often referred to as the 'mother' of all other Extraordinary Vessels, as the one that 'gives birth' to the other seven. It is also thought that the Ren and Du vessels are aspects of the Chong itself; not three separate vessels, but three aspects of one vessel. From this perspective, the Chong Mai is a vessel of 'integration,' merging the self-love and stability learned through proper bonding (Ren) and the strength to be one's self in the face of external pressure (Du).

3. Harmonizing the Lower *Dan Tian* and the 'Ancestral' Vessels

In Classical Chinese Medicine, the Ren, Du, and Chong are known as the Ancestral Vessels. These pass through the center of the Lower *Dan Tian* and form the 'blueprint' for the development of the physical form and the Primary Channels. They also guide the Cycles of 7 and 8 which dictate overall growth and development in one's life, including the maturity to face spiritual challenges related to gender and sex.

When the Ancestral Vessels are not properly functioning, a mix of Yin and Yang, deficient and excess pathology will present. There will be a variety of systemic symptoms involving multiple, unrelated organs and/or channels, extreme temperature variations, neurological/sensation issues, emotional lability or mental health concerns, and complex health conditions. Harmonizing the Ren, Du, and Chong Vessels will clear obstructions in Lower *Dan Tian* and allow the 'flame' to flourish.

- Treatment Principles: Harmonize the Ren, Du, and Chong Vessels *(Note: Treatment of these three vessels will reappear many times throughout this book, as they are intertwined with any issues that obstruct the Constitution and/or the fulfillment of Destiny. Be careful not to damage these structures through aggressive or excessive Acupuncture treatment).*

Primary Modalities

- Acupuncture – *choose from:*

  - Taiji pole: KI 1–KI 16–Du 20 in combination (can substitute Ren 8 with Moxa for KI 16)

  - Chong Vessel: LV 3–SP 4–PC 6 in combination; KI 11–21, ST 30, Ren 1, 7

- Ren Vessel: LU 7–KI 6 in combination, Du 1, Ren 15; palpate for other points along the trajectory

- Du Vessel: SI 3–UB 62 in combination, Du 1, Ren 1, 24; palpate for other points along the trajectory.

- Medical Qigong:

  - Hold the EV Master-Couple pairs to visualize and activate the individual Vessels

  - Circling the Abdomen: Circling the palm over the abdomen counterclockwise and clockwise (may be the opposite order), ending with the palm over Ren 8

  - Taiji pole activation (see treatment 2 above).

- Qigong: Microcosmic Orbit; Hun Yuan Gong–Opening and Closing Heaven and Earth.

Secondary Modalities

- Herbal Formulae for the Ren and Chong: (Nu Ke) Ba Zhen Wan, (Tao Hong) Si Wu Wan, Er Xian Wan, Fu Ke Zhong Zi Wan, Wen Jing Wan, Dang Gui Jing, (Wu Ji) Bai Feng Wan.

- Gemstones:

  - Chong: Alexandrite, Amethyst, Ametrine, Chrysoprase, Coral, Epidote, Spinel, Topaz, Unakite

  - Ren: Diamond, Moonstone, Morganite

  - Du: Beryl, Meteorite, Ruby.

- Lifestyle: Client may need to be counseled regarding the amount and regularity of their sexual practices, as well as the components of healthy sexual activity (see Chapter 7).

SUMMARY

» *Dao* is the 'way' of one's Destiny; *De* is the individual's capacity – their original nature – to follow the *Dao*.

» Nine Palaces are the life challenges that must be addressed by each person throughout their lifetime to avoid reincarnation.

» Health is the palace of self-care. Its lessons are self-knowledge, self-acceptance, and self-worth.

» The Relationship palace includes all forms of relationship: intimate partners, friends, co-workers, etc. It requires the ability to enter relationship freely and without hesitation while maintaining healthy sense of self.

» Travel and Adventure is also the palace of Opportunity. The lesson of this palace is engagement with the unknown and the willingness to change while maintaining healthy sense of self.

» Home is the final palace where one feels they belong and is content in the *Dao*. To attain this palace requires learning all eight lessons: Health, Wealth, Prosperity, Relationship, Creativity and Children, Travel and Adventure, Career, and Wisdom.

» Extraordinary Vessels can be mobilized to help face the challenges of the Nine Palaces, but caution should be exercised to not damage them.

» The Ancestral Vessels – Ren, Du, and Chong – pass directly through the Lower *Dan Tian* and can be used to realign the Three Treasures.

» The Three Treasures of Jing–Qi–(*Wu*) Shen are found in the three *Dan Tian*, and align with the forces of Heaven–Humanity–Earth.

» Anatomical sex is associated with Jing-Essence in the Lower *Dan Tian*. It corresponds to the force of Earth, the flames of the Water Element, and the spirit of the Po (Metal Element).

» Gender expression is associated with Qi in the Middle *Dan Tian*. It corresponds to the force of Humanity (culture), the cooking pot/Post-Natal Qi of the Earth Element, and the Shen-Spirit (Fire Element).

» Gender identity is associated with the (*Wu*) Shen in the Upper *Dan Tian*. It corresponds with the force of Heaven and the spirit of the Hun (Wood Element).

Chapter 5

SPECIAL TOPIC: TRANSGENDER HEALTH CONCERNS

- Binding and Tucking

- Hormonal Homeostasis

- Sex Reassignment

- Emotional Transitioning

Table 5.1 should look familiar. It reappears here because transgender people have a unique experience of the Three Treasures: the anatomical sex they were born with *does not match* the gender identity that they know to be true. 'Transgender' is the best language we have available *at this time* for understanding this particular iteration of Yin and Yang. It is critically important for all practitioners to know that *this is not a disagreement, confusion, or misalignment* of Heaven and Earth. There should be no assumption of conflict for transgender people between their *Wu Shen* and their Jing. Instead, this is a purposeful juxtaposition coming through the Nine Palaces, offering a specific and unique challenge to be addressed in this lifetime: the opportunity to examine the physical body as a journey within itself.

There is no one way this challenge is presented. Transgender, gender-fluid, gender-non-conforming, butch, femme, drag, and transsexual identities may be stable, but they can also shift over time. The level of gender dysphoria distress will also range greatly between individuals, and not every transgender person is looking to transform their body.

If a person does decide to pursue physical transformation, contemporary society fortunately offers many options. This chapter looks at health issues specific to the process of transitioning for both Male-to-Female (MTF) and Female-to-Male (FTM) people: binding and tucking, hormones, medical/surgical scarring, and the emotional journey. Covering these topics in detail is truly a textbook unto itself, so only the basics are addressed here. If a practitioner wishes to work extensively with the transgender population, especially in regard to hormone balancing, further training with an experienced Chinese Medicine mentor is necessary.

Table 5.1: The Three Treasures

Force	Location	Treasure	Influence	Aspect
Heaven	Upper *Dan Tian*	(Wu) Shen Spirit	Self-perception, awareness and acceptance	Gender identity
Humanity	Middle *Dan Tian*	Qi Post-Natal Qi and Emotions	Cultural expectations and day-to-day decisions	Gender expression
Earth	Lower *Dan Tian*	Jing Essence	Physical form	Anatomical sex

The *Dao* of Gender

Having genitalia that does not align with one's gender identity *does not signify lack of alignment* between the Three Treasures. The *Dao* for Transgender people is to examine the physical body as a journey within itself; a great challenge to explore through the Nine Palaces and one's comprehension of Home.

BINDING AND TUCKING

Breast binding and genital taping/tucking are the most basic techniques used to transform gender. Fortunately, online do-it-yourself videos and commercially made products have helped make the process easier, faster, and a lot safer over the years. When individuals don't use the right product or have access to good information, problems can easily arise.

With binding, i.e., flattening the breasts to create a more masculine appearance, FTMs need to avoid products that tightly wrap the entire ribcage as this can easily cause diaphragmatic constriction, bruising, and in extreme cases can contort the shape of the ribs. For MTFs that are taping/tucking their genitalia posteriorly for a smooth frontal pelvic region, product choice is critical to avoid skin damage from adhesives, and most people need to shave the genital area. From a Chinese Medicine perspective, both MTFs and FTMs need to spend time every day with their tissues fully unbound, allowing free movement to reduce the chance of developing Qi and Blood Stagnation in the Channels, which is the primary pattern of disharmony associated with binding or tucking.

Breast Binding

The biggest concern with breast binding is the channel and energetic alignment issues caused by flesh constriction, but there is potential for injury to the San Jiao, Zheng Qi, and Extraordinary Vessels as well. As practitioners, we are already aware of the Qi Stagnation caused by inappropriately fitted women's bras, resulting in varying degrees of:

- Chest tightness and diaphragmatic constriction

- Shortness of breath and accompanying fatigue

- Emotional lability, especially anxiety and worry.

These symptoms are no different from those associated with binding, and clearly exhibit constriction of the *Zong*/Chest Qi acutely impacting the Heart and Lungs. With chronic wear, localized stagnation is also likely in the Stomach, Liver, Pericardium, Gallbladder, and Urinary Bladder Channels, with a high incidence of musculoskeletal excess in the intrascapular and suprascapular regions (GB 21, SI 11–15, UB 11–17, UB 42–46), accompanied by musculoskeletal deficiency in the lower thoracic and lumbar area. This adds the following possible symptoms: neck and shoulder tension, headaches, sinus congestion, numbness and tingling in the hands and fingers, lower back pain, and bowel issues (atonic constipation or diarrhea).

Improper binding remains a serious problem for do-it-yourself FTMs wrapping multiple bands around the ribcage. As a horizontal interruption to overall movement, excessive binding can also injure the body's major energetic horizontal pathway: the Dai Mai. Overly aggressive constriction (too tight or for too long) creates stagnation in the EV that 'binds' all the other channels, leading to classic Dai Mai symptoms such as vaginal discharge and menstrual complications as well as poor circulation to the legs, leg edema, and difficulty turning at the waist. Figure 5.1 offers a visual representation for likely symptom areas from both the physical binding at the diaphragm and Upper Jiao, and the energetic binds that reverberate superiorly and inferiorly.

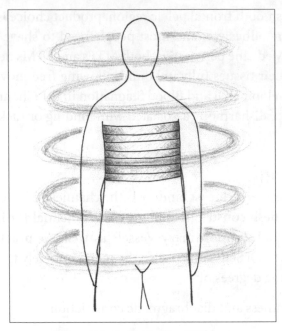

Figure 5.1: Basic Binding Problems

Gender dysphoria issues may also cause FTM individuals to sit in a 'forward slump' in order to hide their breast tissue: an intentional suppression of both the physical body and the energetic fields that surround it. The diaphragm is one of five Ancestral Sinews which interconnect and stabilize the torso, also including the sternocleidomastoid, psoas, paravertebrals, and abdominal rectus. Obstruction of the Diaphragm (through Zong Qi impact, poor posture, etc.) creates stagnation that eventually leads to deficiency and collapse of this core musculature, affecting the stability of other Ancestral Sinews as follows:

- *Sternocleidomastoid* will become overstretched, allowing compression at the occiput and misalignment of the cervical vertebrae; symptoms may include upper neck tension and stiffness, occipital headaches, tonsil stones, and 'Plum Pit Qi.'

- *Paravertebrals* will be forced to overstretch as well, while the *Abdominal Rectus* is allowed to slack, creating upper and mid back pain, hypotonicity of the abdominal flesh, as well as a host of digestive complaints.

- *Psoas* will likely shorten to stabilize the torso to the legs; this can torque the hips and pelvis, create tension in the hamstrings, iliotibial (IT) band, and/or gluteal muscles, and create bowel or menstrual difficulties.

The overall posture will become impacted over time, affecting the operation of the Qi Mechanism, the *Zheng*/Upright Qi, and the body's ability to fight off external illnesses. Figure 5.2 shows some the postural effects of improper binding on the Ancestral Sinews.

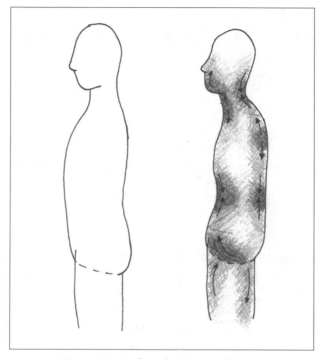

Figure 5.2: Binding the Ancestral Sinews

Beyond injuries to local organs and channels, the Dai Mai, and the Ancestral Sinews, deep impact on fluid movement and San Jiao functioning cannot be ignored. Fluid movement (lymph, blood, etc.) will be obstructed within the bound area, allowing Dampness, Blood Stasis, and/or Phlegm to accumulate in the Upper and/or Middle Jiaos. Yin Stasis could settle into any of the deficient organs or channels that were damaged in the local area, or it could be absorbed by the Extraordinary Vessels as the 'ditches' that collect excess from the Primary Channels. By moving the Yin Stasis into the EV, the body may be working to clear the chest cavity and help protect the Heart-Emperor, but the symptoms of Yin Stasis can appear anywhere system-wide, and could take years of treatment to fully resolve.

In summary, improper or extensive breast binding without appropriate opportunity for Qi and Blood to properly flow through the tissues is associated with multiple patterns of disharmony:

Acute patterns:

- Zong Qi Stagnation (affecting the Lungs, Heart, Pericardium)

- Stagnation in the Channels: Stomach, Liver, Pericardium, Gallbladder, Urinary Bladder.

Additional chronic patterns:

- Dampness, Blood Stasis, or Phlegm in the Upper Jiao (especially affecting the Heart)

- San Jiao obstruction and fluid accumulation (especially in Upper and/or Middle Jiaos)

- Dai Mai obstruction

- Ancestral Sinew and postural alignment issues with Zheng Qi Deficiency

- Yin Stasis in the Extraordinary Vessel(s).

Breast Binding Treatment Options

One must always look to the prevailing symptomology to alleviate suffering, but there are a few common treatment principles:

- 'Opening the Chest' or 'Unbinding the Heart' to clear Qi Stagnation (and/or Blood Stasis) in the Upper Jiao.

- Harmonizing the San Jiao and Dai Mai.

- Clearing Dampness, resolving Blood Stasis or Phlegm (local, systemic, or EV).

- Realigning the Ancestral Sinews and rectifying the Zheng Qi.

Primary Modalities

- Cupping *to clear Qi Stagnation, Phlegm, or Blood in the Upper Jiao and diaphragm*: Stationary/running Cupping in the intrascapular and suprascapular regions; flash Cupping in the intrascapular and supra-scapular regions and the upper chest.

- Qigong *to open and regulate the Zong Qi (generally, use open arm movements)*: Eight Brocades–Archer; Sheng Zhen Qigong: Heart Spirit as One/Jesus Sitting; Five Animal Frolics–Crane.

- Lifestyle: Advise clients to spend many consecutive hours without tissue constrictions, especially during sleep; stretching for the pectoralis, intrascapular, and latissimus dorsi regions; mild to moderate cardio-vascular exercise and core strength training (sit-ups, push-ups, plank pose, etc.).

Secondary Modalities

- Acupuncture: Ren 14–17, LU 1, 2, SP 21, PC 1, 6, ST12–18, LV 14, GB 21, 26–8, UB 13–18, 42–47; also consider applicable channel obstructions, etc.

- Herbal Formulae: Xue Fu Zhu Yu Tang Wan, Er Chen Wan, Nei Xiao Luo Li Wan, (Jia Wei) Xiao Yao Wan, Bu Zhong Yi Qi Wan.

CLIENT EXAMPLE

A lesbian female in her mid-20s presents with anxiety, diffuse musculoskeletal pain, and daily 'digestive attacks' of cramping pain and diarrhea between 7 and 10 am. She hates the cold, has allergies to pets and foods, and is being evaluated for IBS and fibromyalgia. She is thin, walks her dogs for an hour or more daily, is happy in her current relationship, but also has a history of abusive and co-dependent relationships and a very stressful job. In evaluating for the musculoskeletal pain, she flinches frequently, especially when touched on her arms, upper chest, and middle–upper back. She wears very tight athletic bras and tank tops under baggy layers. Her tongue has a large dip at the rear, is pale, swollen, and wet. Her pulse is weak and deep. She is diagnosed with *Zong*/Chest Qi Stagnation, Stagnation in the Channels (Stomach, Liver, Pericardium, Lungs, Gallbladder, Urinary Bladder), San Jiao obstruction with Dampness, and *Zheng*/Upright Qi Deficiency (i.e., Spleen, Kidney, and Lung Deficiency). Treatments included Acupuncture, Cupping, Herbs, Qigong, and Lifestyle counseling to 'unbind' the tissues, along with diet recommendations to clear Dampness and fortify the Spleen and Kidneys. The anxiety, pain, and digestive symptoms disappeared for days after each treatment, but even after three months they continued to reappear within seven to 14 days. She associated the return of symptoms with job stress and dietary 'indiscretions.' This client was kept on a management program for over one year in conjunction with psychotherapy and EMDR, but the allergies and food sensitivities never went away during this time. *Note: This client eventually revealed memories of early childhood incest. Soon after this, they realized they were transgender. They are still married, but now doing FTM hormone therapy.*

Taping and Tucking

When not done properly, strong adhesives from taping can damage the delicate genital flesh, creating rashes and skin sores. External poultices and salves may provide relief from the skin damage, but new ways of tucking must be explored to prevent recurrence. Here too, commercially made products and online videos have made a world of difference in reducing incidence of harm for those that have access.

Tight taping/tucking can easily create pain: the first sign of Qi and Blood Stagnation in the Channels. The channels primarily impacted by tucking are the Liver whose path 'winds' the genitals (penis and testicles), and the Ren Mai which flows directly through the penis as the channel ascends the abdomen. Qi and Blood Stagnation in the Liver Channel can trap both Qi and fluids, creating stagnation anywhere along the trajectory of the channel as well as a localized build-up of Damp-Heat. This may encourage frequent flare-ups of STIs (such as herpes, genital warts, etc.), candida, or other genital rashes. Over time, the obstruction in the Liver Channel can also lead to problems in the Liver organ.

The Ren Mai is an Extraordinary Vessel (EV) so its pathway lies deeper than that of a Primary Channel. It starts in the Lower *Dan Tian* within the 'Room of Essence,' then descends through the Lower Jiao to the pelvic floor before ascending the low abdomen. Obstruction along the Ren Mai can lead to the formation of Qi and Blood Stagnation anywhere in this region. This will most likely affect the prostate, but could also settle into other local organs (Urinary Bladder, Large Intestine, Small Intestine) depending on Constitution or other patterns. As the *Bao Mai* connects the 'Room of Essence' directly to the Heart, stagnation in the Lower Jiao can also transfer to the Upper Jiao, creating Zong and/or Heart Qi related symptoms including anxiety, depression, chest constriction, and palpitations.

There are two other vessels that may be impacted due to their connection to the Ren Mai: the Du and the Chong. The Du Mai is the Yang pair (Sea of Yang) to the Ren (Sea of Yin), so obstructions in the Ren can cycle directly from Yin into Yang to manifest in the Du. This could present as sacro-lumbar pain and intrascapular tension based in Qi and Blood Stagnation. The penis and testicles are considered Yang tissue as they are exposed and upright (compared to the more concealed Yin of the clitoris and vagina), so localized Qi and Blood Stagnation may also directly impact the Du Mai without any obstruction in the Ren.

The Chong Mai is thought to be the 'mother' of all Extraordinary Vessels, so any impact to the Ren or the Du Mai can affect the Chong as well. As the Chong is the Sea of Blood, symptoms are likely to be based in stubborn, intractable Blood Stasis, and can follow the Chong trajectory to appear anywhere in the body.

In summary, genital taping and tucking is associated with the following primary patterns:

- Qi and Blood Stagnation in the Liver Channel

- Damp-Heat in the Liver Channel

- Obstruction of the Ren Mai.

And the following secondary patterns:

- Qi Stagnation in the Chest (Zong Qi) and/or Heart

- Obstruction of the Bao Mai, Du, and/or Chong Vessel.

Taping and Tucking Treatment Options

- Move Qi and Blood in the Lower Jiao.

- Course Qi/Clear Damp-Heat in the Liver Channel.

- Harmonize the Ren (and Bao Mai, Du, and /or Chong as applicable).

Primary Modalities

- Lifestyle: Spending *many consecutive hours* without tissue constrictions, especially during sleep; lavender or salt baths may prove helpful to soothe injured tissue – *exercise caution with Damp-Heat conditions*.

- Topicals: Single herbs such as Bo He can be used to gently clear Heat; Yin-Care Herbal Wash is indicated for issues with Dampness causing rash or irritation; Zheng Gu Shui, Yunnan Bai Yao (topical) or Springwind's Amber Massage Salve for Blood Stasis.

- Acupuncture: LV 2–6, 8–12, ST 29–31, SP 8–13, KI 11–13, Ren 2–6, sacral *Ba Liao* points.

- Herbal Formulae: Huo Luo Xiao Ling Wan, Jin Gu Die Shang Wan, Yan Hu Suo Zhi Tong Wan.

HORMONAL HOMEOSTASIS

When a person has decided to physically alter their body beyond the use of prosthetics (see Chapter 3), the first step on the journey is typically the use of hormones. Both hormone suppression and augmentation strategies are undertaken, and these must be continued indefinitely to maintain the new gender characteristics. In general, hormones are an aspect of Yin which directly impacts the Yin and Yang 'tides' that regulate many physiological processes through the spreading of Yuan Qi and *Ming Men* Fire. As Leslie Franks noted, 'Lung Yin and Stomach Yin relate to the hormones secreted by the thyroid gland, Kidney Yang is analogous to adrenaline, and Kidney Yin is analogous to the gonadal hormones, such as estrogen' (2016, p.371). It is important to note that gonadal hormones include both androgens and estrogens (produced by male and female bodies, respectively) with varying degrees of Yin–Yang balance within the principle of infinite divisibility.

Most practitioners have witnessed the effects of hormone use. Oral contraceptives (OC), IVF protocols, and hormone replacement therapy (HRT) for women provide an inkling of what patterns and symptoms to expect for those making the MTF transition. Edema, weight gain, depression, emotional lability, gastritis, nausea or vomiting, diarrhea, rash, headache, and hypotension are all common side effects. In the simplest Chinese Medicine terms, the reduction of androgens and increase in estrogens present as Yang Deficiency with Excess Yin. This combination easily depletes Spleen and/or Kidney functioning and can extinguish the *Ming Men* and 'digestive fires' while accumulating fluids only increase the burden on the Spleen and Kidney (Qi or Yang) and disrupt proper Qi flow.

On the other side, the testosterone regimen prescribed to FTMs can cause hypertension, anxiety, irritability, emotional lability, acne, polycystic ovarian disease, fluid retention or weight gain, liver function and lipid abnormalities, and liver tumors. Again, using a very basic Chinese Medicine perspective, testosterone acts like an injection of pure Yang, adding a significant amount of Heat to the system. The acute overacting Yang will excessively stir the *Ming Men* Fire, driving up the libido and potentially depleting the Jing-Essence. Any Excess Heat from the Lower Jiao will naturally rise to the Middle and Upper Jiao, affecting other systems. The Heat will primarily affect the Liver Organ as it attempts to regulate the overall Qi Mechanism, but it can also 'cook' or 'scorch' the body fluids, condensing healthy *Jin Ye* into Phlegm.

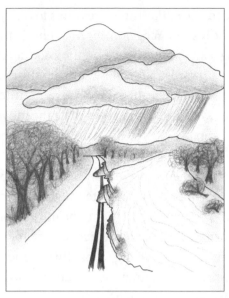

Figure 5.3: MTF Hormones – simplified

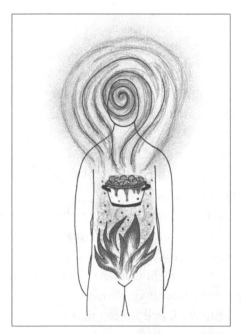

Figure 5.4: FTM Hormones – simplified

Figures 5.3 and 5.4 reflect the hormonal impact that is referred to above. In Figure 5.3, the Sun has been completely blocked by rainclouds; the Earth cannot dry out and the rivers are breaching their banks, washing out roads and impeding traffic flow. The lack of Sun represents the Yang suppression, the overflowing water is the Excess Yin creating Dampness in one form or another, and the damaged roads represent the obstruction of Qi that occurs with Excess Yin.

Figure 5.4 uses the image of the Three Treasures to demonstrate the impact of Excess Yang Energy. The Kidney Yang or *Ming Men* Fire of the Lower Jiao has been turned to *high*, putting way too much heat on the cooking pot of the Middle Jiao and forcing movement upwards in the body, stirring the Liver Yang. The quickly congealing fluids represent the healthy *Jin Ye* turning into Phlegm, which will further impact the Liver system as it tries to regulate the movement of Qi. The high temperature also creates an excess of steam rising to the Upper Jiao, bringing Yang energy (and potentially Phlegm) upwards to affect the head and the Shen-Spirit.

Again, these are simplified representations. It is important to remember that client Constitution will naturally dictate the way an individual responds to hormone therapy. Two versions of the client's health history (prior to hormone use, and then after hormone regulation reached efficacy) must be obtained in order to fully understand the underlying Constitution and any patterns that may be 'disguised' by the hormone regimen. Any pattern of imbalance that existed prior to starting hormones may get aggravated *or could be ameliorated* by hormones, depending on the nature (Hot, Cold, Damp, Dry, etc.) of that pattern and the influence of more Yin (MTF) or Yang (FTM) therapy.

Treatment Options

Regardless of the way in which hormones are impacting the individual, Chinese Medicine treatment for transgender individuals must focus on creating a new homeostasis for the client. As with any pharmaceutical side effects, patterns created by the hormone therapy *will not be cured* unless the hormone therapy is completely stopped. Therefore, the goal is not to cure, but to develop the most appropriate management strategy.

Many of the side effects from hormone therapy can be managed with Acupuncture and small diet changes, but the primary treatment modalities for addressing more aggressive side effects will be Diet and Herbal Formulae. *(Note: Advanced training or further study in Chinese Herbal Formulae is required to work with hormone management, so that information is not included here.)* Essential Oils, Gemstones, and Qigong all work well as secondary approaches. Hormone therapy is associated with the following patterns and treatment principles:

MTF

- Spleen and/or Kidney Yang Deficiency.

- Accumulation of Dampness/Damp-Phlegm/Damp-Cold.

- Qi Stagnation (due to Dampness or Phlegm obstruction).

General Treatment Principles: Warm the Yang, resolve Dampness (or clear Phlegm), course Qi

- Diet: Eating foods that warm and clear Damp (cardamom, cinnamon, garlic, ginger, fennel, onion, rosemary, tea, walnut, etc.); 'Hot flame' cooking (broiling, grilling, etc.).

- Acupuncture – *Moxabustion is applicable:* Ren 4, 6, 12, ST 25, 36, SP 6, 9, LV 3, GB 34, 40, UB 20, 22, 23.

- Gemstones: Amber, Dolomite, Nephrite Jade, Rose Quartz, Smoky Quartz, Sunstone, Yellow Quartz/Citrine.

- Essential Oils: Basil, Cinnamon, Clove, Fennel, Ginger, Lemongrass, Rosemary, Pine, Spruce.

- Qigong – *active, moving postures in general:* Five Animal Frolics–Bear; Gathering the Rice.

- Lifestyle: Walking, biking, or any other light to moderate cardiovascular exercise.

FTM

- Kidney Yang Exuberance with Jing-Essence (Yin aspect) Depletion.

- Liver Patterns: Qi Stagnation with Heat/Liver–GB Damp-Heat/Liver Yang Rising.

- Damp-Heat/Phlegm/Phlegm Fire.

General Treatment Principles: Descend Yang, course Qi, harmonize Fluids (i.e., transform Phlegm and nourish Yin)

- Diet: Avoid warming foods and spices (alcohol, caffeine, sugar; cayenne, chili, clove, etc.); incorporate foods that cool, nourish Yin, and clear Damp/Phlegm (aduki bean, apple, celery, grapes, lemon, parsley, peppermint, watercress, etc.); 'moist' cooking (steaming, soups, etc.).

- Acupuncture: GB 21, 31–34, Four Gates (LV 3–LI 4 in combination), LV 8, SP 6, KI 1.

- Gemstones: Amethyst, Aquamarine/Blue Beryl, Emerald, Green Garnet, Howlite, Moonstone, Opal, Pearl.

- Essential Oils: Angelica, Chamomile, Jasmine, Rose, Sage.

- Qigong – *lying and slow-moving postures in general:* Five Animal Frolics–Crane; Qi Circulation/Tai Yang Circulation (lying); Hun Yun Gong–Descending the Yang, Ascending the Yin.

> Transgender clients *do not* want to return to the homeostasis that existed prior to starting hormone therapy. It is a delicate balance to manage side effects without undoing the desired effect of hormones, so advanced training is required for most practitioners.

SEX REASSIGNMENT

Chapter 2 discussed office forms, including health history questions about scars and surgical history. Any good interview process must cover this information, as the channel obstructions caused by scar tissue can create a whole host of conditions, both local and distal. For transgender individuals, scars resulting from sex reassignment surgery (SRS) can have emotional connections as well, so a gentle approach to these discussions is recommended.

All surgery results in acute, localized Qi and Blood Stagnation. Not all SRS procedures are able to be done at the same time, and there are typically multiple surgeries to complete a full transformation. Just one surgery can cause acute swelling, and if not healed properly will develop chronic stagnation. The more surgeries performed in a certain area, the greater the likelihood of chronic Qi and Blood Stagnation.

Top Surgery

For FTM individuals this includes the removal of breast tissue (mastectomy) along with chest reconstruction or contouring. There may be a second procedure for more extensive chest reconstruction or if pectoral implants are to be inserted; this second procedure is similar to the breast augmentation (mammoplasty) that MTF individuals undergo. For both FTM and MTF clients undergoing top procedures, the primary issues that arise are either acute swelling and pain from surgical recovery, or chronic complications from scar tissue. Local channel impact includes Liver, Stomach, and Pericardium; only rarely will organ systems become involved.

If left untreated, scar tissue adhesions can lead to sensitivity changes in the area (numbness, increased sensitivity, or a mixture of the two), and could lead to postural changes as the person attempts to protect this area (such as the forward 'slump' of the shoulders). Figure 5.5 shows the standard treatment for scar tissue adhesions, with needles inserted at the two ends of the scar and along the sides to create a 'feather' pattern. This technique works incredibly well, and is easily adaptable for almost any type of scar shaping. If the sensitivity changes are chronic, it can be assumed that Primary Channels in the area are also involved; in this case, the 'Above and Below' technique shown in Figure 5.6 should also be used to re-establish proper channel flow.

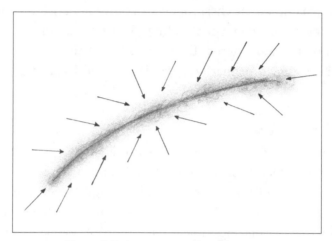

Figure 5.5: Acupuncture Scar Treatment

The primary modality for clearing local stagnation is the Acupuncture Scar Treatment shown in Figure 5.5 combined with external poultices or liniments. Surgical incisions must be fully sealed before using any primary or secondary modality, with the exception of indirect Moxa and Qigong.

- Acupuncture:

    - Plum blossom needle at the area of injury

    - Local points: Ren 17, LU 1, 2, SP 21, ST 12–18, PC 1, LV 14, GB 21, UB 13–18, 42–47

    - Systemic healing and fluid management: SP 3, 6, 9, 10, KI 3, ST 36.

- External poultices or commercially prepared liniments: For physical Trauma – Zheng Gu Shui, Die Da, Wan Hua; to clear Heat and swelling – White Flower Oil.

Secondary modalities can be used in conjunction to help promote faster healing:

- Cupping: Flash Cupping on the upper chest and/or intrascapular area; flash or running Cupping on the intrascapular area.

- Moxabustion: Pole Moxa over the scar can clear fluid stagnation by transforming Dampness; direct Moxa over any scar tissue that is hard, nodular, or extremely flaccid.

- Qigong to unbind the chest (open arm movements): 8 Brocades–Archer; Heaven Nature/Kuan Yin Standing–Boat Rowing in the Stream of Air, Traveling Eastward Across the Ocean; Five Animal Frolics–Crane; Five Healing Sounds – primarily Metal, Wood, and Heart movements.

CLIENT EXAMPLE

A post-operative transgendered male (FTM) in his mid-30s presents with daily chest scar pain from mastectomy and chest reconstruction surgery over two years ago. The sensations are aching and 'pulling.' He has also noticed a subtle shift in his posture over time: his shoulder joints seem 'slumped' forward. He has tried massage and topical liniments (arnica gel, jojoba oil, etc.) without much relief. He has an athletic build, exercises daily at the gym, meditates for stress, is a healthy eater (except the occasional pizza and beer night), and just finished his graduate degree. His tongue shows signs of Spleen Qi Deficiency and Dampness (pale, swollen, thin yellowish coat), and his pulse is wiry. *Note: This is a perfect candidate for Acupuncture Scar Treatment (Figure 5.6) and the other protocols listed above.*

Bottom Surgery

This is always a multi-step process involving both urological and cosmetic surgeries. These are commonly split into multiple procedures, and the financial and emotional expense can be daunting. For reasons such as these, not every transgender individual chooses to complete this set of surgeries. As practitioners, it is critical to know what procedures have *and have not* been done to best assist transgender clients, as gynecological organs (uterus, ovaries, etc.) still in place may contribute to a whole range of health issues.

For MTF individuals, SRS can be a one- or two-step process involving vaginoplasty (the creation of the vaginal canal with tissue from the penis, scrotum, or colon) and labiaplasty (the creation of the labia). For FTM individuals, the completion of a full sex reassignment is commonly a three-step process involving hysterectomy (removal of the uterus, ovaries, and fallopian tubes), vaginectomy (removal of the cervix and vagina), urethroplasty (lengthening the urethra), metoidioplasty (relocating the enlarged clitoris), phalloplasty (tissue graft creation of a penis), and scrotoplasty (creation of the scrotum from the enlarged labia majora, often with the insertion of prosthetic testicles which may or may not require tissue expansion).

Bottom surgeries affect local Primary Channels, the Lower Jiao, and the Lower *Dan Tian*. In terms of the Primaries, impact to the Liver Channel is assumed as this channel 'winds' the genitals, but other pathways that parallel the Liver can be affected such as the Spleen, Kidney, or Stomach Channels. Pericardium and Small Intestine Channel extensions also connect through this area, so distal Acupuncture points along these channels should be considered (such as pairing Liver 3 with Pericardium 6 to affect the Chong Mai and Blood movement in the area). Fortunately, many Primary Channel issues do not require direct scar treatment, and are instead treated with an 'Above and Below' technique that encourages proper coursing of Qi and Blood in the channels. Figure 5.6 shows the basics of this technique.

Above	Point located on the channel 'prior' to the area of injury Needle is directed toward the area of injury	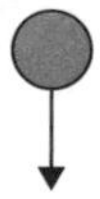
Adjacent	Point located on the channel 'adjacent' to the area of injury – *not in the area of injury!* Needle is directed toward the area of injury	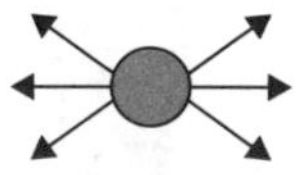
Below	Point located further along the channel Needle is directed with the flow of the channel (or according to regular needling instructions)	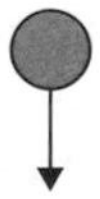

Figure 5.6: Basic 'Above and Below' Technique

Both Top and Bottom scars impact the Primary Channels. Two Acupuncture techniques – *Scar Treatments* (Figure 5.5) and *Basic 'Above and Below' Technique* (Figure 5.6) – can help alleviate the majority of discomfort. Adjunctive techniques such as external salves, Moxa, Cupping, and Essential Oils can help provide relief between treatment sessions and promote faster healing.

'Above and Below' Treatment Examples

- Liver Channel: Liver 8 (He Sea point) needled proximally along the channel pathway to target the genital region and help relieve pain from either Damp-Heat or Blood Stasis inflammation, combined with Liver 10/11/12 for local pain (palpate to determine which, if any, of the three are indicated) and Liver 13/14 (shallow needling) to encourage flow through the area.

- Spleen Channel: Spleen 10 when there is predominant and extreme Heat, or Spleen 11 when there is predominant Dampness (needling can be proximal along the channel, or perpendicular), combined with Spleen 12/13 (superficial and shallow needling directed toward the genital region) to target the treatment locally, and Spleen 14/15/16 (palpate for tenderness) to encourage flow.

- Kidney Channel: Kidney 10 needled proximally along the channel pathway to target the genital region, combined with Kidney 11 to target the local area, and Kidney 12–21 (palpate for tenderness) to encourage flow.

- Stomach Channel: Stomach 25/26/27/28 needled inferiorly along the channel pathway to target the lower abdomen and pelvic bowl, combined with Stomach 29/30/31 to target the specific area, and Stomach 32/33/34 (shallow needling) to encourage flow through the channel.

Using the Above and Below technique can be a welcome relief for clients that experience post-surgical sensitivity, or who already feel over-exposed from medical treatment. In these cases, it is important to remember that the client's preference regarding needle location takes precedence over palpatory findings to ensure their comfort and ability to relax, letting the treatment work. Reconstructed tissues, especially genital tissue which is already sensitive, must be treated with gentleness, compassion, and whole-hearted presence. For this reason, I often start clearing obstruction using only the Above and Below points, omitting the Adjacent point to avoid over-stimulation. I also inform the client of this choice so that if it is not effective, they not only understand why but can actively participate in deciding how they want their body to be treated.

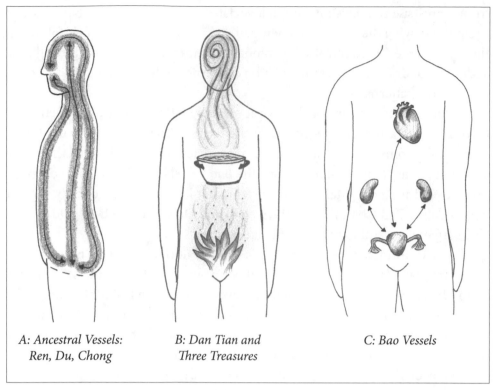

A: Ancestral Vessels: B: Dan Tian and   C: Bao Vessels
 Ren, Du, Chong   Three Treasures

Figure 5.7A–C: Lower Jiao Structures

With SRS procedures, even more important than the external Primary Channel impact is the impact of internal scar tissue on the Extraordinary Vessels (EV). Figure 5.7A–C provide a reminder of the energetic structures that originate or pass through the Lower Jiao and are deeply connected to the sex organs: the Ancestral Vessels (Ren, Du, Chong), the three *Dan Tian* with their Three Treasures, and the *Bao* Vessels (*Bao Mai* and *Bao Luo*), which directly link the Heart and Kidney organs to the Lower Jiao.

For FTMs, the removal of the Uterus has a particularly strong impact on all three systems: EV, *Dan Tian*, and *Bao* Vessels. These will be affected in a similar way to hysterectomy or traumatic C-section, so post-surgical regulation is required to ensure that any damage is repaired before system-wide problems have a chance to develop. The Shen-Spirit has great potential for healing any disruptions to these deep systems, so for those who find spiritual peace from sex reassignment surgery, it is possible that pathology may never appear. When symptoms do occur, they initially appear in the local area; one common complaint is a deep sensation of aching or distention within the lower pelvis, similar to a chronic UTI or cystitis. Due to the energetic pathways, development of emotional symptoms is even more common, including anxiety, depression, and sleep disturbances. Even during the acute healing phase, any severe obstruction from scar tissue can develop pain in associated areas, such as mid-back, jaw, or occiput following the Ancestral Sinew pathways, or in the leg channels following the sacral nerve. There can also be numbness in nearby channels of the thighs or abdomen, or dramatic thermoregulation concerns, such as seen in Heat Above–Cold Below patterns.

In terms of treatment for the Extraordinary or *Bao* Vessels, one method is through the Master–Couple points of the Extraordinary Vessels, paired with other body points along the channel trajectories that are close to the lower abdomen, or are tender on palpation. The *Bao* Vessels are aligned with different portions of the Chong Mai in some systems, but local and energetically aligned points on the Ren Channel (Ren 17, Ren 4) and Du Channel (Du 4, Du 11) are also extremely useful to regulate the Bao pathways.

One Extraordinary Vessel that hasn't been mentioned needs to be addressed here: the Dai Mai. A common side effect of hysterectomy and other lower abdominal surgeries is lower abdominal swelling, and the Dai Mai is intimately involved with fluid regulation in the pelvic bowl. If the Dampness formed by post-surgical swelling is not cleared properly, or is transformed into Damp-Heat or Phlegm by existing patterns or Constitutional concerns, the Dai Mai could become overwhelmed. As the Dai Mai is in charge of maintaining conditions of latency, latent illnesses and unprocessed memories could surface, creating post-surgical physical illnesses or emotional Trauma. *If a client has a history of multiple severe illnesses and/or Trauma, working with the Dai Mai prior to surgery is critical for prevention.*

In terms of the three *Dan Tian*, there is some good news. As the person's anatomical sex is at last coming into alignment with their gender identity, any obstructions impeding the alignment of the three *Dan Tian* and their Treasures will typically not last. Only in the case of existing Jing-Essence or Kidney Deficiency will it take a bit longer for re-alignment to take place, but there are Qigong exercises that can help speed up this process (see below). Unfortunately, the Spirit can also thwart the healing process if the individual's gender identity is not satisfied by their physical transformation. Symptoms to look for include body dysmorphia issues, such as obsessive attention to weight or other physical appearance concerns, or debilitating anxiety, depression, or unusual isolation behaviors that extend beyond the normal phase of surgical healing. Unexpected grief or a sense of loss post-surgery is normal, but if the joy and contentment of transformation are missing or relatively minute in comparison with the grief, pay close attention to interrupt the development of harmful emotional states.

> ### Qigong to Align the *Dan Tian*
>
> Hun Yuan Gong movements specifically target the three *Dan Tian*, and can be easily performed by novices. Opening and Closing the Three *Dan Tian* as well as Opening and Closing Heaven and Earth are perfectly suited for this purpose. If there is any issue with Dai Mai obstruction that is affecting the emotions, Grinding the Corn is another good movement to incorporate. *Note: These and many other Qigong exercises are contraindicated in the case of acute infection or physical illness!*

EMOTIONAL TRANSITIONING

When considering the emotional journey of transitioning, there are two facets to examine: the *personal feelings* one has about their experience, and the transition in *relationships to others*, including one's family of origin, spouse, children, and community. Most people think that once transgender individuals are able to live openly as their new sex or gender, they will suddenly be free of any uncomfortable emotions that plagued their 'previous' existence. This is sometimes, but not always, the case. As Nigel Ching (2016) states: 'Many patients, not just transgendered, invest their sense of happiness in an idealized physical body and hope they will feel harmonious, content and free when they have achieved this. Unfortunately this contentment does not always arise post-operation.'

Transgender individuals may have a history of gender dysphoria (GD), a form of clinically significant distress that develops from the very real difficulties they experience with cultural oppression. For young people, common symptoms of GD include feelings of disgust with their own genitalia, social isolation from their peers, anxiety, loneliness, and depression. Adults with GD are at higher risk for stress, isolation, anxiety, depression, poor self-esteem, and suicide (Davidson 2012). Transgender individuals at any age are also at higher risk for developing eating disorders and other mental health concerns (Diemer *et al.* 2015; Doyle 2015). Examining GD-associated symptoms through the perspective of Chinese Medicine, we can see that gender dysphoria is clearly a form of psychological Trauma.

To reiterate, the discordance of Jing/Anatomy with Shen/Identity is a lesson of the Nine Palaces and *is not in itself the cause* of gender dysphoria (see Chapter 4). The Trauma that transgender people are subject to is caused by the cultural prejudice and oppression that all gender non-conforming people face. The impact of Trauma is covered in Chapter 11, but it is important to note that other deep-seated emotions such as Fear, Shame, Guilt, and Self-Loathing are likely at play (see the appropriate chapters in Section IV). The longer someone has lived with GD, the more ingrained the emotional roots are likely to be, and the inner peace and contentment of living fully as one's true gender may not be enough to clear them.

Transitioning can also bring loss of sexual identity (i.e., heterosexual, lesbian, etc.) or dramatic change to family identity (i.e., daughter/son, etc.) which can bring up unexpected grief. It may also adversely impact intimate relationships and/or one's greater community, affecting the sense of belonging that all human beings need. If any of these losses are combined with a sense of Guilt from the impact of one's actions, or a sense of Self-Loathing that wasn't 'fixed' by transitioning, this can lead to deep depression or even a suicidal state (see Chapters 12, 15). For others, the contentment of transitioning may instead transform into a pathological euphoria, as pent-up Desire and Craving for the 'new self' is released from the state of Repression (see Chapters 13, 14). Varying degrees of mania may ensue, with great potential for self-harming behaviors such as unsafe sexual practices or shopping beyond one's means for new clothing.

Combining Chinese Medicine treatment with mental health counseling is the correct protocol to address the many risk factors that can develop from intense levels of unmitigated emotions. In my own practice, I weigh heavily the value of emotional support under the principle of 'first, do no harm.' Recognizing that Chinese Medicine treatment may 'lift' emotions to the conscious level, I have at times mandated proof of ongoing therapy be provided in order to continue care, even when a client currently appears emotionally stable.

General treatment considerations related to emotional transition can be guided by Five Element associations, by the technique chosen to address these concerns, or a combination of the two. In terms of Five Element associations, the primary elements to work with are:

- *Wood*: The element of courage, direction, and focus.

- *Earth:* The element of self-acceptance, and transformation.

- *Water*: The element of will, self-knowing, the drive to 'get through this.'

Fire and Metal are used to harmonize the actions of the other three, as Fire controls the Shen-Spirit, aligned with both gender identity and expression, and Metal controls the Po, the spirit of the physical body that is aligned with one's anatomical sex and influences how a person feels 'in their own skin.'

In terms of techniques, almost any modality can be used. Techniques may be chosen based on the Five Element association (i.e., sitting Qigong or meditation for the Water element, Gemstones for the Metal element, etc.), the emotional states present (see Section IV), by practitioner preference, or by client Constitution. For emotional conditions and issues of spiritual transformation, I rely heavily on Essential Oils, Gemstones, and Qigong. Here are some treatment options to consider:

- Acupuncture or Moxabustion:

  - UB 60 and GB 40 for enacting the will with direction and focus (Water–Wood)

  - LV 3, 8 to support and encourage courage and focus (Wood); can be combined with KI 6, SP 6, or KI 10 (Water)

  - Du 20 and Sishencong: all five points directed anteriorly (also known as the 'Princess Crown') to activate the Ancestral Vessels (Ren, Du, Chong) and the seventh Chakra, that one may receive guidance from Spirit Guides/Ancestors and remember one's divine nature (Water)

  - ST 36 to help with general transformation, and to 'go the extra mile' even when the toil of the journey makes one weary (Earth)

  - SP 3, 6, 9, 10, Ren 12 to help with general self-acceptance and transformation (Earth).

- Essential Oils:

  - *Wood*: Anise, Chamomile, Geranium, Lavender, Lemon, Melissa, Rose, Vanilla

  - *Earth*: Bergamot, Bitter Orange, Caraway, Cardamom, Clove, Fennel, Ginger, Grapefruit, Lemongrass, Lime, Neroli, Savory, Patchouli

  - *Water*: Basil, Black Spruce, Cinnamon, Clove, Fennel, Geranium, Jasmine, Rose, Sandalwood, Vanilla, Ylang Ylang.

- Gemstones:

  - *Wood*: Amazonite, Amber, Blue Beryl/Aquamarine, Emerald, Green Jade, Petrified Wood

  - *Earth*: Alexandrite, Yellow/Golden Beryl (Heliodor), Yellow Jade, Malachite, Turquoise, Variscite

  - *Water*: Amazonite, Amber, Black Jade, Blue Lace Agate, Black or Red Garnet, Ruby, Sodalite.

- Meditation or Qigong:

  - Seated forms: Warrior Attendant; Sheng Zhen Qigong–Heart Spirit as One/Jesus Sitting

– Standing forms: Wuji Pose; Five Animal Frolics–Crane; Sheng Zhen Wuji Yuan Qigong: Releasing the Heart/Mohammed Standing–Pure Heart Descends

– Affirmation: 'I am exactly who I am meant to be. I belong.'

SUMMARY

» There is no conflict between the Three Treasures of transgender individuals, specifically between the Jing-Essence of anatomical sex, and the Shen-Spirit of gender identity.

» Binding obstructs the *Zong*/Chest Qi, local Primary Channel pathways, the San Jiao and the Dai Mai. This can develop Qi and Blood Stagnation or Phlegm (especially in the Upper Jiao and Heart organs), fluid and Dampness accumulations in the Middle or Upper Jiaos, misalignment of the Ancestral Sinews, the collapse of *Zheng*/Upright Qi, and stagnation of the Extraordinary Vessels.

» Ancestral Sinews include the diaphragm, sternocleidomastoid, psoas, the paravertebrals, and the abdominal rectus muscles.

» Taping/tucking practices can lead to Qi and Blood Stagnation or Damp-Heat in the Liver Channel, and obstruction of the Ren Mai. It can also impact the *Zong*/Chest Qi and the Heart, as well as the Du and/or Chong Mai.

» When considering hormonal homeostasis strategies, the goal is management, not cure.

» Constitution dictates a client's response to hormone therapy. Two versions of health history will clarify the underlying Constitution and any 'hidden' patterns.

» The MTF regimen of estrogen and anti-androgens frequently leads to Spleen and Kidney Yang Deficiency, accumulation of Dampness/Damp-Phlegm/Cold-Damp, and Qi Stagnation due to both fluid obstruction and lack of Kidney Yaun Qi.

» The FTM testosterone regimen frequently leads to Kidney Yang 'exuberance' and Jing-Essence depletion, along with Liver Heat (Qi Stagnation-Heat, Liver–GB Damp-Heat, and/or Liver Yang Rising) and Damp-Heat/Phlegm/Phlegm Fire conditions.

» Sex reassignment surgery scarring can create localized numbness or sensitivity changes, postural changes, and other conditions associated with damage to the Primary Channel pathways, the Lower Jiao, or the Extraordinary Vessels.

» Transgender individuals may experience emotional issues at any point of their transition. The most common response is unexpected grief associated with shifting of sexual identity or loss of a pre-transition sense of community. Emotional support through counseling or psychotherapy in conjunction with Chinese Medicine treatment is strongly recommended to address any emotions that may arise during the healing process.

» Wood, Earth, and Water are the primary elements to address for smooth emotional transitioning.

THE SEXUAL JOURNEY

Realize that bodies are only a fraction of who we are
They're just oddly-shaped vessels for hearts
And honestly, they can barely contain us.

– Gabe Moses 2009

TERMINOLOGY: SEX, SEXUALITY, AND RELATIONSHIP

(an incomplete list)[1]

–   **Asexual** a person that either does not experience sexual feelings or desire, or chooses to not act on those feelings

–   **Bisexual** a person that is not limited in sexual or relationship preference in regard to the traditional binary gender system (i.e., a female-identified person attracted to both male- and female-identified people, and vice versa) – *see also Pansexual*

–   **Gay** a male-identified person that is only attracted to other male-identified people

–   **Heterosexual** a person that is limited in sexual or relationship preference by their exclusive attraction to people of the 'opposite' sex or gender (i.e., a female-identified person attracted only to male-identified people) – *see also Straight*

–   **Homosexual** a person that is a limited in sexual or relationship preference by their exclusive attraction to people of the 'same' sex or gender (i.e., a male-identified person attracted only to male-identified people) – *see also Gay, Lesbian*

–   **Lesbian** a female-identified person that is only attracted to other female-identified people

–   **Marriage** the recognized union (legal or otherwise) of two people in an emotionally intimate, and presumably sexual, relationship

–   **Monogamy** the practice of being sexually and/or intimately involved with only one person at a time

–   **Open relationship/Open marriage** the practice of engaging in an emotionally intimate, and presumably sexual, relationship with one person, while having sexual relationship(s) with other partner(s)

---

1   More definitions are found at the beginnings of Sections I and II.

- **Pansexual** (also called Omnisexual) a person that is not limited in sexual or relationship preference in regard to another person's anatomical sex, gender, or gender identity – *Note: Compared with 'Bisexual,' Pansexual/Omnisexual identity is perceived by some as more inclusive, gender-blind, or rejecting of binary gender*

- **Polyamory** the practice of being sexually and/or intimately involved with more than one person at a time, with the knowledge and consent of all parties

- **Polygamy** the union (legal or otherwise) of multiple people in emotionally intimate, and presumably sexual, relationship

- **Relationship anarchy** a form of polyamory with no formal distinction between sexual, romantic, and platonic (i.e., friendship, asexual) relationships

- **Sex** the act of physical, sexual intimacy between consenting adults

- **Sexuality** a person's preference for specific styles of sexual contact, and their capacity for sexual feelings, desire, and activity

- **Sexual identity** a person's chosen label or language for their own sexual preferences

- **Sexual orientation** a person's sexual identity in relation to the gender(s) to which they are attracted (i.e., heterosexual, homosexual, bisexual) – *Note: This term is considered both binary gender and 'other' focused, and has generally been replaced with 'Sexual identity'*

- **Straight** a heterosexual person; someone attracted to the 'opposite' sex based on anatomical differences or gender identity (i.e., a female attracted to a male and vice versa)

- **Swinging** the practice of swapping sexual partners or engaging in group sex activities (typically without emotional intimacy)

- **Queer** (similar to Genderqueer) a person whose gender, sexual identity, and/or orientation does not correlate with heteronormative or binary gender expectations; also used as an umbrella term for the entire LGBTQ+ community

- **Questioning** a person that is unsure of their sexual or relationship preferences; often used by young people that are not yet ready to declare a firm identity

Chapter 6

ENERGETIC PHYSIOLOGY OF SEX

- The Tides of Yin-Yang: Arousal and Orgasm

- Sexual Alchemy: Entering Wuji

- A Balancing Act

Those who take the 'great elixir,' engage in breathing exercises and internal circulation…but do not know the root of life, are like trees who have ample branches and luxuriant leaves but are without roots. The root of life is the business of the bedroom.

– Yang Xing Yan Ming Lu[1]

Sex is an act of physical intimacy between consenting adults, which may or may not include arousal, orgasm, or emotional intimacy. The act of sex is separate and distinct from both sexuality and sexual identity, but is often conflated with the two.

Sexuality is defined as a person's preference for specific styles of sexual contact. It also includes a person's capacity for sexual feelings or desires and sexual activity, but it does not include the act of sex itself. Sexual identity is a person's chosen label or language for their own sexual orientation or preferences, which also has nothing to do with sexual activity. From a Three Treasures perspective, the physical act of sex requires the Jing-Essence of the Lower *Dan Tian,* where the Heat of Desire stirs the *Ming Men* Fire and stimulates the genital region. Although the healthiest sex utilizes all Three Treasures, sex only *requires* the physiological and energetic responses within the physical body, and is therefore anchored to one's physical anatomy and the force of Earth.

---

1   As quoted in Cohen 1997, p.318.

Sexuality and sexual identity can also be related to the Three Treasures. An individual's sexual identity is how they currently perceive their own sexuality and desire for sexual contact. This involves self-knowledge as well as awareness of linguistic options. Language reflects and is dictated by one's culture, and therefore sexual identity is related to the force of Humanity and the Post-Natal Qi of the Middle *Dan Tian*. Sexuality on the other hand involves relationship: it is how one wishes to relate to one's self or to others, either temporarily or long-term. Relationships of any sort involve the Fire Elements and correspond to the Shen housed in the Heart organ. Sexuality is based in the force of attraction and the capacity or drive for sex (i.e., the Jing-Essence and Lower *Dan Tian*), but it is also a fluid quality that can easily fluctuate. Being anchored to the Lower *Dan Tian* while remaining a fast-moving Qi relates sexuality to the force of Heaven and the Shen-Spirit. Table 6.1 shows the alignment of the Three Treasures, Jing–Qi–Shen, in relation to sex, sexuality, and sexual identity.

Table 6.1: The Three Treasures of Sex, Sexuality, and Sexual Identity

Force	Location	Treasure	Influence	Aspect
Heaven	Upper *Dan Tian*	Shen-Spirit Heaven	Desire for relationship Self-knowledge	Sexuality
Humanity	Middle *Dan Tian*	Qi – Post-Natal Humanity	Language and culture Self-perception	Sexual identity
Earth	Lower *Dan Tian*	Jing-Essence Earth	Anatomy Drive for sex	Sexual activity

There are many ways of having sex, being sexual, or engaging in relationship between people of all sexual orientations and identities. Intimacy can range from physical to emotional to spiritual, with various combinations in-between. Issues relating to sexuality, identity, and emotional or spiritual relationships are covered in Chapter 8; this chapter focuses on the energetic commonalities related to sex, regardless of anatomy, gender, or sexual identity. Although most forms of sex involve physical contact by oneself or with others, *not all sex does*. Arousal and orgasm follow the same energetic pathways during solo sex or partnered play, and these paths can be stimulated by either external/physical or internal/non-physical stimuli.

THE TIDES OF YIN–YANG: AROUSAL AND ORGASM

Healthy sex involves two distinct phases: arousal and orgasm. Arousal is a state of excitation caused by physical contact or non-physical stimulation, such as fantasy or memory. Orgasm is the climax of excitation. It is characterized by feelings of pleasure centered in the genitals accompanied by any combination of neuromuscular tension release, vaginal contractions, or the release of sexual fluids. Neither arousal nor orgasm are *required* for sex to happen, but both are necessary for the important health-promoting aspects of sex to occur.

The process of healthy arousal and orgasm is vital to proper physiological functioning of the human body. Sex can regulate the Three Treasures, the Extraordinary Vessels, the Primary Channels, and all movements of the Qi Mechanism: in, out, up, and down. In general terms, arousal is an expansive Yang process where energy goes up and out through the Extraordinary Vessel (EV) pathways. The Heat of arousal originates in the *Ming Men* where it stimulates the Jing-Essence and flows into the Ancestral Vessels (Ren, Du, Chong) that traverse the 'Room of Essence' in the Lower Jiao. These EVs will assist Heat to rise upward along the Taiji pole, connecting the Jing-Essence of the Lower *Dan Tian* to the Qi and Shen-Spirit levels of the Three Treasures.

Orgasm is a primarily contractive Yin process, where energy goes in and down, promoting fluid movement through the genitals (i.e., ejaculation). As arousal and orgasmic states shift back and forth during sex, the tides of Yin–Yang energy help regulate any EV 'effulgence,' moving the surplus outward to fill the Primary Channels.

Arousal

Arousal begins in the Lower Jiao where Desire stirs the *Ming Men* Fire, expanding its energy to the Ren, Du, and Chong Vessels that flow into the anterior, posterior, and internal aspects of the pelvis. This causes the initial stages of genital swelling and any small release of vaginal lubrication or ejaculate (i.e., pre-cum). The expansive nature of arousal also brings Qi to the surface of the body, increasing skin sensitivity, while the warming nature softens tendons and warms the muscles, allowing for greater physical flexibility and strength for the act of sex itself.

The Chong Mai directly intersects with the energetic centers for the Three Treasures, so as the Chong gets warmed from the ongoing expansion of *Ming Men* Fire, Heat rises into the Middle Jiao and impacts the Post-Natal Qi. This Heat helps to regulate various digestive processes in the Stomach, Spleen, Liver, Gallbladder, and Large Intestine. In the acute phase of arousal, digestion will slow and the appetite dim, but appetite and bowel movements will overall become better regulated through regular, healthy orgasmic sex:

- The Stomach feels 'full' from the presence of physiological warmth that is stimulated by arousal; some of this warmth remains after orgasm and helps curb overeating.

- The Gallbladder has more support from *Ming Men* Fire to spread warmth to the internal organs, enabling them to more effectively perform their overall digestive functions.

- The healthy warmth from the Gallbladder specifically supports Spleen Yang, helping transform Dampness and regulate all aspects of digestion.

- The healthy warmth from the Gallbladder also helps discharge stagnation from the Liver–Gallbladder system, regulating not only the digestion, but the movement of all Qi.

As the Heat of arousal spreads upward along the Chong Mai, it enters the Upper Jiao, where the Shen-Spirit and *Zong*/Chest Qi are stimulated. The eyes and complexion reflect the impact of warmth on the Shen-Spirit through pupil dilation and facial flushing. As the Zong Qi is warmed, there will be signs of Qi Stagnation releasing from the chest: relaxed sighs, deeper breath sounds, and vocal expressions.

When the arousal state escalates toward orgasm, the upward and outward movement of *Ming Men* Fire expansion becomes more extreme: this could be seen as the *Ultimate Yang* state of sex. Eventually, the Yang energy will reach a peak and start to shift toward Yin energy. During this *Yin within Yang* phase, arousal stops steadily building and transforms instead into short waves of rising expansion (i.e., Yang energy) alternating with periods of inward contraction and downward movement (i.e., Yin energy). This pre-orgasmic state often occurs during a sexual act, with breath sounds and body movements shifting back and forth between loud and expansive to more quiet and contractive forms. The shifting of Yin and Yang tides from one state to another is visualized in Figure 6.1 by a sine wave that arcs between the two states over an undefined period of time.

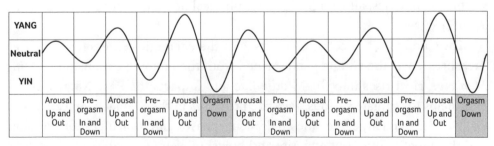

Figure 6.1: Yin and Yang Tides

Orgasm

Eventually the *Yin within Yang* transformation will shift fully to the *Ultimate Yin* state, where a strong downward push of energy stimulates vaginal contractions and glandular or ejaculatory release. If the intensity of the inward and downward contraction of orgasm is prolonged, or the individual has multiple orgasms in succession, it is likely that a simultaneous release of Yang energy will occur in other areas of the body. This *Yang within Yin* phase allows Yin substances to flow out through the orifices as sweat, tears, and deep vocal utterances.

The pre-orgasm phase that shifts between rising expansion – Yang – to downward contraction – Yin – is rooted in the bi-directional flow capability of the Extraordinary Vessels. The four movements of the Qi Mechanism – in, out, up, and down – are regulated by these same processes. The multi-directional movements of the arousal, pre-orgasm, and orgasm states are visualized in Figure 6.2A–C.

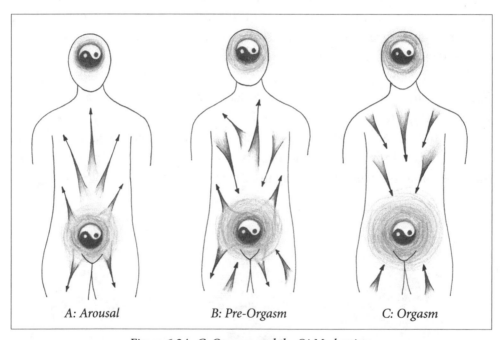

A: Arousal   B: Pre-Orgasm   C: Orgasm

Figure 6.2A–C: Orgasm and the Qi Mechanism

Internal regulation

The tides of Yin and Yang allow the Three Treasures and the Extraordinary Vessels to flow freely during sexual activity, encouraging EV excess to fill the Primary Channels. If there is no surplus of Yin, Yang, or Blood to be shared, the EVs will hold on to these substances to preserve them. Individuals may experience diminished vaginal secretions or ejaculate volume, but not show any general signs or symptoms of deficiency. There is one situation that can undermine the EV control mechanism and force substances to leave the EV even when there is no excess: multi-orgasmic women that have intense orgasms in quick succession. This is a common cause of acute, extreme fatigue and dehydration after sex, and a factor in sexual taxation for women (see below).

The amount of fluid released during sex and orgasm has a lot to do with the internal fluid balance of the individual. Applying the questions of the Nine Palaces, is there enough Abundance to share? This is primarily dictated by the state of the Chong and the Ren Vessels, which store the abundance of Blood and Yin respectively. It is also important to note that not all fluids released during sex are *physiological*, i.e., Blood or Yin. Fluid release (through vaginal lubrication, male or female ejaculate, sweat, tears, etc.) may also be reflective of *pathological* Dampness that has built up in the system, being forcibly expelled by the Qi Mechanism and Extraordinary Vessels to maintain balance. The tides of Yin–Yang are a self-regulating system that moves Qi, Blood, Yin, and Yang very strongly; in this way, a healthy, balanced sex life can promote self-healing.

Figures 6.3A and 6.3B demonstrate the flow of 'effulgence' from the Extraordinary Vessels into the Primary Channels. The Ren 'spills over' to the Kidney Channel, then to the Stomach, Spleen, and Liver Channels as they follow the Ren's trajectory on the torso. The Du Mai flows into the Urinary Bladder, Small Intestine, San Jiao, and Gallbladder Channels on the back. The Ren and Du Mai also help fuel the internal organs as well, through the *Mu* points on the abdomen, and the *Shu* points along the Urinary Bladder Channel.

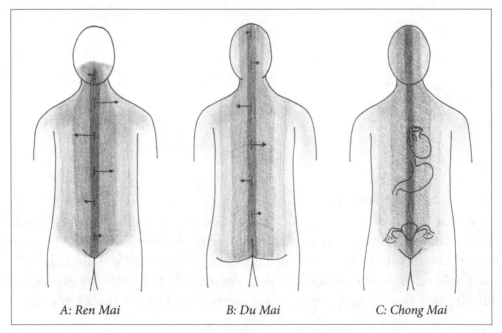

| A: Ren Mai | B: Du Mai | C: Chong Mai |

Figure 6.3A–C: Extraordinary Vessel Effulgence

The effulgence of the Chong Mai is shown in Figure 6.3C. As it is a deep vessel, it internally regulates the vertical movements of the internal Qi Mechanism, interconnects the Three Treasures, and directly connects to the Uterus, Stomach, and Heart. For this reason it is the most important of the EVs in proper orgasmic functioning, especially for women. If the Chong is not properly aligned with the Three Treasures, or if any EV is obstructed (by Qi Stagnation, Blood Stasis, Dampness, or Phlegm), orgasms may become painful, incredibly difficult to achieve, or even non-existent.

SEXUAL ALCHEMY: ENTERING WUJI

Daoist alchemy is based on the mixing of substances to promote longevity, cultivate virtue, or create external wealth. It is divided into two basic types: outer and inner. Outer alchemy traditionally focused on the ingestion of substances that could guarantee immortality (gold, cinnabar, etc.) or the external creation of precious metals (such as gold or silver from mercury). Although outer forms of alchemy have fallen out of favor, inner alchemy is still practiced today. Inner alchemy focuses on the cultivation and mixing of internal substances – specifically the Three Treasures – through breathing, meditation, and movement to cultivate virtue and promote long-life. Most commonly found in certain forms of Qigong, Tai Chi, Yoga, and meditation, anything that focuses inward and helps cultivate the Three Treasures would be considered an alchemical practice.

Healthy sexual practices help to not only mix and cultivate the Three Treasures, but also regulate the Extraordinary Vessels, the Primary Channels, and the entire Qi Mechanism. This is incredibly similar to the effects of internal alchemical practices. One of the principal goals of Qigong is to experience the Wuji state of 'one-ness' (see Chapter 3); this is done through simultaneous settling of mind and Spirit, softening of the physical body, and stimulation of energetic flow through the Three Treasures and the Taiji pole. This requires the ability to tune out external and internal distractions (worry, stress, physical pain, etc.) and be completely present in each moment of one's existence. These abilities are also required to attain the health-promoting qualities of sex.

Each person is a unique blend of Yin–Yang energies (i.e., the Taiji), manifested through the balance of Qi and the Five Elements. Medical Qigong texts frequently refer to the Taiji pole that exists within the physical body, anchored to the pelvic floor at Ren 1 and to the top of the head at Du 20/Bai Hui. In sex, as the tides of Yang (arousal) and Yin (orgasm) wash back and forth, this Taiji pole of energy activates. The Three Treasures and their respective *Dan Tian* are located along the trajectory of the Taiji pole, so they too become roused in this process. As sex progresses, the physical, emotional, and spiritual delineations between the Treasures begin to blur, and all three will eventually blend into the Taiji. If these tides and the blurring of lines is unobstructed both physically and emotionally (i.e., no fear of loss of control, no distractions from other rooms, etc.), then the interconnected Yin–Yang energies will fully merge into a state of pure Qi, allowing the individual to enter the Wuji space.

Figure 6.4A–C show the basics of this transformation within the human body, where the Three *Dan Tian* that store the Three Treasures each have a small Taiji – blending of Yin and Yang – along the Taiji pole. As already discussed, the first Treasure to activate is the Jing-Essence in the Lower *Dan Tian*. The Chong brings the Heat of arousal up to the Post-Natal Qi and then the Shen-Spirit. As each Treasure activates, the Yin–Yang energies in that area begin to meld. Eventually, all three *Dan Tian* are churning, and the three small Taiji can form the whole-person Taiji. If allowed to continue, the Yin–Yang energy of the whole body will actually merge into non-duality, forming the pure Qi state of one-ness, the Wuji.

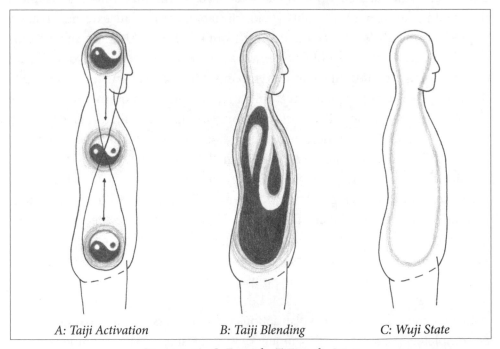

A: Taiji Activation   B: Taiji Blending   C: Wuji State

Figure 6.4A–C: From the Taiji to the Wuji

Figure 6.4A–C show only what is happening for the individual. This is a pre-cursor to Figures 6.5 and 6.6, which illustrate two people merging together in Wuji.

In partnered sex, participants start out as individuals (Figure 6.4). As arousal states increase, the churning of Yin and Yang energies inside of each person creates two individual Taijis. If there is a strong physical, emotional, and spiritual connection between sex partners, their Taiji poles can align, synchronizing the Yin–Yang tides. This is shown in Figure 6.5, where infinity symbols represent the synergy of the three *Dan Tian* and the Taiji poles. If this level of interconnectedness is entered into willingly, freely, and allowed to thrive, a somewhat hypnotic state will ensue. This is the joining of the two people, i.e., two Taijis, into one Taiji, which is shown in Figure 6.6. At this level of sexual connection, sensing a partner's arousal state, 'loss' of time and place, and simultaneous orgasm are all commonplace. This is the attainment of sexual one-ness, the pure Qi state of Wuji.

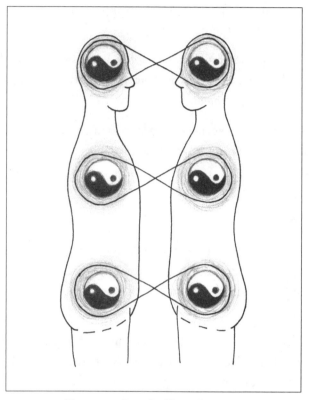

Figure 6.5: Jing-Qi-Shen Alignment

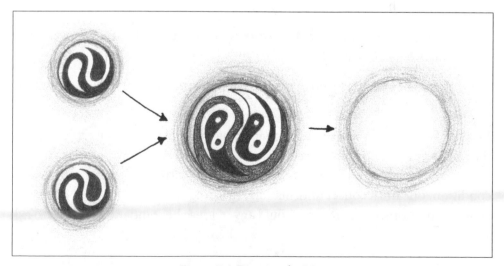

Figure 6.6: Entering the Wuji

Notes about Sexual Alchemy

- The energetics mentioned are not specific to gender, anatomy, or a particular sex act.

- Number of participants is not limited. Sexual alchemy can occur between multiple partners when each person is fully emotionally and spiritually present.

- *Taiji* 'mixing' may be easiest to obtain when partners are face to face and pelvis to pelvis, as this encourages EV and *Dan Tian* alignment, *but this is not a requirement*.

- Physical contact is not necessary for sexual alchemy to occur, especially for those with extensive experience in energy practices (Qigong, Yoga, Tantra, etc).

Obstructions

The unfortunate reality is that sexual alchemy is experienced by far too few individuals. When a client is struggling with libido (arousal), inability to orgasm, or simply feels disconnected during sex, there are some principle areas to examine:

- The Extraordinary Vessels (Ren, Du, and Chong especially, but also the Dai Mai) must be 'effulgent' and clear of obstructions (i.e., Qi Stagnation, Blood Stasis, Dampness, Phlegm).

- The Three Treasures must be properly aligned and in easy communication with each other.

- The Qi Mechanism must be working properly via the four movements: in, out, up, down.

- The San Jiao must be free of obstruction, with free flow of substances: Qi, Blood, Yang, Yin.

When a client is seeking treatment for any major sexual health concern, it is likely that one or more of the above require treatment.

To investigate the physical, emotional, or spiritual roots of a sex-related condition, one must collect information regarding the client's masturbation and genital sensations. By no means should any of these be standard questions to ask every client, but for those struggling with specific sexual concerns a few simple, respectful questions might include:

- Are there any areas of numbness or lesser sensation in the genital region?

- Do you have any desire to masturbate or self-stimulate?

- What gets in the way (i.e., time/scheduling, kids, alone time, emotions, etc.)?

Physical obstructions typically present as localized pain or numbness. This requires targeted treatment for Qi or Blood Stagnation with Acupuncture or another deep tissue modality (such as Myofascial Release (MFR)), often combined with Herbal Formulae.

Emotional obstructions include Anger, Grief, Embarrassment, Shame, or Fear, often related to being 'caught' in a sex act or labeled as a sex or gender deviant. Spiritual obstructions include the repression of fantasies or more taboo sex or gender practices, and likely include elements of emotional obstruction as well. Both emotional and spiritual obstructions can thwart an individual's ability to engage in sexual experimentation, effectively communicate desires, fantasies, and needs, and thwart the development of truly intimate connection.

Treatment for emotional obstruction requires attention to internal and oppressive thinking patterns, such as gained through talk therapy or mental health counseling. Spirit obstructions require transformation through 'lifting' issues to the surface. This is best addressed through Gemstone or Essential Oil treatments and mindful movement practices, such as Yoga and Qigong; talk therapy may also prove useful here (also see Section IV).

CLIENT EXAMPLE

A queer-identified female in her early 30s presented with headaches during sex (penetrative and non) that started a few months prior. The pain is centered at the occiput, with palpable tension and tenderness at and between GB 20, UB 10, and Du 15–6. The headaches start during arousal, worsen just prior to orgasm, and have become so painful that she often has to discontinue sexual activity. She is getting (understandably) frustrated and angry. She also complains of chronic tension in the upper back–neck–shoulders due to excessive computer use at work. Her pulse is wiry and thin, her tongue is pale, slightly quivering, and dry. A 'whiplash pattern' (Yang Qiao–Du and Yang Wei–Dai obstruction) is confirmed by Manaka-style Japanese Acupuncture Hara Diagnosis. Initial treatment involved the following:

1. Ion discs (no needles) placed at SJ 5–GB 41 and UB 62–SI 3 bilaterally.

2. Points on the UB Channel (UB 14, 43, 15, 44, 18, 19, 48, 22, 51, 27, 28) selected based on palpation, then shallow-needled and retained until the *Sha*/redness disappeared.

3. Sotai stretches and resistance exercises to release the pelvic floor/hip muscles along the anterior superior iliac spine (ASIS).

4. Korean Hand Therapy using stainless steel press beads, located on the bilateral 3rd fingers between and on the inter-phalangeal joints.

Herbal Formulae were incorporated into the treatment plan to address underlying issues from Blood and Yin Deficiency and to encourage free flow in the Channels and Collaterals:

- Jia Wei Xiao Yao Wan and Xue Fu Zhu Yu Tang Wan for 8–10 days

- Jia Wei Xiao Yao Wan and Gui Pi Wan for one month.

After the first Acupuncture treatment, the headaches completely disappeared and did not return. Two more treatments were done to ensure full-body healing and prevent relapse.

Types of Sexual Activity

Although the general energetics of arousal and orgasm are consistent, individual sexual practices can more strongly stimulate specific Elements, Primary Channels, or Extraordinary Vessels. When someone has a strong preference for only one type of sex, this information can be used diagnostically to develop a Chinese Medicine treatment.

Anal Stimulation: Receiving

- Stimulates and relaxes the Metal Element and the Large Intestine Channel.

- Stimulates the Du Mai, Upper *Dan Tian*, and the Sea of Marrow/Brain.

- Harmonizes the Du–Ren connection.

Oral-Genital Stimulation: Giving

- Stimulates and relaxes the Earth Element and the Stomach Channel.

- Stimulates the Chong Mai and the Middle *Dan Tian.*

- Harmonizes the Ren–Du connection.

Oral-Genital Stimulation: Receiving

- Stimulates and relaxes the Wood Element and the Liver Channel.

- Stimulates the Ren Mai and the Lower *Dan Tian.*

Vaginal Stimulation: Receiving

- Stimulates and relaxes the Wood Element and the Liver Channel.

- Stimulates the Chong Mai, all three *Dan Tian,* and the flow of the Three Treasures.

- Harmonizes the Ren–Chong connection.

A BALANCING ACT

The best sexual practices are those in which the Three Treasures are fully engaged and the individual experiences physical, emotional, and spiritual connection both internally and to any other person/people present. This is where the Taiji pole and North–South axis may flow unencumbered, and the internal alchemy of Fire and Water can occur.

Fire and Water are the respective *Ultimate Yang* and *Ultimate Yin* states of the Five Elements. Respectively they relate to the Heart/Pericardium in the Upper Jiao and the Kidneys in the Lower Jiao. In order for an inner alchemical reaction to occur during sexual practices, the two regions must be able to easily communicate. Again, this requires free flow through the San Jiao and the Ancestral Vessels (Ren, Du, Chong), as well as proper alignment and communication between the Three Treasures along the Taiji pole. There are also two energetic vessels, the *Bao Mai* and *Bao Luo*, that help connect these areas and their organ systems, routing Fire and Water energies through the 'Room of Essence' which the Ren, Du, and Chong Vessels traverse. The overlap of terminology is emphasized here because these are not distinct parts; many practitioners of Medical Qigong see the Taiji, the Three Treasures, the *Bao* Vessels, and the Chong Mai as phenomenal aspects of the same energetic structure.

Regardless of one's perspective on the North–South axis, there are three Elements that are part of this flow: Fire, Earth, and Water. The root of any Fire–Water disharmony affecting sexual arousal, orgasm, and/or connection to one's self or sexual partner(s) commonly stems from issues with the middle: the Earth Element. Earth, firmly situated in the Middle Jiao, is primarily responsible for the creation of Post-Natal Qi, which supports the needs of daily life. Post-Natal Qi is created through the basic necessities of sleep (preservation of Kidney energy), good food and drink (preservation of Stomach/Spleen Qi), and the air we breathe, including basic cardiovascular activity (preservation of Lung and *Zong/* Chest Qi). These three components – Kidney, Spleen and Stomach, and Lung and Chest Qi – form the basis for all Qi and Blood in the human body. Without proper sleep, food and drink, air and cardiovascular activity, the Post-Natal Qi and Middle Jiao will suffer, creating poor digestion of any sort and also obstructing the energetics of sex. These conditions may be acceptable for a casual sex experience where the Shen-Spirit or the Qi-Emotions may not be involved, but this is not recommended for health-promoting sex in general, or for the creation of a new and healthy human being.

Even when there is not an underlying obstruction, if a person chooses to regularly engage in casual sex that does not include emotional and spiritual connection, obstructions between the Three Treasures can form. The manifestation of these obstructions will initially be seen in the flow of the Chong Mai and the intercommunication of the San Jiao cavities. Fluid transformation issues involving Blood or Yin in any Jiao can also stem from this lack of intimacy, and consistent lack of psycho-spiritual engagement may create bigger problems with long-term sexual satisfaction and relationship choices.

There are other ways obstructions can form. One of the biggest concerns is the timing of sexual activity. Damage can result from sex that occurs before the Extraordinary Vessels have matured, sex during menses that impacts the proper functioning of the Qi Mechanism, and sex during pregnancy causing 'Restless Fetus Syndrome' or other issues.

Premature Sex

Premature sexual activity includes any form of stimulation or penetration that can damage the Extraordinary or *Bao* Vessels. Premature sex affects all sexes and gender identities equally, but the state of physical 'readiness' is easiest to pinpoint in cis females because of menstruation. Menarche – the first menstrual period – indicates that the maturing of the Extraordinary Vessels has begun, but full maturation of the EVs can take approximately two years after menarche to complete.

In developed nations, menarche normally occurs between the ages of 10 and 16; adding the two years of maturation therefore offers a range from 12–18 years old. Another guideline is to assume sexual maturity only after the second Cycle of 7 and 8 is complete. Combining the two indicators, physical readiness occurs between ages 14–18, *but only after menarche* and the stabilization of the menstrual cycle (timing, flow, etc.). If sex is engaged in before the body is physically ready, damage to the Ren, Du, and/or Chong Vessels is almost inevitable. If a practitioner can learn what sex acts were engaged in prematurely, this points toward the area of damage (see 'Types of Sexual Activity' in this chapter).

Figures 6.7–6.9 show the physical damage of premature sexual activity to the EVs. The Ren Mai is easily damaged by penetrative oral sex, such as with fellatio. This sex act is practiced by many young people, and can have lasting damage on the mouth, throat, esophagus, and Stomach when premature. This may present as thyroid imbalances, acid reflux/gastroesophageal reflux disease, food allergies or intolerances, or metabolic syndrome issues. The Du Mai will be easily damaged by anal penetration; another popular sex act among young people that wish to 'remain virgins' while experimenting with sex. Damage to the Du Mai primarily affects the anus, Large Intestine, and Spleen. Beyond any hemorrhoids caused by acute physical damage to the anal sphincter from improper sex practices, damage to the Du may present as digestive complaints (chronic constipation, diarrhea, IBS, intestinal polyps, inflammatory bowel disorders), issues with the spine and postural alignment, chronic sinus congestion, or headaches.

The Chong Mai can be damaged by any form of premature vaginal or anal penetration. In cases of a pre-existing Constitutional condition or forced sex (see Chapter 9), the Chong might be damaged by premature oral penetration as well. As the Chong traverses the center of the body, flowing up the anterior spine and penetrating multiple organs, symptoms of Chong damage will be widespread and involve many systems. The most common areas of damage will include two or more of the following: the cervix, Uterus, Kidneys, Intestines (Small or Large), Stomach, Spleen, Liver, or Heart. Symptoms might include cervical or uterine polyps, endometriosis, menstrual cycle irregularities, mixed Hot–Cold syndromes, digestive complaints (especially food allergy/intolerance or IBS), anxiety, insomnia, heart palpitations, and any condition related to Liver Qi Constraint or Stagnation.

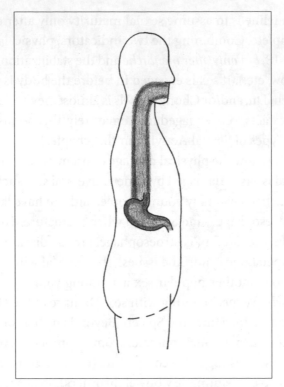

Figure 6.7: Damage to the Ren Mai

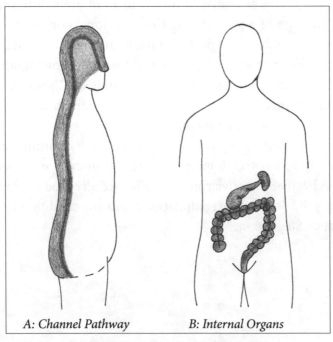

A: Channel Pathway   B: Internal Organs

Figure 6.8A–B: Damage to the Du Mai

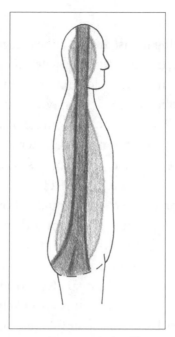

Figure 6.9: Damage to the Chong Mai

The age guidelines mentioned are clearly oriented toward *physical* readiness and do not take into account *emotional* or *spiritual* readiness. When the person is not psycho-spiritually ready for sex to occur, the symptoms of physical damage will likely combine with:

- Earth Element dysfunction from lack of acceptance and integration, the 'transformation and transportation' of the experience

- Heart–Kidney Disharmony, either from lack of acceptance affecting the Earth Element, Post-Natal Qi, and the Middle Jiao, or from direct damage to the Shen-Spirit and Jing-Essence

- Heart pathology – Blood/Yin Deficiency or Blood Stasis – from the over-churning of emotions such as seen in Trauma (see Chapter 11)

- Dai Mai obstruction created by emotional churning focused on the Lower *Dan Tian*, Jing-Essence, or the 'Room of Essence.' This can appear in Above and Below imbalances, Heart–Kidney Disharmonies, and the creation of latency issues including auto-immune conditions.

Menstrual Sex

Warnings against sex during menstruation appear regularly in Chinese Medical gynecological texts, suggesting that the 'jade gate' (cervix) is more easily invaded by external pathogens when 'open,' a clear implication of increased vulnerability during menses. This implies that it is simply easier for a woman to contract gynecological and sexual diseases – including invasions of Damp-Heat, Cold, and Wind – into the vaginal and uterine areas when menstruating. In a contemporary culture of strong hygiene practices, protected sex, and greater awareness of sexually transmitted infections (i.e., STIs, STDs) however, the more common problem seen in clinical practice is that of counter-flow Qi.

In a general arousal state, Heat expands upward and outward from the Lower Jiao, dramatically lifting the Qi. This is in direct opposition to the flow of menstrual Blood, which is inward and downward. As Qi is the Commander of Blood, the opposition creates counter-flow that can temporarily or completely arrest the menstrual flow of the current cycle. It is also likely to create Blood Stasis in the Uterus that presents as large clots, painful cramping, and 'searing' low back or sacral pain for one to two cycles that follow. If menstrual sex is repeatedly engaged in, Blood Stasis in the Uterus can expand into the entire Lower Jiao with endometriosis, fibroids, or cysts. The Blood Stasis could also travel directly through the *Bao* Vessel to the Heart, or obstruct the flow of the Extraordinary Vessels that go through the Uterus, especially the Chong Mai, Sea of Blood.

Some female clients have described that the orgasms during menstrual sex help push out clots and stop any menstrual cramping or low back pain during the current cycle. They may be loath to stop having sex during their menses for this reason. Lifestyle counseling will only work when combined with Herbal Formulae to heal the condition as fast as possible. Both Yan Hu Suo Zhi Tong Wan and Tong Jing Wan are excellent patent formulas for this situation. Other lifestyle suggestions include a heating pad or hot water bottle for the low back or lower abdomen, a pillow or other light weight on the abdomen itself (if there is underlying deficiency or a mixed pattern), increased physical activity for one to two days prior to the start of menses, and 'blood-moving' foods (eggplant, eel, etc.).

Special Attention for FTM Clients

Clearly both menstrual sex and sex during pregnancy only affect cis females, but attention must also be given to these issues when working with transgender FTM individuals. FTM clients may have engaged in these sexual practices prior to transitioning and the cessation of menstrual flow. This information may help pinpoint root etiology or pre-existing patterns.

Pregnant Sex

Pregnancy is viewed as another time of vulnerability for the jade gate. Gynecology texts advise pregnant women to be cautious about sexual activity, especially what we might now describe as 'rough' sex. In this context, exuberant sexual activity is potentially too much for the 'House of the Fetus' (Uterus), with the potential to cause 'Restless Fetus Syndrome,' a precursor to the more modern term of miscarriage. Because of increased vulnerability, extra hygiene precautions should be taken for anything that may come in contact with a pregnant woman's genitals during sex, including her own and any partner's hands, teeth, genitals, or sex toys. Any form of infection could cause a ruptured placenta, putting both mother and child at extreme risk.

Rough sex and hygiene concerns are two topics covered extensively by Gynecology, Infertility, and Obstetrics texts, but these are not common concerns of pregnancy in my own clinical practice. Among the typically educated women that seek Acupuncture, problems with sexual activity during pregnancy more commonly stem from either Kidney exhaustion or lack of sex. Kidney exhaustion is especially common among those who get pregnant after the age of 35, when the Spleen has begun its natural process of decline. This Chinese Medicine concept aligns well with the allopathic view of older pregnant women – over age 35 – being in a high-risk category for birth defects and other complications. What was once a normal and health-promoting amount of sex for a 35- to 40-year-old woman may have to be dramatically curtailed in order to prevent symptoms of sexual taxation during pregnancy. In other words, the woman that enjoyed sex twice a week prior to pregnancy may now only be able to enjoy sex twice a month.

Kidney exhaustion is more likely in older women, but can happen to women of any age if there are pre-existing Kidney issues, such as those caused by excessive mental work, caffeine intake, or sleep deprivation (i.e., the modern worker). The most common initial symptom of Kidney exhaustion is extreme fatigue. When pre-existing, this will appear early, in the first or early second trimester. Even though this is the most common timeframe, Kidney exhaustion can appear at any time during gestation, along with other sexual taxation symptoms as well. Reduction of sexual activity – but not complete cessation – is the most important lifestyle adjustment, along with increased mental and physical rest. Treatment to reverse the Kidney Deficiency focuses on strengthening the Kidneys, and can be as simple as daily self-treatment with pole Moxa on Stomach 36 and Kidney 3 when combined with lifestyle recommendations.

Lack of sex during pregnancy is also a concern, especially when entering the final months of pregnancy. This is a time when the Fluids (Jin Ye, Yin, Blood) are at their most 'effulgent' with plenty to spare! Unfortunately, many women experience the symptoms of Dampness and Damp-Phlegm during this time, even if they were not heavily overweight pre-pregnancy. These heavy, sinking pathological fluids can obstruct the libido, making it difficult to become aroused or to orgasm properly. Lack of sex during pregnancy can contribute to prolonged labor, which is a common cause of Cesarean section deliveries. It is critical for women to remain physically active throughout pregnancy, and health-promoting sex is a vital component to keep the stamina strong, the pelvis open, and the Qi Mechanism ready for the process of labor and delivery.

Sexual Taxation Redefined

Texts that refer to an 'appropriate' amount of sex are typically directed at cis-gendered males. They suggest that only men may suffer from too much sex or masturbation, as men lose Jing-Essence with ejaculate and women do not. With a more inclusive perspective on gender, and a contemporary understanding of female anatomy, orgasm, and ejaculate, these guidelines are inappropriate. When considering the amount of sex that is right for any individual, the symptoms associated with sexual taxation prove more helpful than any gender-based rules.

The symptoms themselves remain consistent for any gender, as they describe damage being done to the Kidneys and the Jing-Essence:

- Low back pain – mild to extreme

- Knee and ankle joint weakness

- Dizziness.

In my own practice I have encountered many women that are happily enjoying the sexual peak of their 30s and 40s. But they are also experiencing the known symptoms of sexual taxation listed above, as well as:

- *Acute:* Fatigue, dehydration (can last two to five days)

- Chronic fatigue

- Dehydration

- Headaches – especially deficient type, mild to extreme

- Vaginal dryness – mild to extreme

- Symptoms of premature ageing – graying hair, skin pigmentation (i.e., age spots).

In every person's life there are times of increased sexual activity. These periods are most common with new relationships, during Spring and Summer seasons, and for some people at times of extreme stress (such as the death of a loved one). If Kidney pulses are depleted (i.e., deep and weak, hidden, or faint) *but there are no presenting symptoms*, it is appropriate to ask the client about any recent increase in sexual activity and to advise them of symptoms that could indicate they've reached their physical limit. Approach any lifestyle guidance with care as it is common for people to feel Shame around 'excessive' sexual activity. Instead, focus on Herbal Medicine, Diet, and restful movement (Qigong, restorative Yoga, short walks, etc.) that could strengthen and nourish the Kidneys to prevent symptoms from developing. In other words, educate the client about self-care so that they can enjoy this phase of life!

Taxation of the Three Treasures

Avoiding symptoms from 'too much' sexual activity is an issue of managing Jing-Essence depletion and balancing the Three Treasures. Damage to the Three Treasures is an indication that the individual has performed well beyond any abundance of Jing, Kidney energy, or EV substance. If over-engaging in sex, the EVs will attempt to hold on to their substances, making orgasm or ejaculation incredibly difficult. Excessive orgasm and ejaculatory release can create a whole host of health concerns for multi-orgasmic women that 'force' substances to leave the EVs, leaving even more Deficiency in the wake. Taxation can occur at any level – Jing, Qi, or Shen – but is most commonly addressed only at the Jing level, as demonstrated by the classically identified symptoms.

Jing Taxation

Jing-Essence rules a person's *capacity* for sex, including the sexual release of Kidney Yin (i.e., ejaculate) and the stamina needed to engage in the physical act of sex, provided by Kidney Yang. The symptoms already listed are an accurate reflection of damage to the Jing level. It is always appropriate to strengthen the Kidneys (both Yin and Yang) for any individual showing these symptoms, combining treatment with compassionate lifestyle guidance to reduce sex and increase physical rest until symptoms resolve. For women, proper regulation of sexual activity may also include guidance to engage in activity primarily around ovulation and pre-menstruation, with less sexual activity at other times during their cycle. As the Jing-Essence level is best supported by physical substances, Herbal medicine and Diet are the most critical ingredients for a comprehensive treatment plan:

- Treatment Principle: Nourish and tonify Kidney Yin, Yang, Qi, and Essence.

- Herbal Formulae: Zuo Gui Wan, You Gui Wan, Wu Zi Yan Zong Wan, Lu Rong.

- Diet – Jing-Essence-nourishing foods: beans, eggs, seeds, nuts.

- Acupuncture – *Moxibustion is applicable*: KI 3, Ren 4, UB 23.

- Lifestyle: Reduce sexual activity and increase physical rest; restorative Yoga, meditation, and short, slow walks may be useful to stay active.

Qi Taxation

The Qi-Emotion level is intimately involved in one's ability to connect or relate to the person and act of intimacy itself. Sexual taxation affecting this level typically presents as resistance to partnered sex itself, or willingness to engage only in quick, orgasmic-focused sexual acts. If someone is emotionally exhausted from life stressors, these symptoms can appear on their own, without any prior sexual taxation; however, they are more likely to occur in combination with sexual indulgence, including excessive masturbation. As the Qi level is related to the Post-Natal Qi supported by daily life, it is a mixture of Diet, rest, and fresh air or deep breathing that helps this area to heal fastest. Advising clients to eat well (i.e., timing, types of foods, etc.), along with easy exercise (i.e., Qigong, restorative Yoga, short walks, etc.), and mindful breathing techniques may be all they need to transform this condition. When this condition is severe, partnered clients are advised to sleep alone for one to two weeks to ensure full rest at night for the body and the Hun.

- Treatment Principle: Tonify Post-Natal Qi (Spleen, Stomach, Lungs, Kidneys).

- Diet: Advise clients about healthy eating habits in regard to timing, emotions, smaller meals, specific foods related to organ concerns (i.e., rice and honey for the Spleen, seaweed and fish for the Kidneys).

- Lifestyle: Rest, mindful breathing, and easy exercise.

- Acupuncture – *Moxibustion is applicable*: Ren 4, 6, 12, 17, LU 1, 2, ST 36, KI 3; UB 13, 20, 21, 22, 23.

- Herbal Formulae: Nu Ke Ba Zhen Wan, Si Jun Zi Wan, Bu Fei Wan, Ba Ji Yin Yang Wan.

Shen Taxation

Shen-Spirit controls aspects of pleasure and desire, and it can easily outweigh the influence of Qi or Jing in determining the frequency of sex. The Shen's desire to sexually connect is the most common etiology for taxation; both 'honeymoon syndrome' and 'new relationship energy' are terms used to describe this phase. As discussed, it is common for people to engage in increased sexual activity at various points in their life, especially when the Spirit is excited about a new relationship. It is extremely unlikely that sexual taxation would be allowed to impact the Spirit level in a normal adult client, as the lack of stamina (Jing level) and desire to interact (Qi level) would prevent this from occurring. The few cases of Spirit level taxation I have witnessed were situations where the client had been subjected to extreme, ritualized sex abuse as a child, leaving their Spirit scarred by incurable mental illness rooted in all Three Treasures of Jing–Qi–Shen.

The Spirit is best supported by more energetic modalities, such as meditation, Essential Oils, and Gemstone therapy. Acupuncture and moxibustion are indicated to harmonize the Qi Mechanism and heal any energetic 'holes.' Herbal medicine may be used at a low dose, for three to 36 months depending on the duration of the condition.

- Treatment Principle: Harmonize Heart and Kidney, the San Jiao, and the Sea of Marrow.

- For treatments, look at Section IV, especially Chapter 11 on Trauma.

CLIENT EXAMPLE

A bisexual, pregnant woman in her late 20s presented with inability to orgasm, low libido, and difficulty becoming aroused for the past two to three months. She is obese with dark rosy cheeks, and in her third term of her first pregnancy (female sex child). Her only other pregnancy difficulties include extreme fatigue and scent-sensitivity that both appeared in the third month. She cancelled work travel and has been telecommuting two to three days per week to rest more, which has balanced the fatigue. She is still taking 15- to 30-minute walks and doing a 20-minute Yoga practice daily to keep active. Her tongue is swollen, pale, scalloped, with a red-dry tip, thin greasy coat and large red dots at the rear, and thick-dark sublingual veins at the root. Pulses are strong, slippery, wiry overall, but weak-deep in the rear position on the right. She was treated for Damp-Phlegm and Blood Stasis obstructing the Lower Jiao, the Du and Chong Vessels, the San Jiao, and Kidney Yang. The client was not open to taking herbs during pregnancy, so primary modalities were Acupuncture, Diet, and Qigong.

- Initial Acupuncture treatment focused on the Du Channel and the Ba Liao points with needle-Moxa on UB 20, 22, UB 23, UB 31–35, bilaterally. Other points included DU 4, UB 14, 15, SP 3, 9, ST 40, GB 40. Press seeds were placed on SI 3 and UB 62 bilaterally.

- Diet: Avoiding Damp-aggravating foods (dairy, wheat, bananas, yeast, fatty meats, peanuts, etc.); focus on Damp- and Phlegm-clearing foods (apples, almonds, celery, green tea, mustard greens, onion, parsley, scallions, etc.); client was also instructed to make water from Yi Yi Ren/ job's tears to drink throughout the day.

- Qigong: Wuji – moving. *Note: Client was unable to perform more moving Qigong as the Damp-Phlegm would rise from the Lower Jiao, creating extreme nausea.*

After two treatments the client noticed a significant increase in libido, ability to walk more vigorously, and more willingness to engage in sexual activity, but the Damp-Phlegm continued to obstruct orgasm, feeling 'difficult and muffled.'

- Treatment for frustrated Liver Qi was incorporated, using GB 20, 34, Yintang–Du 24 (in combination, and PC 6).

- After 38 weeks' gestation, GB 21, LV 3, LI 4, and SP 6 were added to the protocol.

Energy was greatly improved with treatment, but orgasm was only occasionally better and still felt 'muffled.' Labor was delayed (after 41 weeks) and prolonged (over 24 hours), leading to a Cesarean section.

SUMMARY

» Sex is separate and distinct from both sexuality and sexual identity.

» The general energetics of sex are not specific to gender, anatomy, or a particular sex act.

» Symptoms of sexual taxation apply to any gender or anatomical sex, and can lead to taxation for any of the Three Treasures.

» Jing taxation requires physical nourishment that supports the Kidneys (especially Herbs, Diet, and physical rest). Qi taxation requires mental and emotional nourishment that supports the Post-Natal Qi (especially Diet, mental-emotional rest, and fresh air). Shen taxation requires energetic nourishment (especially meditation, Gemstones, or Essential Oils).

» The process of healthy arousal and orgasm can regulate the Three Treasures, the Extraordinary Vessels, the Primary Channels, and all movements of the Qi Mechanism.

» Arousal is an expansive Yang process where Heat stimulates the Jing-Essence and the Ancestral Vessels (Ren, Du, Chong), uniting the Three Treasures along the Taiji pole.

» Pre-orgasm is the phase of *Yin within Yang*, where the tides of Yin–Yang alternate.

» Orgasm is a contractive Yin process that promotes fluid movement through the genitals (i.e., ejaculation). If there is no surplus, the EVs will hold on to their substances, making orgasm or ejaculation difficult.

» As arousal and orgasmic states shift back and forth during sex, the tides of Yin–Yang regulate Extraordinary Vessel 'effulgence' by moving it into the Primary Channels.

» Not all fluids released during sex are *physiological*, i.e., Blood or Yin. Pathological Dampness can also be forcibly expelled by the Qi Mechanism and EVs to maintain balance.

» Multi-orgasmic women can 'force' EV substances to move. This can cause extreme fatigue and dehydration after sex, and is an important factor in sexual taxation for women.

» Premature sex can damage the Extraordinary and *Bao* Vessels, the Earth Element, the North–South axis, and the Heart–Kidney connection. Look also for evidence of Trauma.

» Menstrual sex causes counter-flow Qi and Blood Stasis in the Uterus, leading to clots, cramps, and other Lower Jiao stasis. It can also flow through the *Bao Mai* to the Heart.

» Pregnancy sex concerns include infection, Kidney taxation, rough sex, and too little sex.

» Obstructions to internal sexual alchemy are common. Physical obstructions create numbness or pain. Emotional and Spiritual obstructions can thwart experimentation, communication, and more intimate connection.

Chapter 7

SPECIAL TOPIC: SEXUAL HEALTH

- Masturbation

- Asexuality

- Obsession with Sex and Pornography

With regard to sexual health, one of the most important questions is 'How much sex is too much, or too little?' There are general classical guidelines regarding the amount of sex, but, as already noted, these can be problematic. In *The Web That Has No Weaver*, Ted Kaptchuk wrote:

> Like any society, China's relationship to sexuality has been complex. Attitudes toward various forms of sexual behavior – such as same-sex relationships (ancient China's elite, like classical Greece, was often homosexually centered), sexual versus reproductive relationships, autoeroticism, masturbation, transsexualism, fetishism – and the essential question of how to balance duty and pleasure varied tremendously and differently influenced medical texts. The discussion of what is 'proper' sexuality often merges with what is 'healthy' sexuality; medical knowledge often masks social constraints and culturally contrived norms. (1983, pp.162–163)

Kaptchuk is not alone in acknowledging the cultural influence on what is deemed medically 'proper.' Chapter 6 covered the energetics of sex, along with the potential for problems in regard to quantity, quality, and timing of sexual activity. It is worth reiterating here that *only the state of the individual* – viewed without prejudice or judgment – is the determining factor of health.

- Is the general system healthy?

- Are there any physical or emotional symptoms of sexual taxation?

- Are the Kidneys strong, as evidenced by the pulse strength or presenting symptoms?

These questions are primarily oriented toward identifying symptoms of too much sexual activity. But what about when there is *too little* sexual activity? Texts often point out the dangers of long-term sexual abstinence, where arousal is present but there is no opportunity to act upon it. In contemporary society, where eroticism and sex are constantly advertised, *excessive arousal with lack of sexual activity* has become a far more common cause of disease than overdoing it.

When a person experiences sexual arousal and is unable to express those feelings, the Lower Jiao Heat is suppressed, creating acute Qi Stagnation with Heat. If one is able to have satisfying sexual activity within a reasonable timeframe, or is able to re-route that energy into other physical exercise to adequately course the Qi and Heat (i.e., running, yardwork, certain Yoga or Qigong practices, etc.), the acute pattern will be easily dispersed. Unfortunately, the sedentary lifestyle of a modern worker does not promote physical movement, so this situation will likely become compounded by multiple instances of unexpressed arousal. Chronic repetition of this experience binds Qi Stagnation-Heat in the Lower Jiao and genital region, mimicking Repression along with the potential to transform healthy Desire into Craving (see Chapters 13, 14). Heat tends to rise and Qi Stagnation anywhere in the body affects the Liver, so the Middle and Upper Jiao are more likely to exhibit initial symptoms: recurring temporal or occipital headaches, migraines, upper chest, back, or facial acne, rosacea, chronic shoulder and neck tension, and TMJD (temporomandibular joint disorder) can all stem from chronic arousal and long-term lack of sexual expression.

Liver Qi Stagnation-Heat is one of the most commonly seen patterns in clinical practice, easily combining with (or creating) patterns such as Spleen Deficiency, Blood Deficiency, Dampness, and Damp-Heat. William Maclean has explained the entwined nature of these patterns and their ability to engender each other through his theory of the 'Primary Pathological Triad'/PPT (see Chapter 13). As these issues are sexual in nature, the Stagnation-Heat that is bound in the Lower Jiao will eventually show symptoms as well. For women, menstrual difficulties like uterine cramping, irregular timing (early and/or delayed), and a mixture of bright red (Heat) and dark red or brown blood (Fluid Stasis) are incredibly common. If Dampness is present, leukorrhea or vulvar cysts may develop as well. In men, testicular swellings and elevated prostate levels are common. For both sexes, dark, blood-filled hemorrhoids or unusually dark-pigmented genital tissue areas[1] may develop.

---

1   It is important to note that genital tissue pigment varies greatly, and that recent fads such as genital and anal 'bleaching' are indications that many people experience insecurity around this issue. Caution must therefore be exercised when approaching this topic.

This chapter dives into the health-promoting and pathological potential of masturbation and asexuality, as well as the unique pathology stemming from sexual or pornographic obsession. Because as Kaptchuk also noted, 'The bottom line…is that the East Asian physician recognized sexuality as a basic and fundamental force in the human landscape' (1983, p.163).

MASTURBATION

The various physical and energetic effects of arousal and orgasm on the Three Treasures, Extraordinary Vessels, Primary Channels, and Qi Mechanism have already been discussed (see Chapter 6). Masturbation is one of the best ways for any individual to address the arousal that naturally comes from being a healthy, aware, sexual human being. Unfortunately, many people engage in only one form of masturbation, or are focused solely on quick orgasmic release. Although solo sex play can address the Heat that comes with acute arousal, the use of one standard, fast-paced orgasm-focused technique is not sufficient to release the Stagnation-Heat that is created from chronically contained and suppressed arousal. Good masturbation, after all, should resemble good partnered sex, where the waves of arousal and pre-orgasm are allowed to build again and again until the blending of Yin–Yang allows the individual to enter the time- and space-lessness of the Wuji.

On the emotional and spiritual level, the act of masturbation is highly self-serving. Solo sexual practices can support and encourage a healthy sense of self-acceptance, self-worth, love, and compassion for one's self. Engaging in a variety of solo sex practices promotes intimate knowledge of one's own genitalia and sexual preferences, which will assist in the ability to communicate one's needs with sex partners, creating more connected and satisfying experiences. Unfortunately, many families still punish children for self-stimulation, teaching them it is wrong to touch themselves. These inappropriate beliefs can continue well into adulthood, greatly limiting one's sexual expression.

The most common emotions that get in the way of healthy solo sex are Shame, Guilt, Anxiety, and Fear. The etiology and treatment of these emotions is more extensively covered in Section IV, but solo sex practices can pinpoint the impact of these emotions on arousal and orgasm to identify the correct etiology. For any client, talk therapy should be considered a complementary treatment option to help unwind cultural mores and taboos.

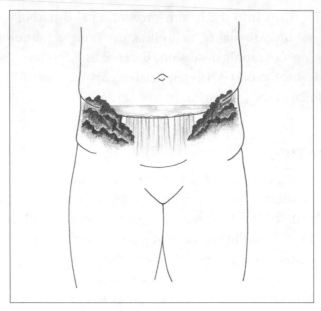

Figure 7.1: Fluid Obstruction

Shame and Guilt

Shame and Guilt are categorically paired because they share certain similarities: they are both heavy and descending in nature, and they both engender stasis of Fluids. Figure 7.1 shows the Heavy, Descending, and Fluid Stasis aspects of these conditions, which typically impact the Lower Jiao. In chronic cases, one may also see weight gain centered in this area from the accumulations of Fluids (Dampness, Damp-Phlegm, or Blood), along with other pattern-related symptoms. Over time, Fluid Stasis will impact the functioning of the Dai Mai. Because of these characteristics, there are two typical problems:

- Heavy and Descending: It may be difficult to obtain or maintain an adequate arousal state, leading to erectile dysfunction or generalized lack of libido.

- Engender Fluid Stasis: It may be difficult to adequately move fluids or experience sufficient 'release,' leading to either unsatisfactory or complete inability to orgasm or ejaculate.

Guilt will present with Blood Stasis, whereas Shame will show more Dampness or Phlegm; they can, of course, appear together. To best discern the differences and treatment options for Shame and Guilt, see Chapter 12.

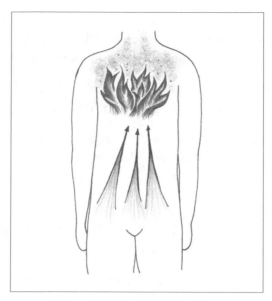

Figure 7.2: Anxiety Obstruction

Anxiety and Fear

Embarrassment and sexual shyness in an otherwise outgoing or extroverted personality is perhaps the most common symptom of Anxiety and Fear related to sex/masturbation. Anxiety is an unrooted emotion that strongly holds energy upward; it is associated with the Heart and Fire Element, and is the predominant emotion in this situation. Fear pulls strongly inward and downward, and is associated with the Kidneys and Water Element. Fear and Anxiety are located at the respective North–South poles of the Taiji, which blends Yin–Yang during arousal and orgasm. The opposing movements of this combination may stem from – or easily create – Heart–Kidney Disharmony and Heat Above–Cold Below patterns, but the symptoms of Heat and upward movement will always predominate. Figure 7.2 shows the extreme Heat and upward movement, with the flames of anxiety holding and drawing the Qi upward. Figure 7.3 shows the impact of Fear as a knot forming in the Lower Jiao. In general, Anxiety and Fear create these specific energetic patterns.

- Upward: This Yang motion may make it easy to get aroused (perhaps too easy), but difficult to maintain the 'waves' that create orgasm or promote ejaculation, leading to headaches, anxiety attacks, and frustrated orgasm.

- Heat: Although Heat is primarily in the Upper Jiao, it can impact sexual activity by diminishing the overall amount of Yin substances (Water controlling Fire) or by over-quickening sexual response time, leading to vaginal dryness, diminished ejaculate, low sperm count, and premature ejaculation.

- Bound Qi: Fear in the Lower Jiao may create diminished sensation, difficult ejaculation or even complete lack of orgasm. There will likely be menstrual irregularities and low back or sacro-illiac joint pain as well.

Treatment is focused on Anchoring Qi, Clearing Heat and Lower Jiao Obstructions, and Harmonizing Heart and Kidney Yin. Treatment options might include:

- Acupuncture: KI 1, 2, 5, 6, 10, HT 3, 6, 8, PC 8, LI 11, LV 2, 3, 5, 8, SP 6, GB 21, 26, 44, Du 20, Sishencong (directed away from Du 20), Chong Mai (SP 4–PC 6), and local points found by palpation on the lower abdomen or sacrum.

- Herbal Formulae: Tian Wang Bu Xin Wan, An Shen Bu Xin Wan, Suan Zao Ren Wan, Jia Wie Xiao Yao Wan, Long Dan Xie Gan Wan.

- Essential Oils: Frankincense, Lavender, Mimosa, Narcissus, Vetiver, Violet, Ylang Ylang.

- Gemstones: Amethyst, Bloodstone, Hematite, Lavender Jade, Red Jasper, Black Obsidian, Red Garnet, Coral, Meteorite, Moonstone, Pearl, Pink Topaz, Pink Andean Opal, Sapphire (Blue Or Pink), Carnelian/Red Chalcedony.

- Also see treatment options under Fear below.

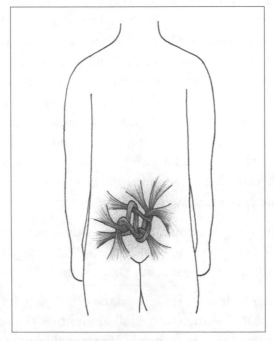

Figure 7.3: Fear Obstruction

Fear

Fear is the emotion of the Water Element rooted in the *Zhi*/Will to survive of Kidney Yin–Yang in the Lower Jiao. Fear is a binding emotion that forces energy downward and inward, the exact opposite direction of the expansive and upward energy of arousal. In regard to sex and sexuality, Fear is common among sex abuse survivors (see Chapter 9), and if not properly managed can easily deplete the overall energy of the Kidneys (also see Chapter 10). There are two common characteristics of Fear:

- Downward and Inward, Binding

- Kidney Depletion.

When Fear is at play, it becomes difficult for the Jing-Essence level to engage in sexual activity, which begets complicating factors for the Three Treasures and Extraordinary Vessels. It may be difficult for an individual to get or maintain arousal, to have the sense of Abundance necessary to engage in sex (Nine Palaces), or to adequately achieve orgasm, leading to pathological asexuality (see below in this chapter), low or repressed libido, erectile dysfunction, difficult ejaculation or even complete lack of orgasm. Some people are able to energetically 'cut off' from their Fear to engage in sex, but this creates problems with the Qi-Emotion level of the Three Treasures, prevents the Taiji pole from full internal movement, and denies the Yin–Yang blending that provides access to the Wuji.

Besides sexual functioning, other signs of Lower Jiao 'binding' are expected: constipation, alternating bowel habits, IBS, hemorrhoids, menstrual irregularities (delayed, irregular timing, clots, cramping pain, low back pain), low back/sacro-illiac joint pain, and vaginismus or infertility. Appropriate treatment is focused on:

- Lifting and Unbinding Qi from the Lower Jiao

- Nourishing and Tonifying the Kidneys.

As Fear binds both Qi and Fluids, Dampness, Damp-Phlegm, or Blood Stasis may also develop and should be addressed where appropriate. Extraordinary Vessels may be incorporated to activate the deep energy pathways in the Lower Jiao, but care should be taken to not overtreat them. Clients should be advised to increase expansive whole-body movement to counteract the 'pulling in' of Fear. Treatment options might include:

- Acupuncture: Ren 4, 6, Du 4, 20, LV 3, 5, 8 (directed toward the Lower Jiao), GB 26, ST 36, KI 3, 5, 7, UB 23, 31–34, 52, Dai Mai (GB 41–SJ5), Du Mai (SI 3–UB 62), Ren Mai (LU 7–KI 6), palpate for lower abdomen points (KI 11–16, ST 25–28, Zigong, etc.).

- Herbal Formulae: Er Xian Wan, Ba Ji Yin Yang Wan, You Gui Wan, Zuo Gui Wan.

- Essential Oils: Frankincense, Vetiver, Ylang Ylang.

- Gemstones: Amazonite, Blue Beryl/Aquamarine, Mahogany Obsidian, Red Garnet, Tourmaline (Black Or Yellow).

- Qigong: Five Animal Frolics–Bear and Crane; Hun Yuan Gong–Opening and Closing the Lower *Dan Tian*, Opening and Closing Heaven and Earth.

- Lifestyle: Regular, whole-body physical movement (walking, dancing, swimming, etc.).

CLIENT EXAMPLE

A heterosexual female in her late 30s was recently diagnosed with vaginismus. She is suffering from painful intercourse with vaginal dryness and inability to orgasm for the past six to eight months (previously healthy sex life with her husband of 5+ years). Recent life stressors include trying to sell their house, wanting to move, and trying to get pregnant. They have already done IVF twice, and are doing Acupuncture before the third (and final) round. She has a lot of anxiety about not getting pregnant at her age, and is already seeing a therapist for stress management. Other symptoms include fatigue, low back pain, scant menstrual blood, and the lower abdomen is cold on palpation. Pulse is weak overall, especially in right rear position. Tongue is slightly pale and thin, with dark sublingual veins. She is diagnosed with fear obstructing the Kidneys and Blood Deficiency–Stasis caused by chronic emotional stress (see Chapter 11). She is treated as follows:

- Acupuncture: Ren 2–6, 12, KI 11–16, ST 25–28, Zigong, LV 3–PC 6 (in combination), LV 8 (directed toward the Lower Jiao), ST 36, Du 20, Dai Mai (GB 41–SJ 5).

- Moxibustion: Ren 4, 6, ST 27, 36, Zigong.

- Herbal Formulae: Fu Ke Zhong Zi Wan, Xiao Yao Wan.

- Lifestyle: Establish a regular exercise routine – 15–30 minutes daily preferably in nature/outside (walking, biking, etc.); stop IVF and all penetrative sex for three months minimum; experiment with masturbation (solo and partnered) to best determine energetic, emotional, or physical obstructions – allowing plenty of time for relaxed sex play.

ASEXUALITY

This text defines Asexual as 'a person that does not experience sexual feelings or Desire, or chooses to not act on those feelings.' This includes those that don't engage in any sexual activity, as well as those that consistently have very little desire to engage in sex.

There are three types of Asexuality that must be addressed: voluntary, involuntary, and pathological (i.e., a symptom of an underlying imbalance). From a clinical perspective, what must be first discerned is the issue of pathology: is there an obstruction, deficiency, or excess that is preventing the true expression of the individual's sexuality? One must also look to the individual's overall zest for life: how is their libido beyond the act of sex? Also, how is their ability to connect with others: are they engaging with other people in meaningful and intimate ways outside of sex? When a person is present and mindfully engaged in their life, with creative aspirations and goals, intimate and meaningful connections, healthy pulses, a thriving spirit, and no presenting symptoms of sexual repression, they are clearly making the correct choice for their Constitution and life curriculum.

Voluntary Asexuality

During arousal, Heat expands and rises from the Lower Jiao through the Extraordinary Vessels. This brings Jing-Essence in contact with the Qi-emotions and Shen-Spirit, helping to combine and mix the Three Treasures. As arousal and pre-orgasm states blend, energy moves upward and downward through the 'waves' of Yang and Yin energies, promoting interaction of the Upper, Middle, and Lower *Dan Tian* along the Taiji pole, and rectifying the entire Qi Mechanism. With orgasm, the strong downward movement releases excess Fluids through ejaculation. This entire process was thoroughly covered in Chapter 6.

For those that choose to not engage in sex (either complete avoidance or infrequent contact), it is very difficult to encounter the symptoms of sexual taxation. It is a mistake, however, to assume that asexuality implies a complete inability to become aroused. Arousal has been referred to in this text as a sexual state, but the word 'arouse' simply means to evoke, awaken, or become excited. Asexual people may experience arousal on a frequent basis, but it might not be *sexual* in nature.

Most commonly, asexuality as a lifestyle choice is a way for the individual to support either intellect or spirituality. During intellectual or spiritual arousal, such as what happens with passionate and respectful academic discourse, intense prayer, or deep meditation, the Heat of arousal does not expand to the genital region or to the surface of the body (such as with sexual arousal). Instead, it becomes much more strongly focused in the upward direction, bringing

Jing-Essence directly into the Sea of Marrow, circulating throughout the brain. This re-routing of Jing is shown in Figure 7.4, where the flow of energy rises up through the Extraordinary Vessels and the cerebrospinal fluid, flooding the Sea of Marrow and the ventricular spaces of the Upper *Dan Tian*.

Anyone can practice re-routing Jing-Essence in this way for intellectual or spiritual growth. However, individuals can excessively focus on re-routing the Jing-Essence if they do not have proper training through Qigong or other meditative arts. Symptoms to watch for are due to either excessive flow of Extraordinary Vessel energy to the head or the 'wasting' of Primary Channels and overall physical strength due to EV surplus being re-routed. Common symptoms are insomnia, headaches, flaccidity of muscle or flesh, diarrhea or atonic constipation, fatigue, anemia, and prolapse. Treatment options might include:

- Excessive flow of Extraordinary Vessel energy to the head: Du 20 and Sishencong (directed away from Du 20), Du 20 with Kidney 1, UB 1 with UB 60, GB 21, Kidney 3.

- 'Wasting' of the Primary Channels and physical strength: Ren 12, Ren 6 – with Moxa, Lung 7 with LI 4, LI 10 with Stomach 36 – with Moxa.

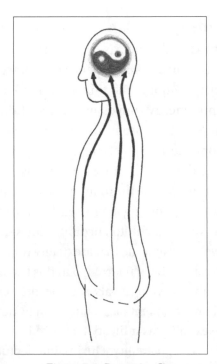

Figure 7.4: Rerouting Jing

Involuntary Asexuality

When the physical expression of sexuality becomes extremely limited or impossible, either due to oppressive cultural influence or a cramped living situation, this is involuntary asexuality. Even for those who chose their situation, such as military personnel or celibate priests, when both sex and masturbation are denied to someone that *wants* to participate in sexual activity, chronic obstruction of the libido creates both Qi Stagnation-Heat and stagnation of Jing-Essence.

If arousal in any form – sexual, intellectual, or spiritual – is not allowed to regularly spread Jing-Essence, it will stagnate. As Jing is both Yin and Yang in its nature, this will create conditions of Lower Jiao Dampness, Damp-Heat, or Phlegm-Heat. As the *Ming Men* Fire is obstructed from its proper flow, Lower Jiao Heat will continue to build. This can transform a healthy libido into a pathological Desire or Craving (see Chapter 14). If this condition becomes chronic or is combined with the extreme Stagnation caused by Repression or Secrecy (see Chapter 13), the creation of Phlegm-Heat or Phlegm-Fire is inevitable. This will likely lead to misplaced judgment and reason, increased sexual distress, pathological or abusive sexual behaviors, or could even turn on itself to create Self-Loathing or Suicidal Ideation (see Chapter 15).

Figure 7.5 shows the problems caused by the obstruction of proper flow in the Lower Jiao, with both Fluid Stasis and accumulating Heat visualized as an active volcano. Scorching hot steam will rise to harass the Qi-Emotions and Shen-Spirit levels, creating irritability, insomnia, and other emotional Heat signs. The hot and slow-moving lava can easily impact the skin level as the Heat not only rises, but expands; there can be a tendency to eczema, rashes, herpes outbreaks, etc. It is important to note that active volcanoes are ready to erupt at any time, so Heat and hot Fluids (i.e., Phlegm-Heat or Blood-Heat) can spew in any direction at a rapid rate if provoked by other triggers (alcohol, spicy foods, etc.).

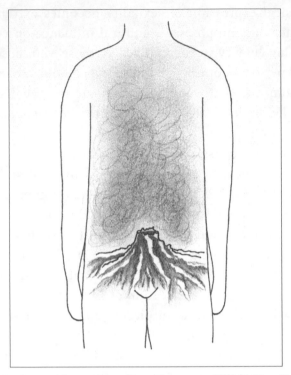

Figure 7.5: Obstruction of Jing-Essence and Ming Men *Fire*

To review, involuntary asexuality always forms Qi Stagnation-Heat in the Lower Jiao which obstructs flow of Jing-Essence and *Ming Men* Fire, leading to varying degrees of localized Dampness and Heat. The pulse will always be wiry to some degree due to the stagnation and/or Phlegm, but it may not express a rapid quality if the Dampness or Phlegm predominates (this may change during a treatment session as the Dampness and Phlegm lift). Emotionally, it is very likely for mood swings (anger, frustration, depression, etc.) and passive-aggressive behavior to develop. Physical symptoms to watch for include:

- Qi Stagnation-Heat: Tension or pain in the Liver/GB Channel regions (hip/IT band/psoas area, vaginismus), menstrual irregularities (irregular timing, cramping, extreme irritability/emotional upset, bloating), endometriosis.

- Dampness/Phlegm (obstructed Jing-Essence–Yin aspect): Menstrual irregularities (delayed flow, cramping, clotting, brownish color) leukorrhea, fertility issues (men and women), ovarian cysts and fibroids, weight gain in lower abdomen/high hip region/along the Dai Mai, genital rashes, vulvar cysts, Dai Mai obstruction patterns (Heat Above–Cold Below, etc.).

- Heat/Fire (obstructed Jing-Essence–Yang aspect): Genital rash or herpes symptoms (recurring outbreaks, prodromal symptoms), prostatitis, menstrual irregularities (early flow, excessive or scant bleeding, bright red color), vaginal dryness, fertility issues (men and women).

The primary focus of treatment is to Course Qi, Clear Heat, and Resolve Dampness/Phlegm in the Lower Jiao. The use of Extraordinary Vessels may prove helpful to move 'surplus' out to the Primary Channels, but care should be taken to not overtreat them. Treatment options might include:

- Acupuncture: Four Gates (LV 3–LI 4), KI 2, LV 2, 3, 8 (directed toward the Lower Jiao), LI 11, ST 36, 40, 44, SP 3, 6, 9, UB 18, 19, 22, 31–34, Du Mai (SI 3–UB 62), Ren Mai (LU 7–KI 6), Chong Mai (SP 4–PC 6), palpate for lower abdomen points (Ren 2–7, KI 11–16, ST 25–28, Zigong, etc.).

- Herbs: Jia Wei Xiao Yao Wan, Long Dan Xie Gan Wan, Chai Hu Long Gu Mu Li Wan, Bi Xie Sheng Shi Wan, Huang Lian Jie Du Wan.

- Essential Oils: Cedarwood, Chamomile, Fir, Peppermint, Jasmine, Lavender, Lemon, Lemon Verbena, Marjoram, Melissa, Rose, Sandalwood, Tea Tree.

- Gemstones: Amethyst, Rutilated Quartz, Agate, Jasper, Chalcedony, Amber, Calcite, Tourmaline, Aventurine, Green Garnet, Malachite, Prehnite, Chrysoprase, Lepidolite.

- Qigong: Pounding and Scrubbing–Gallbladder Channel; Hun Yuan Gong–Grinding the Corn, Opening and Closing the Three *Dan Tian*.

- Lifestyle: Ensure adequate exercise; encourage physical motion in the pelvis (dancing, running, Yoga, Qigong, etc.).

Pathological Asexuality

This type of asexuality stems from either an underlying obstruction or a deficiency that is preventing the individual's libido from fully manifesting. When considering etiology, one must discern physical versus emotional causes to create an appropriate treatment plan:

- Is there a *physical obstruction* to the Lower Jiao flow (*Ming Men* Fire and Jing-Essence) thwarting the natural process of arousal? This could have been caused by internal or external Trauma causing Qi and Blood Stasis (i.e., injury, surgical scar tissue, etc.).

- Is there *un-manifested desire* causing obstruction to the Lower Jiao flow? This could be the result of emotions that create Stagnation, such as Shame, Guilt, Repression, or Secrecy.

- Is there a *physical deficiency* such that arousal cannot be supported? Most commonly this is the Kidneys, but a Spleen or Liver Deficiency could also 'over-draw' on the Kidneys for support.

- Is there an *emotional concern* that is excessively depleting the Kidneys? Fear, Anxiety, Anger, and Grief are the most common issues, often with roots in Trauma (see Section IV).

- Is *'over use' of the intellect or spirit* drawing too much Jing-Essence to the Sea of Marrow, so there is inadequate supply to support sexual arousal?

Besides a generalized lack of libido, symptoms will clearly vary based on the root cause: deficiency or obstruction.

- Deficient presentation: Menstrual difficulties (delayed menses, amenorrhea, anovulation, scant flow), infertility, low sperm count, erectile dysfunction, miscarriage; along with other signs of Kidney Deficiency (fatigue, low back pain, knee weakness, vaginal dryness – mild with no rash, depression, etc.).

- Obstruction presentation: Menstrual difficulties (delayed or irregular cycle, cramping, clots, dark or brownish flow, bloating, low back pain), leukorrhea, infertility, endometriosis, cysts and fibroids; along with other localized signs of Qi Stagnation-Heat (mild) and Fluid Stasis (digestive difficulties, recurring UTI symptoms, etc.).

Contrary to the strong Kidney pulses found with voluntary asexuality, pulses here will be deep and wiry, hidden, thin, or empty. Deficient pathology is typically based in Kidney Deficiency (Yin, Yang, Jing, or a combination), but there may be other systems involved as noted above. Obstruction pathology is based in Qi Stagnation-Heat as discussed above, but there will likely be Fluid Stasis (Blood, Dampness, and/or Phlegm) as well, 'locking in' the obstruction. Symptoms of Heat will be mild, as this obstruction lacks the emotional triggers seen with involuntary asexuality. Etiology dictates the treatment, and as with any chronic condition, there is the possibility of *both* patterns occurring simultaneously.

The basic treatment for pathological asexuality is to tonify the Kidneys and Jing-Essence, harmonize the Extraordinary Vessels (Ren, Du, Chong, and Dai), and to rectify the Qi Mechanism as needed. Each client will be a unique presentation based on etiology; many of the necessary treatment strategies are found in this chapter and in Section IV.

CLIENT EXAMPLE

A heterosexual male in his mid 20s is looking for seasonal adjustment treatments to prevent illness. He is a vegetarian, Yoga instructor (two to three classes six days per week), and also meditates at home, typically cross-legged on the floor. He is thin but not muscular, with thin hair and 'spacey' eyes. He credits his excellent meditation and low sexual activity (about once a month) for his ability to sleep only one night a week. He is not complaining about the insomnia; he likes the productivity and spends his nights walking, meditating, reading, or playing music. He gets mild headaches every couple of days, which he blames on negative energy fields. His pulses are thin-weak overall and non-existent in either rear position. His tongue is pale and dry, with peeled sides and fine red dots at tip. He is diagnosed with incorrect re-routing of Jing-Essence into the Upper *Dan Tian* and concurrent Liver Blood Deficiency (Water not nourishing Wood). He is treated as follows:

- Acupuncture: Du 20 and Sishencong (directed away from Du 20), Yintang, GB 20, 21, UB 60, KI 3, ST 36, SP 6, LV 3, 8, PC 6, Ren 4, 6, 12.

- Moxbustion: Ren 4, 6, 12, ST 36, KI 1, 3.

- Herbal Formulae: Liu Wei Di Huang Wan, Si Jun Zi Wan.

- Diet: Blood and Jing-Essence-nourishing foods (sweet potato, molasses, eggs, nuts, etc.).

- Lifestyle: Advised that too much focus on Upper *Dan Tian* is known to cause psychosis, and that he needs to focus on Lower *Dan Tian* cultivation to ensure proper health; advised to meditate by sitting in a chair or lying down more often than cross-legged.

OBSESSION WITH SEX AND PORNOGRAPHY

The term 'sex addict' first appeared in the United States starting in the 1980s, but it did not originate within the psychiatric or addiction counseling communities. The origins of an addiction model trace to the evangelical Christian movement's attempt to define what is considered normal in regard to sexual behavior.

This perspective continues to focus on traditional, binary gender concepts and roles, with conservative, homophobic, and 'slut-shaming' limits.

Scientific research into a model of 'sex addiction' has *not* consistently demonstrated neurochemistry changes similar to traditional substance addictions (i.e., alcohol, drugs, smoking), and the American Psychiatric Association (APA) does not identify addiction to either sexual activity or pornography as a mental health disorder. In 2016, the American Association of Sexuality Educators, Counselors, and Therapists (AASECT) released a position statement against the addiction model, noting that current research lacked definition or methodological rigor, reflected sociocultural biases, and did not include a wide range of sexual behaviors, identities, or sexual rights (Aaron 2016; AASECT n.d.).

Meanwhile, it is interesting to note that Internet Addiction Disorder (IAD), a pathologically intense level of internet use that includes internet pornography, gaming, and social media exposure, is gaining ground as a valid medical concern. The symptoms of IAD match those from the sex and porn addiction models: concentration difficulties, emotional distress (anxiety, depression), and erectile dysfunction. This is important to note because most people now access pornography through the internet; one must therefore ask if these symptoms are sex- and porn-related, or if they are *internet*-related. Regardless of potential cause, medical practitioners must assume a perspective of cultural objectivity and non-moral judgment. From this stance, the real concern with excessive exposure to sexual activity or pornography is not necessarily quantity, but obsession.

Certain Constitutions focus more on sexual activity and imagery than others. For example, the Water Constitution is known for being more sexually explorative in general, and both Water and Wood Elements are known for having an excellent sex drive. To avoid the trappings of cultural bias around sex and pornography, remember that *symptoms of pathology must exist* before etiology of disease can be determined!

Moderation – the avoidance of excess or extremes in any activity or belief – is a value espoused by Daoism, Buddhism, and other spiritual traditions. Obsession is moderation's opposite: it is preoccupation with an idea, thought, or behavior that is allowed to constantly intrude on a person's conscious mind. In Chinese Medicine, obsessive thinking injures the Earth Element, but preoccupation with sexual activity and erotic or explicit imagery creates two other problems: excessive stirring of the *Ming Men* Fire, and desensitization of the Shen-Spirit. Therefore, there are three patterns that could arise separately, or coincide:

- Earth Element dysfunction from obsessive thought depleting the Yi-Intellect (this will usually appear in conjunction with one or both of the following).

- *Ming Men* Fire being allowed to 'run amok' from unbridled arousal.

- Shen-Spirit pathology from misalignment of the Jing-Essence to the Taiji pole.

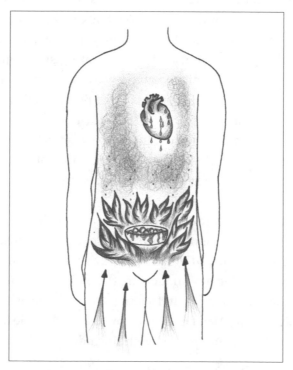

Figure 7.6: Stirring the Ming Men *Fire*

Unbridled Obsession: Stirring the *Ming Men* Fire

The Heat of arousal starts in the Lower Jiao, spreading *Ming Men* Fire into the 'Room of Essence' before entering the Ren, Du, and Chong Vessels. When a person is in a state of constant arousal, this Heat is continuously released until the exhaustion of the *Ming Men* and Kidney Yang. Simultaneously, the extreme Heat 'cooks' the Kidney Yin aspect of Jing-Essence, while also rising upward to disturb the Heart and Shen-Spirit in the Upper Jiao. Between the depletion of Water energy and the overstimulation of Fire energy, a disconnect will occur between the two. The split between Heaven and Earth creates an 'inability to ground' which only further depletes the Water Element and the three Leg Yin Channels (Water, Earth, and Wood) as well.

This situation is the most common problem with excessive amounts of sexual activity or pornography exposure, but it is not limited to these interests alone. Online social media and dating websites, with a constant stream of new people, information, and 'likes,' also stimulate the Heat of excitation from the *Ming Men*. This can be a cause of extreme, unidentified emotional stress and anxiety as Heat consistently rises to harass the Shen-Spirit, while depleting the Water Element that would help cool the internal Fire.

Figure 7.6 shows the unbridled blazing of Obsession Heat. Heat in the Lower Jiao 'cooks' the Jing, leading to fatigue, low back or knee weakness, a strong libido with lack of desire to engage in sex, limited ejaculate, or infertility (in men especially). The flames of Heat also rise up, creating symptoms in the Upper Jiao region: headaches, insomnia, or anxiety are common, but Heat can also appear as acne in those prone to Dampness in the flesh. As Obsession is a chronic condition, energy remains upward, away from the leg Yin Channels, which will eventually suffer from lack of Qi and Yang. Impact is likely more intense on the Yin Channels, but can also show up in malnourishment of the large tendons along the GB and UB Channels (iliotibial band, hamstrings), or in the joints of the hips, knee and/or ankle.

The combination of upward-focused energy and depletion of the Lower Jiao – including the leg channels, and Kidneys – will eventually cause a Heat Above–Cold Below pattern. Once the *Ming Men* Fire is exhausted, complete inability to become aroused and erectile dysfunction are the major symptoms. For the initial stages of this condition, appropriate treatment would nourish Kidney Yin and Jing-Essence, anchor *Ming Men* Fire in the Lower Jiao, clear Heat, and harmonize Heart and Kidney. Treatment options might include:

- Acupuncture: KI 1, 2, 3, 7, 10, Ren 4, 6, UB 23, 52, Du 4, PC 8, HT 3, 8, LV 2, 3, 8, SP 3, 6, LI 11.

- Moxibustion – *with caution*: KI 1, Ren 4, UB 23, Du 4.

- Herbal Formulae: Er Xian Wan, Zhi Bai Di Huang Wan, Tian Wang Bu Xin Wan, Wu Zi Yan Zong Wan, Liu Wei Di Huang Wan, Zuo Gui Wan.

- Essential Oils: Clary Sage, Fennel, Geranium, Jasmine, Melissa, Mimosa, Rose, Vetiver, Ylang Ylang.

- Gemstones: Optical Calcite, Zircon, Rainbow Obsidian, Green Beryl/ Emerald, Lepidolite.

- Qigong: Qi Circulation/Tai Yang Circulation (laying); Five Animal Frolics–Crane.

- Diet: Kidney- and Jing-nourishing foods (eggs, seeds, nuts, beans, etc.), and Cooling foods (bamboo shoot, lettuce, millet, mung bean sprouts, peppermint, etc.); avoid Hot foods (spices, sugars, shellfish, lamb, alcohol, etc.).

- Lifestyle: Avoid or greatly cut back on stimulation activities for treatment to have beneficial effect. *Note: Meditation will generally not be applicable, as the mind will likely use the opportunity to wander back to the obsession.*

Lack of Presence: Absent Shen

Obsession with sex or pornography can also encourage the Shen-Spirit to disconnect from the intensity of the experience, allowing cultural tendencies of objectification and dehumanization to flourish. This occurs most easily with anonymous sex, 'one-night stands,' prostitution, strip clubs, and internet pornography. Unfortunately, because of the extensive use of erotic and sexualized content in advertising, desensitization has become a far-too-common problem across cultures on all continents, and it is truly our entire planet and all species that now suffer from the consequences of disconnected relationship. Of course, the concern as healthcare practitioners is regarding the creation of pathology.

The problem begins in the flow of the Three Treasures, where the force of Humanity connects with the forces of Heaven and Earth. This connection is critical to enter any healthy relationship, but in this case arousal Heat is *not permitted* to travel upward and link the Jing-Essence with the Qi-Emotion and Shen-Spirit levels. Instead, Qi follows intent, so obsession with the external and objectified stimulus disperses the Jing-Essence outward toward the source of arousal. The lack of Qi-Emotion and Shen-Spirit participation is what allows a person to become desensitized to the needs of any 'other.' For most people, this is an occasional occurrence; if balanced with connected forms of arousal and sex, there will be no lasting repercussions. However, when one is chronically aroused by excessive, external-focused, 'distanced,' or disconnected stimuli, the Jing-Essence and Lower *Dan Tian* will lose their Taiji pole alignment.

Any form of sex that follows, whether solo or partnered, will suffer from misalignment, with both Qi-Emotions and Shen-Spirit struggling to be a part of the experience; over time the Middle and Upper *Dan Tian* will also falter. This makes it extremely difficult for the root of Desire – i.e., the very real human need to connect and relate to another human being in a deeply emotional and spiritual capacity – to be satisfied, leaving greater longing, loneliness, and obsession in its wake.

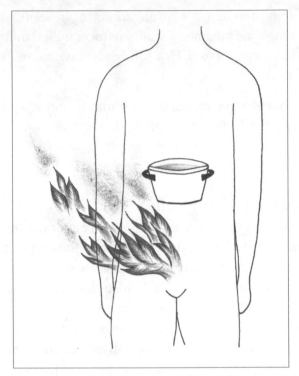

Figure 7.7: Displacement of the Jing-Essence

Displacement of the Jing-Essence toward the external stimuli is shown in Figure 7.7, where the flames of arousal are displaced from the Taiji pole. No matter how high these flames burn, they simply cannot adequately warm the cooking pot, leading to diminished Qi and Shen, and a huge impact on one's overall health. In their attempt to support other internal systems, the Kidneys and *Ming Men* will be forced to overwork, which will eventually exhaust the Jing-Essence and Kidneys, as well as the arousal response. This is a common root cause of low libido and erectile dysfunction, making any form of sexual activity – solo or partnered – increasingly difficult to engage in. Obstruction of the Extraordinary Vessels and Qi Mechanism that are partially regulated through arousal and orgasm processes is also inevitable (see Chapter 6).

Without Jing-Essence supporting the other Treasures, the Qi-Emotion level will destabilize. Depression is the most common result, as there is no energy to fuel the emotional state or the creation of the Post-Natal Qi. Poor digestion will be the most common early symptom, but Qi or Blood Deficiency could arise in any location based on Constitution and other lifestyle factors. The Shen-Spirit level will suffer as well. Not only has the Shen-Spirit been encouraged to be absent during the act of sex through over-exposure desensitization, now it suffers from lack of support for all of its functioning. If combined with cultural shaming around pornography or sex, the spiritual aspects of self-acceptance, self-worth, and feelings of belonging will become very difficult to maintain. As mentioned above, this will only exacerbate the feelings of longing, loneliness, and obsession.

The Shen-Spirit may also 'lose its root,' becoming un-anchored; the most common presentation is that of anxiety due to Heart Yin or Blood Deficiency. If desensitization to humanity and the 'other' is allowed for many years, the divide between Heaven and Earth forces will expand too far, allowing total dissolution of Qi and Shen. Severe bipolar, schizophrenia and other psychopathic mental illness will result.

Treatment must focus primarily on the re-alignment of the Jing-Essence, the Three Treasures, and the Taiji pole. This is done primarily through Medical Qigong, Qigong, and lifestyle practices. Acupuncture can be used as an adjunctive therapy to nourish and tonify the Kidneys and Jing-Essence, as well as harmonize the Three Treasures and Extraordinary Vessels (Ren, Du, Chong). Treatment might include:

- Medical Qigong – done in the following order:

  - Anchor the Lower *Dan Tian*: Holding the lower abdomen and pelvic region with one palm under the sacrum, the other at Ren 4–6, visualizing the *Dan Tian* into alignment with the 'Room of Essence'

  - Open and align the three *Dan Tian*: Laying one palm over the Lower *Dan Tian*, then linking the three *Dan Tian* between two palms at Lower–Middle, then Middle–Upper, then Upper–Lower, then back to one palm on the Lower *Dan Tian*

  - Rectify the Taiji: Placing a palm two to three inches above Du 20, the other over the Lower *Dan Tian*, then placing a palm at the Lower *Dan Tian*, and the other under Kidney 1.

- Qigong: Hun Yuan Gong–Holding the three *Dan Tian*, Opening and Closing the three *Dan Tian,* Opening and Closing Heaven and Earth; Five Breaths to Dawn; Wuji Pose – standing or moving.

- Lifestyle: Complete abstinence from external stimuli (i.e., pornography, erotic imagery/texts, advertising, casual sex, strip clubs, etc.) is often required for two to 12 months. Depending on the severity of the condition it may need to be consistently regulated for many years. Talk therapy or mental health counseling is strongly recommended.

- Acupuncture: KI 1–Du 20 (in combination), KI 2, 3, 6, 7, 10, Ren 4, 6, UB 23, 52, Du 4; palpate for lower abdomen points – *these will not usually be needled bilaterally* (KI 11–16, ST 25–28, Zigong, etc.).

If Jing-Essence is not just misaligned, but also depleted, consider also:

- Herbal Formulae: Zuo Gui Wan, You Gui Wan, Wu Zi Yan Zong Wan, Lu Rong.

- Diet: Jing-Essence-nourishing foods (beans, eggs, seeds, nuts, etc.).

Re-establishing Relationship

Any lack of Shen-Spirit is resolved by re-establishing proper *relationship*. Therefore, any modalities used (Acupuncture points, Herbs, Essential Oils, etc.) must be considered in terms of *relation* to each other. Does the treatment construct a *whole* picture to counteract the disconnection? Are all three Jiaos and their *Dan Tian* being addressed *simultaneously*? Consider bilateral and paired Extraordinary Vessel needling, or front and back treatment in one session, or full-body massage to reintegrate the entire body–mind–spirit.

CLIENT EXAMPLE

A heterosexual male in his late 20s is suffering from joint pain in the knees, which is aggravated by his construction job. The knees feel warm but deficient. He is thin with reddish cheeks. He also has red patches on the torso and limbs that are warm to the touch which he calls 'heat rash' (it is summer). He is a former alcoholic and cocaine addict, sober for two years. He has a few casual sex partners, has sex five nights a week, and has never had a relationship last more than two to three months. He is diagnosed with excessive stirring of the *Ming Men* and Yin Deficiency–Heat of the Liver and Kidneys.

- Nourish Kidney and Liver Yin, Jing-Essence, clear Deficiency–Heat, anchor *Ming Men*.

- Acupuncture: KI 1, 2, 3, 10, LV 2, 3, 8, SP 6, PC 8, HT 5, 8, LI 11, Du 24, Ren 4.

- Herbal Formulae: Long Dan Xie Gan Wan, Da Bu Yin Wan.

- Diet: Cooling and Yin-nourishing foods (asparagus, bananas, eggs, lemon, mango, watermelon); avoid all caffeine and sugar.

- Qigong: Qi Circulation/Tai Yang Circulation (lying).

- Lifestyle: Client is advised to cut back on sexual stimulation activities (only 2–3 per week, with no pornographic or other aggressively erotic stimuli between) for treatment to have beneficial effect.

SUMMARY

» When determining the amount of sex that is 'healthy,' it is best to ignore classical guidelines and focus instead on the mental and physical state of the specific individual.

» In contemporary culture, excessive arousal combined with *lack* of sexual activity is a more common cause of disease than excessive sexual activity. This situation typically presents with Qi Stagnation-Heat in the Lower Jiao.

» Masturbation is an important component of a healthy sexual life. It is a means to satisfy arousal, cultivate self-acceptance, and expand one's personal knowledge of their genitalia and touch preferences.

» Shame and Guilt are both heavy, descending, and engender stasis of Fluids. Guilt will present with Blood Stasis, Shame with Dampness or Phlegm.

» Anxiety and Fear often occur together, but are energetically opposed. Anxiety is an unrooted emotion that holds energy upward; Fear pulls inward and downward. This opposition easily creates Heart–Kidney Disharmony and Heat Above–Cold Below patterns.

» Fear's inward and downward movement directly obstructs the lifting of arousal. It is commonly present in sex abuse survivors and can deplete the Kidney energetics if left untreated.

» There are three distinct types of asexuality: voluntary, involuntary, and pathological.

» Voluntary asexuality is often done to support the intellect or spiritual life by re-routing the Jing-Essence to the Sea of Marrow and Upper *Dan Tian*. Improper routing of Jing-Essence is a common pathology.

» Involuntary asexuality occurs when an individual wants to participate in sexual activity (sex, masturbation, etc.) but feels unable to do so due to external factors. This situation creates Qi Stagnation-Heat in the Lower Jiao and stagnation of Jing-Essence.

» Pathological asexuality can stem from obstruction or deficiency patterns. Causes include physical Trauma, stagnating or depleting emotions (Fear, Grief, Guilt, Shame, Repression, Secrecy, etc.), Spleen, Kidney, or Liver Deficiency, or the overuse of Jing-Essence to fuel the intellect or spirit.

» Due to the majority of pornography being viewed on the internet, it is difficult to separate excessive pornography viewing from Internet Addiction Disorder (IAD).

» Obsessive exposure to sex or pornography injures the Spleen, excessively stirs the Ministerial Fire, and desensitizes the Shen-Spirit to allow objectification of the 'other.'

Chapter 8

ATTRACTION AND EXPLORATION

- Issues of the Heart

- Elemental Influences

- Nine Palaces Revisited

Cultural limitations on sexuality and sexual identity are one way that people are oppressed all over the globe. Agents of power that attempt to control sexuality were once religious or tribal leaders, but now politicians, educational institutions, and even corporations seek to command the general population. The prevailing psycho-social understanding is that by hindering sexual experimentation (i.e., freeing up the Jing and Qi), one might hamper independent thought as well (i.e., Shen-Spirit). In *The Ethical Slut*, Dossie Easton and Janet Hardy commented on the negative influence of sexual barriers:

> In his lectures to young communists in Germany during the rise of Hitler and the Nazis, psychologist Wilhelm Reich theorized that the suppression of sexuality was essential to an authoritarian government. Without the imposition of antisexual morality, he believed, people would be free from shame and would trust their own sense of right and wrong. They would be unlikely to march to war against their wishes, or to operate death camps. Perhaps if we were raised without shame and guilt about our desires, we might be freer people in more ways than simply the sexual. (2009, p.10)

We are taught what is proper relationship through cultural traditions, family, and advertising, and in contemporary society these messages are predominantly heteronormative and monogamy-focused. Fear, Guilt, Repression, Shame, and other judgmental forces are used to proscribe 'inappropriate' forms of Desire: in other words, they are used to place limits on arousal and the natural spreading of Jing-Essence. Under these strict conditions, any form of sexual experimentation directly challenges the Post-Natal Qi by placing doubt on a person's sexual identity. Without these hinderances, sexuality could be a delightful process of self-discovery that allows one to properly align with the force of Heaven. This concept is built into the spiritual journey of the Nine Palaces through Travel and Adventure, where all forms of experimentation – including sexuality – sit at the very center of awakening.

> From a psychoanalysis perspective, sexual identity, like any identity, is bound by Ego: the place where self-esteem and self-importance are rooted between the conscious and unconscious minds. When the Ego is over-zealous, one's self-esteem is quite fragile, easily 'shaken' by experimentation. To protect the Ego, sexual experimentation under these conditions must be either entirely avoided, or only done with mind-altering substances (alcohol, drugs, etc.) which inhibit consciousness and enable the individual to thwart any challenge to sexual identity.

Chapter 3 examined the Taiji symbol and the spherical movements of Yin–Yang: churning in and out, around and about, just like the movements of the Qi Mechanism. As any possibility may come to the surface of the sphere over time, these movements negate any binary concepts. Chapter 6 discussed the differences between sex, sexuality, and sexual identity as aspects of the Three Treasures and challenges of the spiritual journey. Of course, having minimal options available does not accurately represent the infinite possibilities at the foundation of Yin–Yang. In reality, there are innumerable ways of having sex, being sexual, or engaging in intimate relationship between people of all sexual identities, ranging from physical to energetic to spiritual and everything in-between. It is therefore extremely likely that sexuality and relationship styles are much more flexible than the dominant culture would have us imagine.

Looking back to *The Genderbread Person* (Figure 3.2), Sam Killermann separated sexual attraction and desire for relationship into two distinct categories that do not always overlap: 'sexual attraction' versus 'romantic attraction.' This means that someone can be sexually attracted to a whole range of individuals (such as bi/pansexuality) but may only be romantically interested in pursuing an intimate relationship with a particular set of personal characteristics (such as 'hetero/homo-romantic'). It is also possible for a person to identify as polyamorous – desiring more than one romantic relationship – while also identifying as asexual, with limited to no desire for sexual intimacy in those relationships. In her book *Opening Up*, Tristan Taormino put it this way: 'Each story and each relationship is unique. There are similarities and patterns, but no one does it exactly the same as anyone else' (2008, p.xxiii).

As practitioners, we must dismiss any internal moral judgment regarding sexuality or relationship in order to best support our clients in their pursuit of health and happiness. The overall strength of the Heart-Emperor and the energetics of the Five Elements will take precedence in determining health, but the spiritual journey through the lessons of the Nine Palaces cannot be ignored.

The Truth is in the Tongue

SHAPE = Is there *enough* love?

BLOOD & YIN = Is there the capacity to *experience* love?

HEAT = Is there *Craving* or *Lying* – to one's self or others?

ISSUES OF THE HEART

It is the Fire Element that is in charge of relating to the outside world, and it is the Heart that rules the Fire Element. The overall condition of the Heart organ is therefore the best indicator for one's ability to experience healthy relationship. The state of the Heart can also be used to assess a client's overall well-being, as the Emperor (Heart) can simultaneously *dictate and reflect* the state of the whole Kingdom (body). In relation to sexuality and relationship, important Heart health questions include:

- Does this client feel loved?

- Is their Heart fully satisfied?

- Are they able to honestly communicate their needs and desires?

These questions are critical for both sexually active and inactive individuals, and are actually quite easily diagnosed. Chronic, long-standing lack of love shows up as extreme Deficiency in the Heart. As this is a spirit concern, there may not be any major health complaints: most commonly seen is the *occasional* sadness, heart palpitation (at rest), or sleep disturbance. This Deficiency may manifest as a weak, thin, or floating Heart pulse, but it is far more likely to present in the tissue that corresponds to the Fire Element: the tongue.

In tongue diagnosis the Heart is positioned at the tip, where both shaping and color can indicate pathology. The normal tip should be fleshed out in both shape and color: not too thin, too pale, too red, or misshapen. These are all indicators that the Heart has 'enough.'

The shape of the tongue at the tip indicates the 'fullness' of the Heart, so a thin, dipped, or curled-under tongue tip is an automatic indicator that there is not enough love being received by the individual (see Figure 8.1A–C). This is commonplace among single people that strongly desire intimate relationship, married or partnered individuals that are unsatisfied, and polyamorous people that do not have enough intimate relationships to feel properly balanced. Although this concern can be managed with Chinese Medicine treatments combined with talk therapy, meditation, or other self-care practices, recognizing the etiology and bringing more love into one's life is the best long-term solution.

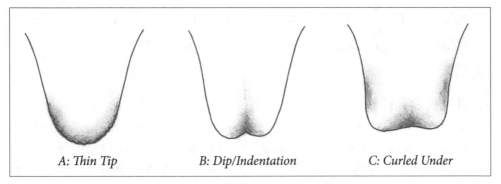

A: Thin Tip   *B: Dip/Indentation*   *C: Curled Under*

Figure 8.1A–C: Shape of Love

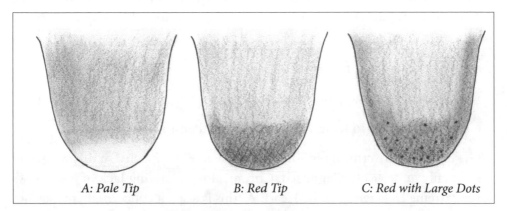

A: Pale Tip   *B: Red Tip*   *C: Red with Large Dots*

Figure 8.2A–C: Color of Love

Another sign of Heart Deficiency is the pale-pink or pink-red tongue, indicating Blood or Yin Deficiency (see Figure 8.2A–B). Whereas the shape of the tongue tip usually indicates the amount of love being received, the color of the Heart position indicates *the capacity of the individual to experience* the love that surrounds them. When there is a Blood or Yin Deficiency, the Heart's capacity to hold on to the feeling of love is diminished. Therefore, the person's experience of Love becomes constricted even if they are already involved in truly loving and fulfilling relationship(s). A simple Blood- or Yin-nourishing Herbal Formula and Diet plan are the best approach for this specific concern, but it may take a long time for the Heart to heal if there are fine red dots combined with the pale-pink or pale-red color (indicating an Empty Heat condition), or if the Blood or Yin Deficiency color is combined with any of the shaping issues described above (indicating the potential for either a life-long concern such as early childhood neglect or an innate Constitutional trait). The following are some treatment options to address the issues of shape and color associated with Heart Blood or Yin Deficiency patterns:

- Acupuncture: Ren 17, PC 1, 3, 6, HT 3, 5, 6, Du 20, Yintang, KI 2, 3, 6, 10.

- Medical Qigong: Holding the Heart:
  - Place palm over Ren 17 and visualize a large, deep red, glowing color (the Heart) enveloped in pink (the Pericardium)
  - Hold until the colors stabilize
  - If this isn't working, try placing one hand over Ren 17, and the other at Du 11 while asking the client to also visualize these colors.

- Herbal Formulae: Nu Ke Ba Zhen Wan, Gui Pi Wan, Tian Wang Bu Xin Wan.

- Diet: Bitter foods to enter the Heart (broccoli, kale, dark chocolate, dark beer, etc.); Blood- and Yin-nourishing foods (spinach, beets, dates, meat, eggs, dairy, etc.).

- Qigong: Sheng Zhen Qigong: Heart Spirit as One/Jesus Sitting.

- Essential Oils: Angelica, Chamomile, Geranium, Jasmine, Rose.

- Gemstones: Amethyst, Quartz (Clear, Rose, or Smoky), Bloodstone, Carnelian, Tiger Eye, Jadeite, Garnet, Hematite, Kunzite, Lapis Lazuli, Peridot, Ruby, Moonstone, Topaz.

There is excess to examine on the tongue as well: the presence of large red dots on the tongue tip, indicating a Full Heat condition in the Heart (see Figure 8.2C). This is common for those that experience Craving for love. The Heat in this case may have begun elsewhere, such as from chronic arousal stirring the *Ming Men* Fire, but the Heat has now settled in the Heart, creating a lust for love that is difficult – if not impossible – to satisfy. In this case, the fluids are likely to also be consumed by the Heat, creating a 'catch-22' situation where the lusting individual cannot truly experience the love that surrounds them, and so they are constantly seeking more. This may be seen in any form of obsession, especially for those that constantly engage in casual sex or cheating (see Chapters 7 and 14 for treatment options).

As the Heart's corresponding tissue, the tongue is not just a good diagnostic tool. The tongue is considered an 'extension' of the Heart itself: it reflects an individual's ability to speak the truth and ask for what they want. Any symptoms of chronic or occasional stuttering, inability to find the right words, or feeling 'tongue-tied' can be another indicator of long-standing lack of love or a diminished capacity to experience love. Most often, however, it is an indicator of the inability to communicate one's needs brought on by either embarrassment or Shame. Stuttering and other tongue-tied conditions where expressions of love become difficult can come from either Heart or Pericardium issues: either the Heart is struggling to express itself, or the Pericardium cannot properly manifest the messages.

A Note on Stuttering

Stuttering that is associated with genetic inheritance or is caused by physical Trauma to the brain clearly did not stem from an emotional root, but it can be the cause of elevated anxiety and stress, creating ongoing communication issues in all relationships.

A Note on Cheating

Cheating is the practice of engaging in sexually or emotionally intimate relationships without the consent of one's other partner(s), which is not an emotionally or energetically health-promoting practice. Cheating involves lying (i.e., going against one's words), as well as Secrecy, Shame, Guilt, or Desire, all of which go against the Upright Qi by obstructing the Qi Mechanism, Five Element cycles, and the lessons of the Nine Palaces. Regardless, the cheating client requires a practitioner's empathy and love as they work to transform these patterns.

CLIENT EXAMPLE

A married bisexual female in her mid 30s has been coming in monthly for management of digestive upsets, alternating bowels, and anxiety related to childhood-onset PTSD for over five years. She also has mild neck and shoulder tension from computer work, sees both a therapist and massage therapist regularly, and is trying to lose 30–40 pounds with exercise. Her tongue is always pale, swollen, curled under at the tip, with a dip at the rear or center. Her pulse is usually slippery-wiry and weak on both sides. She is being treated for Heart–Kidney disharmony, Spleen Qi Deficiency with Dampness, and Liver Qi Stagnation (Liver invading Spleen), which keeps her emotions and digestion stable overall. Her 'go to' Herbal Formulae are Tian Wang Bu Xin Wan, with either Nu Ke Ba Zhen Wan (week 1–2 of menses) or Xiao Yao Wan (week 3–4 of menses); during humid weather she sometimes needs Bi Xie Sheng Shi Wan at ovulation to manage bloating. Today her tongue is a normal color and shape for the first time, except for a slightly thin tip. Her pulse is relaxed and only slightly slippery in the Spleen/Stomach position. When asked about the state of love in her life, her eyes sparkle and she smiles. She met someone new just over a month ago, and although she has 'always known' she was poly, this is the first time she's ever had two lovers in an openly polyamorous relationship: 'I am completely full of love, from two people that accept me for who I really am and accept each other's presence in my life. I truly cannot believe how lucky I am.'

THE ELEMENTS OF ENGAGEMENT

Looking beyond the Heart, issues of deficiency or stagnation in other systems can also wreak havoc on the ability to properly engage in intimate relationship. Five Element cycle interactions help pinpoint some of the factors that contribute to chronically inappropriate relationship choices.

Briefly examining the Five Element generating cycle, it is Water that reflects a person's fears, insecurities, and vulnerabilities, and it takes strong Wood to have the courage to go out into the world and connect with others. Through these interactions one develops Fire's discernment, determining which forms of relationship bring joy, and which do not. Crafting authentic and long-term happiness requires Earth's strong sense of self and ability to transform through the stages of relationship. The changes necessary could bump against cultural mores, pushing Metal to determine what is truly important, and what can be dismissed. When a person is able to determine their own needs without attention to cultural pressure, Water's intuition and will can thrive, boosting the courage to start the cycle all over again.

The essential components that generate appropriate relationships are shown in Figure 8.3. The specifics of each element's actions are further discussed below, along with pathological concerns that can interrupt the process of healthy engagement.

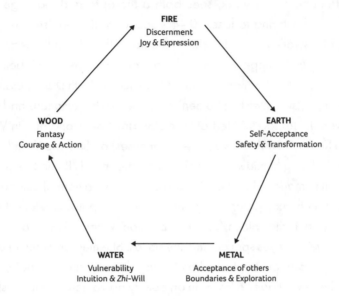

Figure 8.3: The Elements of Engagement

Wood: Fantasy and Courage

The spirit that corresponds to the Wood Element is the Hun, associated with ideas, dreams, and fantasies. A healthy Wood Element combines the Hun's desires with the courage to act on them – a critical component to a healthy sex life. It is Wood that provides courage to get one's needs met in terms of partners, sex acts, fantasies, and other forms of sexual expression. Therefore, any inability to express one's fantasies or to take charge in sexual relationships may be related to Wood pathology.

In Wood pathology, the courage to pursue one's desires and needs is thwarted by either deficiency or obstruction affecting the Liver. Perhaps the individual is exhausted by excessive mental work, leaving no Blood or Yin to nourish the Liver. Arousal may or may not be inhibited, but the expression of one's fantasies, the ability to 'take charge' during sex, or general passivity in choosing sex partners or sex acts will most certainly be impacted. There could be an underlying emotional obstruction preventing the free flow of Liver Qi and the courage to go after one's needs: Repression, Secrecy, Guilt, Shame, Fear, and Trauma are all common etiological concerns (see Section IV).

Fire: Discernment and Joy

Fire contains aspects of both joy and discernment, the respective emotions of the Heart and Small Intestine. Discernment is perhaps the most important of all elemental aspects for creating healthy long-term relationships, as it includes the simultaneous weighing of multiple variables: relationship style preferences, gender and sexuality preferences, and personality or Constitution matching, as well as lifestyle and socio-economic concerns. In terms of Fire Element pathology that contributes to the formation of unhealthy relationships, Small Intestine can be overly discerning, thwarting one's ability to interact with a wide range of individuals for a healthy and broad range of friendships, or it may be non-discerning, mis-identifying 'types' that are right for intimate relationships and allowing a consistent history of poor relationship choices that were 'doomed from the start.'

As the Emperor, the Heart is considered the seat of both the Shen-Spirit and the *Wu Shen*. Belonging to the force of Heaven, the Heart also helps connect the individual to the Divine Emperor, granting each person the ability to see the divine spirit in others. With this enhanced perception the Heart is prone to falling in love; so, like the ancient Kings, the Heart must be protected.

It is the Pericardium that serves as Heart's protector, advisor, and emissary, responsible for filtering information (both external and internal stimuli) before it reaches the Heart, and for externally manifesting Heart's Qi through the expression of love. As such, the Pericardium must identify 'unworthy' or unmatched individuals that made it past Small Intestine's filter, and determine appropriate levels of intimacy in all forms of relationship. Failure of the Pericardium to protect the Heart includes excessive 'falling in love,' entering relationships with inappropriate partners, and not ending poor relationships in a timely fashion (perhaps expecting that it 'might get better with time'). On the other hand, complete inability to fall in love, develop intimate friendships, or ending relationships at the first sign of trouble could indicate extreme rigidity and over-protection of the Heart.

Rarely, complete inability to fall in love is due to obstruction of the Heart that thwarts the ability either to see the divine in others or to experience love. In this case, there will be some of the tongue signs already discussed, as well as physical evidence of Blood Stasis or Phlegm. There may also be a long-standing physical heart condition such as a murmur or congenital abnormality. On the emotional side, there could be severe mental illness such as psychotic or sociopathic behavior.

New Relationship Energy (NRE)

NRE is that euphoric state of love or lust in which the world seems to revolve around the new person. It is both wonderful and dangerous.

– Tristan Taormino 2008, p.185

NRE is a perfectly natural condition that most people have experienced. It is wonderful because of the new-ness of connection. The other person's divine spark is so visible that love ignites Fire, helping course the intellectual, spiritual, or sexual arousal of Jing-Essence. This warmth relaxes Metal, allowing the new person to traverse the outer gate into the Kingdom for closer evaluation. Under normal circumstances, a healthy individual sees their own signs of infatuation and allows time to pass before making any major life changes or inviting the new person further in. However, if Fire burns too hot, Metal's boundaries could 'melt,' permitting Wood's fantasies about this new person to run amok, potentially leading to rash decisions and boundary violations that are later regretted. When a client finds themselves suffering the 'heat' of NRE, general treatment principles include clearing Heat, dispersing Fire, strengthening Metal, harmonizing Metal and Fire, and nourishing Yin substances to better anchor the Shen and Hun.

Earth: Acceptance, Change, and Safety

Earth pathology mainly revolves around acceptance. Yin Earth (Spleen and Pancreas) addresses the ability to adapt, change, and transform, along with the ability to feel safe, confident, and secure during the process of change. Yang Earth (Stomach) addresses the ability to accept, which has multiple applications including food, external stimuli, other people, and one's self. Earth energy overall is also in charge of the Post-Natal Qi; as such, it is related to the day-to-day fostering of Qi and Blood. Regular nourishment and acceptance of transformation are both critical to develop a healthy sense of self, and to support intimate friendships and relationships.

Issues of acceptance and transformation are related to the *security and stability* of Earth – Is it safe to do this? Am I allowed to change? This is highly dependent on Earth feeling nurtured by Fire, but also by the food and drink that form Gu Qi, and through proper alignment of the Middle *Dan Tian*. Problems in Earth can thwart acceptance of personal or cultural differences, preventing opportunities for spiritual growth and the development of discernment. If a person struggles with accepting their own gender, sexual preferences, or relationship needs, they may choose friends or intimate partners that – although good people – are poor matches. Chronic disappointment in others is more likely an inability to accept perceived imperfections (a Metal concern) but could also stem from lack of self-acceptance in Earth.

Earth pathology may also reflect an inability to accept change. Some people cannot manage transformation of relationship, such as a transition from friend to sex partner, or from sexual to non-sexual relationship. Ending short-term relationships at the point of transition from passion to loyalty, playfulness, or enduring love is another, less common, Earth issue. Trouble in the Earth Element typically presents as chronic Worry or mild Fear, poor diet choices, multiple food intolerances, and generalized inability to transform and transport caused by deficiency or obstruction. There will likely be excess weight or poor muscle tone along with signs of excess fluid accumulation (sinus congestion, vaginal secretions, diarrhea, etc.).

Metal: Boundaries and Rules

The Metal Element corresponds to the spirit of the Po, which relates to the physical body and its sensations. Metal is also associated with the skin, including physical sensation, the opening and closing of the pores, and the circulation of the Wei Qi in maintaining healthy boundaries to the external world. Metal is also associated with flexibility and rigidity. In terms of sexuality and relationships, Metal must be relaxed enough to allow for experimentation, but also strong enough to identify areas of potential hazard.

Although sexual and relationship exploration may be exciting, it can also bring up triggers and issues around physical or emotional boundaries. Metal is primarily responsible for ensuring that one's personal boundaries are not violated in the process. If Metal is deficient, boundaries are likely to be poor, allowing co-dependent or abusive situations to develop. If Metal is obstructed or stagnant, then boundaries will be too strong and likely to entirely restrict sexual exploration or relationship styles.

As a cool element, Metal requires the warming of Fire energy and its capacity for love to stay supple and soft, but too much Heat and it can lose integrity. A soft and relaxed – but not deficient – Metal Element is required to help 'trim Wood,' making sure that fantasies and courage do not grow out of control, overshadowing the realities of safe and consensual sex acts. If Metal stagnates and over-controls Wood, a person's authentic fantasies or sexual needs may be completely repressed, and safe sex practices may become unreasonably excessive. If a person is unable to let go of the 'rules' around dating, sex, or relationships, it is likely that Fire is not strong enough to soften Metal; so instead of creating authentic experience, they are engaged in completing a checklist of the 'shoulds.'

Dating 'rules'

Rigid perspectives on friendships, intimacy, sexuality, and relationship styles are related to the Metal Element, but stagnant Metal may be due to a Water Element issue. Any obstruction of Water by Fear can prevent the proper flow of Metal, leading to rigid thinking patterns. When this is the case, treatment principles should include dispersing Metal, nourishing and coursing Water, harmonizing Metal and Water, and 'expanding one's perspective' through Sea of Marrow, Windows of the Sky, or other points that increase access to Heaven energy.

Water: Intuition, Fear, Jealousy, Suspicion

The Water Element controls Intuition, a form of internal knowing or understanding that exists without conscious reasoning or intellectual decision-making process. Intuition is ruled by Water's Yin aspect, the Kidneys, which are also the 'seat' of the *Zhi*-Will aspect of *Wu Shen*, including the drive to live and to reproduce. The Yang Water aspect (Urinary Bladder) is more responsible for the emotion and mobilization of Fear, which includes issues of Jealousy and Suspicion of the unknown. The relationship questions that pertain to the Water Element are in regard to *vulnerability*: Can I stand being vulnerable or exposed? Can I open myself to intimate relationships or connections that could bring me pain? Can I trust this journey to unfold at its own pace?

A strong Water Element will be able to use intuition to guide relationship choices, balancing Fear of the unknown with the trust that is from time and experiences spent together. When Water is suffering, fear can take over with an inward turmoil that prevents the 'gut' from feeling what is right. In a state of extreme Fear, few people will be trusted; the creation of friendships, intimate relationships, or engaging in relationship styles outside the familiar or 'culturally approved' will likely become impossible.

If jealousy and suspicion are allowed to flourish, obstructions are common in the Urinary Bladder organ or Channel, with UTI symptoms and various spinal problems (i.e., musculoskeletal back, neck, or sacral pain, spinal stenosis and/or arthritis, etc.). Digestive symptoms (including cock-crow diarrhea) are also common, as well as incontinence of urine, excessive vaginal discharge, flooding menses, and seminal emissions.

Chronic obstruction by fear will lead to a mixed Deficiency–Stagnation pattern in the Water Element, which will prevent the proper influx of Qi from the Metal Element through the generating Five Phase cycle. Water and Fire, when healthy and aligned, combine intuition and unconscious knowledge of Destiny (Water Element), with the ability to discern another person's true nature (Fire

Element). When all five systems are well harmonized, their combined efforts reveal the best partners and relationship styles for any Constitution, creating meaningful, satisfying, and long-lasting intimacy.

CLIENT EXAMPLE

A heterosexual, re-married female in her mid 40s presents with recurring right hypochondriac pain with lying down at night. This has been going on for over one year and can prevent sleep; she often moves to the other bedroom to not disturb her husband. She also has chronic upper back tension, environmental allergies (year-round), IBS (predominant constipation), and extreme sensitivity to the thoughts and emotions of others. Her stressors include a teenage daughter, recent move to the area (i.e., lack of local community and friendship, navigating the unfamiliar), and a new job. She is treated weekly for Liver Qi Stagnation, Damp-Heat brewing in the Gallbladder, and Wei Qi Deficiency. Acupuncture includes GB 20, 21, 24, 34, 40, LV 3, 8, 13, 14, SP 6, 9, Ren 12, 6, 4, Yintang, Taiyang. Cupping and Tuina to clear obstructions in the upper back and UB Channel are done following Acupuncture treatments, and Essential Oils are frequently used (including Angelica, Eucalyptus, Frankincense, Geranium, Jasmine, Rosemary, Savory, Spruce, and Tea Tree). Li Dan Wan and Shu Gan Wan were taken until the right pain ceased (about six weeks), then switched to Xiao Yao Wan and Yu Ping Feng Wan; Pe Min Kan Wan was used to control allergies throughout. After two months the right side pain was gone, allergies were controlled, and digestion and emotional sensitivity were 50–75 percent improved. Treatments were reduced to a maintenance schedule (every two weeks) for tension and stress management with no further improvement. After five to six months of maintenance she finds a Rose Quartz necklace that helps her feel stronger: 'I like it so much I sleep with it too.' After the necklace purchase she starts taking walks after dinner each night by herself, and is now looking for a different job 'where people treat me better.' Once she completes a few job interviews, she divulges ongoing dissatisfaction with her husband's sex preferences that are prompting her to consider divorce and getting a job 'back home' instead.

NINE PALACES REVISITED

Once again, the Nine Palaces come into play. These are the challenges of one's 'life curriculum' discussed in Chapter 4. As already stated, the goal of these challenges is *not* the attainment of any form of perfection. Instead, each individual must learn to accept their struggles and define their needs without judgment. When an individual cannot 'live up to' the definition they constructed (or was imposed upon them by cultural forces), they will not be able to move through the challenges of that palace with ease.

Two palaces are of greatest interest in the exploration of sexuality and attraction: Relationship, and Travel and Adventure. The Relationship Palace is situated in the fourth position – after Health, Wealth, and Prosperity. These three have a huge impact on an individual's capacity to offer anything of value toward long-lasting friendship or sexual intimacy. They ask: Can I take care of my physical and emotional needs? Can I create abundance (financial, community, etc.) and appreciate what I have? Can I share with others, without sacrificing myself? In order to face the challenges presented via Relationship, each person must address, or at least be in the process of working with, the preceding challenges.

Between Relationship and Travel and Adventure lies the palace of Creativity and Children. This palace asks: Can I trust my own abilities/knowledge in order to offer something to the world? It may require releasing inappropriate belief about self-worth or perceived inadequacies to muddle through this palace, but Creativity starts the process of freeing up innovative thought by recognizing and believing in one's own talents.

The Nine Palaces

1. Health	4. *Relationship*	7. Career
2. Wealth	5. Creativity and Children	8. Wisdom
3. Prosperity	6. *Travel and Adventure*	9. HOME

Relationship Palace

The Relationship Palace includes all forms of interaction, including friendships, lovers, and life partners. Determining the types of relationships one wants to engage in and the types of people that are best suited for those relationships is a big part of the relationship puzzle. The challenges of Relationship integrate those of Health, Wealth, and Prosperity, including the ability to trust, to give and receive, to refrain from judgment, and to balance the needs of multiple individuals without developing co-dependency or sacrificing self-care. The Relationship Palace is about understanding appropriate 'levels of engagement' for different relationships (i.e., work colleague vs. intimate sex partner), and maintaining healthy emotional boundaries in all types of interactions. Questions for this palace include:

- Do I share stories/information at an appropriate level for that relationship?

- Do I have the ability to form intimate friendships or relate well to others?

- Do I maintain my sense of self in relationship, or 'lose myself' in another?

- Do I consistently put other's needs in front of my own?

On a physical level, maintaining a healthy boundary and identifying appropriate interaction pertain to the *Wei*/Defensive Qi, which is ultimately related to the overall state of the *Zheng*/Upright Qi. Any general deficiencies will impact the ability of the Zheng Qi to properly function, but the Metal and Earth organs are primarily responsible for the formation and dissemination of Wei Qi. From a Six Stage perspective, it is Wei Qi circulation within the Small Intestine, Urinary Bladder, Large Intestine, and Stomach Channels that is responsible for protection from the initial states of external penetration. Symptoms of chronic allergies, frequent colds (especially post-menstrual), and chronic upper back/scapula region tension are all signs that the Wei Qi is suffering.

Deficient Wei Qi can lead to co-dependent relationship styles where other people's perceived needs or emotional states take priority over the individual's. On an emotional or spiritual level, Wei Qi Deficient individuals are often highly sensitive to others and their surrounds, and may suffer from anxiety because of the lack of boundary to protect the Heart. On the other hand, an overactive Wei Qi system could prevent proper connection with others by reducing the ability to empathize or consider another's emotions when interacting. That individual may be seen as 'cold-hearted' or have great difficulty allowing emotional intimacy to develop. The Relationship Palace emphasizes communication and connection, so it is critical that the 'sides and chambers' of the body can allow both Wei and Zheng Qi to flow through. Are there any left–right or top–bottom imbalances? Are the San Jiao and overall Qi Mechanism functioning properly? If present, these issues should be addressed in the overall treatment plan.

Wei Qi circulates in the *Cou Li* space between the skin and the muscle layers; therefore, hands-on massage modalities are the primary technique for overall health and regulation. As Wei Qi circulation relies on the spreading function of the San Jiao, special attention to the abdomen and any tension areas that may obstruct proper flow of the Wei Qi is required. Full-body integrative massage can be combined with Cupping, Deep tissue massage, Tuina, Acupuncture, or Qigong to clear channel obstructions, and Herbal Formulae are useful for any underlying deficiencies. In regards to external relationships and boundaries,[1] treatment options for the Wei Qi might include:

- Treatment Principles: Regulate and tonify the Wei Qi, San Jiao, Metal and Earth Elements (as needed); Course and regulate the Tai Yang and Yang Ming Channels.

- Acupuncture: Du 14, LI 4, 10, LU 7, GB 20, PC 6, ST 36; UB 10, 12, 13, 14, 20, 22, 23:

    - Per Trigrams (see Chapter 4): Yin Qiao Mai, Dai Mai.

- Tuina: Scrubbing, pressing, and pushing of the Yang Channels; Arm and Leg Vibrations.

- Medical Qigong: Circulating Abdominal Qi (Large Intestine only):

    - Connect with abdominal Qi at either Ren 12 or Ren 4–6

    - Slowly rotate the Qi – clockwise only – ending at the start point.

- Qigong: Abdominal Round-Rubbing.

- Essential Oils: Bergamot, Ginger, Lavender, Peppermint, Rosemary, Tea Tree.

- Gemstones: Blue Beryl/Aquamarine, Green Tourmaline/Verdilite, Rhodonite (also see Chapter 4).

Travel and Adventure

The following is an excerpt from Chapter 4, which discussed the Travel and Adventure Palace at length:

> This palace represents one's engagement with the external world, learning new ways of doing, seeing, and thinking outside of one's 'comfort zone.' The spiritual journey of gender and sex involves being open-minded, pushing against cultural and personal boundaries, and granting one's self the latitude to engage without judgment. Associated with Yang-Metal, this palace also involves release of one's attachment to the known: once we set out to travel to a new place or learn something new, there is no guarantee of returning the same person as when we left. Curiosity, adaptability, and resilience are all required for Travel and Adventure, especially when we might encounter the unexpected.

---

1   Treatment options that address damage to Wei Qi from Trauma are found in Chapter 11.

Lessons and ideas from one's original culture and any new ideology must be weighed against the knowledge of the authentic self in order to identify concepts or traditions to discard. For a DGS individual coming from conservative religion or another oppressive environment, free determination will likely be met with community disapproval, and in extreme cases a person could be banished or ostracized from their friends and family. The stories of those that lost family or community when they 'came out' are commonplace, and Travel and Adventure is not an easy palace to engage in for this very reason. Questions for this palace include:

- Am I open to learning new ways of doing things?

- Am I willing to see or hear alternative perspectives?

- Am I afraid of losing myself, my family, or my culture if I try new things?

- Am I afraid to face this journey alone, without the support of my community?

As stated, this palace relates to the Metal Element and the release of attachment. It is the Metal Element that is charged with letting go and grieving, but it is the Water Element that is responsible for facing Fear and vulnerability. Harmonizing the Lung–Kidney axis while addressing any deficiency or obstruction affecting these organs and their channels will help a person face challenges of Travel and Adventure, which is best done through Acupuncture and Qigong exercises. Treatment options include:

- Acupuncture:

  - Combinations: LU 5–KI 7, KI 27–LU 1 or 2, LU 7–KI 6 (Ren Mai, associated with deep nurturing to counter Fear)

  - Per Trigrams (see Chapter 4): Chong Mai, Yin Wei Mai

  - Body Points: LI 4, 10, 11, KI 3, 7, 10, ST 36.

- Qigong: Five Animal Frolics–Crane; Healing Sounds and Colors–Metal and Water Elements.

- Essential Oils: Cypress, Fir, Frankincense, Pine, Spruce.

- Gemstones: Blue Tourmaline, Hematite, Smoky Quartz, Stalactite/Stalagmite, Tourmalinated Quartz, Zircon (see also Chapter 4).

CLIENT EXAMPLE

A queer, polyamorous female in her early 30s presents with menstrual irregularities, poor digestion, recurring frontal headaches and sinus congestion, allergies, anxiety attacks with heart palpitations, occasional insomnia, and a history of PTSD. She had experienced all of these symptoms in high school and college, but they had disappeared with previous Acupuncture, massage, and talk therapy, which she did regularly for five years. She is seeking a new acupuncturist to assist, because she has recently moved 'back home' (she left for the 'big city' when she went to college and has lived in two other metropolitan areas since). She is of average weight, exercises regularly, has a happy relationship with a female partner, and would like to date once the new job and health issues are more settled. Her pulse is wiry, thin, and slippery; her tongue is swollen, pale, and dry, with a thin tip and peeled sides. She is initially diagnosed with Liver Blood Deficiency–Qi Stagnation, Spleen and Wei Qi Deficiency, and Heart Blood Deficiency, treated primarily with Herbal Formulae: Gui Pi Wan and Xiao Yao Wan for two months. The digestion, menstrual irregularities, and anxiety attacks improve by 60–75 percent during that time, but the allergies, sinus congestion, and headaches are only slightly improved. Her pulse is now slightly thin in the left front and middle positions, and empty in the right front position. The tongue is a better color and less dry overall. She is treated for Heart–Liver Blood Deficiency and Lung–Kidney Disharmony. Acupuncture includes HT 5, 6, PC 6, LV 3, 8, GB 21, 34, ST 36, LI 10, 11, SP 3, 6, Ren 17, LU 1, KI 3, Ren Mai (LU 7–KI 6), Chong Mai (SP 4–PC 6). Herbs include Nu Ke Ba Zhen Wan and a low dose of Ba Ji Yin Yang Wan. She wants to switch to a monthly maintenance schedule, so Pine and Spruce Essential Oils, Crane Qigong, and Smoky Quartz and Moonstone Gemstones (tumbled) are also recommended. At her next monthly appointment, she comments that the Qigong and Gemstones are her 'new best friends,' that her car smells amazing with the Essential Oil dosing, that she told her family she is polyamorous, and she has put up a new online dating profile.

SUMMARY

» Sexual attraction and desire for relationship are two distinct states that do not always overlap.

» Without Fear, Guilt, Repression, Shame, and other cultural forces that attempt to dictate 'appropriate' Desire, experimentation would not cause a person's identify to come into question, and sexuality could be a process of self-discovery.

» The Heart is the Emperor that rules the Kingdom, so the state of the Heart can assess a client's overall health. Important Heart questions include: Does this client feel loved? Is their Heart fully satisfied? Are they able to honestly communicate their needs and desires?

» The Wood Element provides the courage to act on the Hun's quest to fulfill the individual's sexual needs and fantasies. Wood pathology will likely present as the inability to express one's fantasies or to take charge in sexual relationships.

» In terms of the Fire Element, the Heart provides connection to the divine Emperor through the Shen-Spirit, allowing the ability to see the divine in others.

» The Small Intestine and Pericardium are charged with protecting the Heart. Small Intestine's discernment helps weigh variables to choose appropriate connections, but it can be overly discerning and limit possibilities, or non-discerning with a consistent history of poor relationship choices. Pericardium needs to be flexible enough to allow the Heart to 'fall in love' and develop intimacy, but strong enough to end poor relationships in a timely fashion.

» The Earth Element combines the Spleen's ability to adapt and feel secure during change, with the Stomach's ability for acceptance and evaluation. Pathology will present as an inability to accept change in one's self, including sexual exploration and identity issues related to the Middle *Dan Tian* (see Table 6.1).

» The Po of the Metal Element relates to the physical body and sensation, the skin, the opening and closing of the pores, circulation of Wei Qi, and maintaining healthy boundaries. Stagnant or 'rigid' Metal can restrict sexual exploration for self or one's partners. Metal Deficiency can allow poor boundaries and create a set-up for emotional or physical abuse.

» New Relationship Energy (NRE) is associated with an escalation of Fire, temporarily increasing the 'flexibility' of Metal.

» The Water Element combines intuition and Will from the Kidneys with the Urinary Bladder's ability to manage vulnerability and fear of the unknown. In pathology, Water can be consumed by Fear, jealousy, or suspicion, preventing intuition from properly guiding the individual toward truly satisfying intimate or sexual relationships.

» The Nine Palaces provide each individual the challenge to accept their life struggles and enact behavior reflective of self-worth, able to define their boundaries and needs without judgment or sacrifice.

» The Relationship Palace is about understanding appropriate 'levels of engagement' and maintaining healthy emotional boundaries in all types of interactions. It can be treated by regulating and tonifying the Wei Qi, San Jiao, Metal and Earth Elements, and the channels of Tai Yang and Yang Ming.

» The Travel and Adventure Palace weighs one's birth culture and traditions against new ideology and the authentic self. It involves the Metal Element's ability to let go, grieve, and release attachments, which relies on the Water Element to help face vulnerabilities and Fears. It can be treated by Harmonizing the Lung–Kidney axis to balance Metal and Water.

Chapter 9

SPECIAL TOPIC: POWER EXCHANGE

- 'Safe, Sane, and Consensual'

- Common BDSM Injuries

- Sexual Manipulation and Abuse

All relationships involve an exchange of power and control. Many relationships strive for a sense of equality, where participants feel loved and cherished, but also respected through equivalent rights, status, and opportunities for growth. In other situations, power is wielded without the goal of balance; here it is consent and personal satisfaction that distinguish between health and pathology.

Specifically, *consent is a form of permission* – verbal or otherwise – that can only be granted between mature adults that have informed knowledge of a situation and its potential consequences. As described on rekink.com, 'Consent is at the basis of any healthy power exchange, regardless of whether the exchange lasts an hour, a day, or a lifetime' (Rekink 2018). This chapter outlines two types of power relationships – consensual and non-consensual – and some of the energetic problems that arise when consent is violated.

'SAFE, SANE, AND CONSENSUAL'

The importance of consent has been primarily spearheaded by BDSM communities looking to create safe practices while protecting their members and organizations from legal repercussions. 'Safe, Sane, and Consensual' (SSC) has become widely accepted in the kink communities to describe three aspects of responsible play:

- *Safe*: Identifying and preventing any physical or mental health risks before engaging in an activity, as well as being appropriately trained and choosing the proper tools for the activity.

- *Sane*: Engaging in BDSM activities only while mentally and physically competent to do so.

- *Consensual*: Having the full consent (see above) of all parties to engage in the activity.

Although SSC is widely used, there are other mottos that attempt to communicate similar ideas. Regardless of the chosen catchphrase, the key ingredient is consent. Mistress Tokyo, a professional Dominatrix in Australia, commented in a 2018 interview that BDSM 'is the opposite of sexual misconduct. Everything – no matter how violent or torturous it may seem – is consensual and carefully negotiated before the fantasy takes place' (quoted in Fernando 2018).

Desire to engage in kinky sex play is actually incredibly normal. Some of the most common sexual fantasies noted by sex and relationship experts are BDSM activities, including bondage, Dominance-submission (D-s), and exhibitionism. Portrayal of kink in mainstream media has exploded in the past decade, but cultural prejudice continues to exist. Fortunately, the American Psychiatric Association's *Diagnostic and Statistical Manual of Mental Disorders* most recent publication, the DSM-5 published in 2013, firmly states that participating in BDSM does not require intervention, thus securing the separation of kink from mental illness.

When working with kinksters, there are a few well-established identities to be aware of. Not everyone uses this terminology to define their relationships or sex practices, but they are helpful to understand the energetics of BDSM:

- *Dominance*: The position of power or control within an activity. Individuals that identify with this role are called Dominant, Dom, Domme, or Domina. *Note: Dominatrix and pro-Dom/Domme are considered professional titles for those that provide kink play for financial gain.*

- *Submission*: The release of power or control, allowing a Dominant to hold this position within an activity. Individuals that identify with this role are called submissive or sub. *Note: There are professional submissives as well.*

- *Top, Topping*: The person that initiates or performs an activity.

- *Bottom, Bottoming*: The person that receives or responds to an activity.

- *Exhibitionist, Exhibitionism*: Gaining erotic or sexual gratification from having one's body or interaction displayed in front of others.

- *Voyeur, Voyeurism*: Gaining erotic and/or sexual gratification from witnessing other people's bodies or interactions.

These definitions are easily translated into opposing pairs: Domination versus submission, topping versus bottoming, and exhibitionism versus voyeurism. In Figure 9.1, these pairs are placed into the *Ultimate Yang* and *Ultimate Yin* positions of the Taiji.

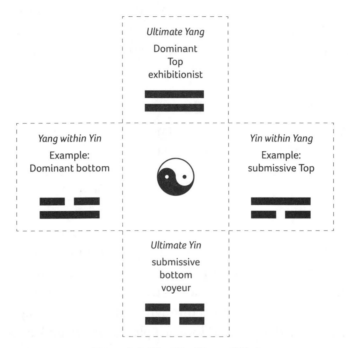

Figure 9.1: The Yin–Yang of Kink

Chapter 3 discussed Yin–Yang Theory and its basic principles. The principle of infinite divisibility states that nothing is ever *all Yin* or *all Yang*, and BDSM is no exception. For example, a Dominant can be the Top in a given activity, getting erotic pleasure from the theatricality of doing their 'scene' in a BDSM club where many people are watching; this would be in alignment with *Ultimate Yang*. However, it is also possible for Yin and Yang to blend, where the Dominant is in charge of what is happening, but is on the receiving end of the action: a Dominant bottom. There are also plenty of 'mixed' identities in BDSM that stand along the horizontal axis of *Yin within Yang* or *Yang within Yin*, including service tops, switches, and brats.

Adding BDSM into one's sex play is becoming increasingly common for a good reason: heightened arousal and orgasm response. Chapter 6 discussed the 'tides' of Yin–Yang that occur with arousal and pre-orgasm states, as well as the merging of the Taiji that can occur. BDSM play accentuates the dynamics of Yin–Yang through the designation of roles. This consensual give-and-take can strengthen the Yin–Yang tides, making a more intense sexual experience, even if sex is delayed until sometime later.

Many kinksters also describe a 'head space' that participants in any role can achieve, with or without sex. Within this head space, everything outside the immediate moment melts away: only the participants remain in an exchange of erotic energy and power dynamics. This perfectly describes the Wuji space of one-ness, where individuals have activated and aligned their Taiji poles. Consent is what allows this heightened experience to flow unencumbered, enabling the safety and capacity to experience the fullness of an erotic exchange.

COMMON BDSM INJURIES

Even when SSC is practiced, there are some common – and expected – injuries for which Chinese Medicine can provide support. This text covers the basics for three major categories of BDSM: impact play, bondage, and bleeding.

Impact Play

Impact includes any act of hitting: spanking, cropping, caning, flogging, punching, and whipping. Impact play is considered one of the most common forms of BDSM, and almost everyone has tried a mild version of it. It can range from a few small flirtatious spanks through clothing all the way to an intense flogging scene. When done *properly*, impact play is known for leaving red marks, scrapes, bruises, and welts, i.e., external Trauma to the musculoskeletal layers and the Primary Channels. In an acute case, blending traditional or modern 'Dit Da Jow' type topicals with light massage to stimulate the area can help repair the local Qi and Blood Stagnation fast, as long as there are no open wounds to consider. Zheng Gu Shui is not only ready-made and low-cost, but it is able to penetrate deeply to address both surface Trauma and any underlying stagnations. Acupuncture can be incorporated around welts or small cuts where massage and topicals are contraindicated, or used with internal herbs to promote general healing.

Channels that are getting injured time and again can translate local Qi and Blood Stagnation deeper into the channel, or start to affect the associated organ. One common problem is the development of Lower Jiao Blood Stasis through repeated bruising to the low back, hips, buttocks, and thighs. The Spleen and Liver organs may also be affected by regular bruising anywhere on the body, through the constant re-healing of flesh and broken Blood.

- Acute treatment principle: Move Qi and Blood Stagnation in the Channels.

- Topical Formulae: 'Die Da' liniments/plasters, Zheng Gu Shui, Amber Massage Salve (Springwind), Po Sum On, Arnica Gel (homeopathic).

- Massage/Tuina: Light pressure to the local area, with stronger stimulation along the channels above and below the area of injury; whole-body treatment is best to take advantage of correspondences, microsystems, and bilateral channel pathways.

- Acupuncture:

  - 'Above and Below' Technique (see Figure 5.6)

  - General healing: ST 36, SP 6, LV 8, Ren 4, 6, 12, KI 3; LV 3–PC 6, LV 3–LI 4.

- Herbal Formulae: Jin Gu Die Shang Wan, Huo Luo Xiao Ling Wan.

> Intense bruising is commonplace in BDSM, and many kinksters feel a sense of pride over the bruises/marks they obtained or inflicted. It is always wise to get client consent before helping bruises heal faster to ensure a lasting client–practitioner relationship!

Bondage

Bondage involves any act of physical restraint or restriction, either full body or partial. This can include handcuffs, clamps, corsets, waist binding, rope, suspensions, and straightjackets. Bondage is another BDSM activity that most sexually active adults have tried, but most people do not get enough training before attempting even mild bondage play. A common problem is excessive constriction affecting proper circulation; if there is lack of sensation or extensive damage to the tissue, refer out for immediate medical attention.

The other form of bondage is that of constraint, where a body part is forced into an awkward or unnatural form. This includes nipple clamps and cock-and-ball torture (CBT) devices which are not designed to be worn for extensive periods of time, and extremely tight corsets and waist-binders/trainers that can be used to forcibly alter the form of the body. The more surface devices will alter the Primary Channel pathways, coursing the channels in an unusual form. Once the constraining device is removed (or dissipates, such as with saline injections), Qi should be able to return to the normal flow. If the device was too tight or there is any local tissue damage, this would be addressed with some of the circulation techniques listed below.

In terms of clothing-style constraints, there is a clear distinction between someone wearing a well-fitted corset to 'look sexy' and a person that has been waist-training for several years. As a practitioner, one must look for signs of damage. When worn regularly, clothing constraints can thwart Qi Mechanism functioning, or even alter the structural alignment of the body and cause internal organ damage. The initial impact of tight constraint is always respiratory, affecting the Lungs and the development of Post-Natal Qi. Short-term use (i.e., for a few hours) will not have any impact that a few minutes of deep belly-breathing and stretching cannot manage. Long-term or regular alteration of diaphragmatic expansion will simultaneously deplete and obstruct both the *Zong*/Chest Qi and the Liver Qi. This will impact the overall *Zheng*/Upright Qi, affecting the erectness of physical posture and the emotional ability to 'stand up for one's self.' As organs become further displaced, proper transformation, transportation, and elimination will be affected, allowing accumulations of Dampness, Phlegm, Blood Stasis, or Blood Heat (from toxicity).

When an individual engages in constraint for the purpose of extreme physical transformation regardless of any health consequences, emotional etiology is at play. There may be an underlying deficiency needing to be 'held' (see 'Diagnosis by Kink' in this chapter), but any willingness to force one's organs into unnatural placement is undeniably related to issues of self-acceptance and Self-Loathing (see Chapter 15). In this situation, collaboration with a mental health professional to help the client consciously address these issues is required.

Techniques to heal surface bondage wounds include topical Herbs and Acupuncture; these can also be used for faster healing of conditions listed under impact play. For local tissue damage and circulation concerns, Acupuncture techniques will be channel focused, and plum blossom technique may prove useful for circulation recovery or to 'flesh out' any areas that suffer from chronic deficiency. Modified scar treatment may also be useful to target any specific area of tissue injury (see Chapter 5). Light massage, heating pads, and wraps are also useful to warm and stimulate the areas of injury and promote healing.

For deeper tissue damage, internal and topical Herbal Formulae are mandatory to repair organ damage or address Vital Substance deficiencies. The other primary treatment modality for internal damage is Qigong, both Medical and self-guided practice. Tuina, other massage work, or Cupping can assist in 'unbinding the chest' and help rectify the emotions. Below are treatment examples for two common injury sites.

Treatment Option: Wrist Binding

- Treatment Principles: Clear obstructions and harmonize channels, Move Qi and Blood.

- Acupuncture: *Select two to four points per channel based on palpation, and needle with the flow of the channel:* LU 1, 2, 5, 7, 10; PC 3, 6, 7, 8; HT 3, 5, 6, 8; LI 3, 4, 5, 6, 10, 11; SJ 3, 4, 5, 6, 10, 14; SI 3, 4, 5, 6, 8, 9, 10, 11.

- Topical Formulae: Surround the entire wrist and one to two inches above and below the area of injury with a broad stroke of Zheng Gu Shui (or other trauma liniment listed under *Impact Play*); instruct client to apply 2–3 times daily.

- Tuina: Arm vibrations, wrist and finger rotations.

- Qigong: Silk-Reeling (especially wrist and ankle joints), Combing the Hair.

Treatment Option: Breast or Nipple Constriction

- Treatment Principles: Course Liver, Stomach, and Pericardium Channels, Move Qi and Blood.

- Acupuncture:

    - Targeting and local: PC 1, Ren 17, ST 18, SP 21, KI 21–27

    - Combinations: LU 1 or 2–LV 14, ST 15–18 (or ST 12–25)

    - General: PC 6, LV 3, 8, ST 36, 40, Yintang, GB 21–24.

- Cupping: Flash on pectoralis, upper chest; flash and running on upper back, intrascapular.

- Moxibustion: Pole Moxa around bruised areas.

- Topical Formulae (on breast tissue only, not nipple): apply a one- to two-inch-wide circle surrounding the affected area; see recommendations listed above, and under *Impact Play*.

- Herbal Formulae: Xue Fu Zhu Yu Wan.

- Qigong: Rotating the Sun and Moon.

Bleeding

This category involves any act designed to penetrate the skin, either to draw blood or leave a lasting mark. It includes cutting, needle play, genital alteration (piercing, stapling, etc.), branding, and abrasion. Although techniques that are designed to interact with the blood are a 'hard no' for many people, bleeding does often – and sometimes intentionally – result from intense impact play as well.

Needle play and stapling leave small bruises and quick-healing puncture sites. Once the acute bleeding has fully stopped, topical formulae, heating pad, and massage techniques already recommended for general impact and bondage healing are likely sufficient for any residual surface injury. Deeper cuts or burns that break the skin barrier will naturally take longer to heal, so any topical or massage techniques will be contraindicated during initial healing stages. If any cuts or burns go well beyond the skin with extensive damage to the tissue or lack of sensation, immediate medical attention is required.

Primary techniques to heal surface wounds include Acupuncture and Herbal Formulae. Acupuncture is used to promote faster healing of affected channels with 'Above and Below' or scar treatment techniques (see Chapter 5). Internal Herbal Formulae should be focused on nourishing the Blood and/or healing Blood Stasis; these same formulae can also be used to promote even faster healing for Bondage and Impact injuries.

- Treatment Principles (surface wounds): Nourish Blood, Move Blood Stasis, Move Qi and Blood Stagnation in the Channels.

- Topical Herbal Formulae: see *Impact Play*.

- Internal Herbal Formulae: Jin Gu Die Shang Wan, Huo Luo Xiao Ling Wan, Tao Hong Si Wu Wan, Si Jun Zi Wan, Nu Ke Ba Zhen Wan.

- Acupuncture:

  - Channel specific: 'Above and Below' Technique

  - Scar Treatment (if needed)

  - General healing: ST 36, SP 6, LV 8, Ren 4, 6, 12, KI 3.

- Gemstones: Amethyst, Bloodstone, Carnelian, Garnet, Hematite, Lapis Lazuli, Meteorite, Rose Quartz, Tiger Eye.

A cutting fetish is very different from a desire to self-harm, even though the way they manifest is similar. People with a cutting fetish often have healthy self-confidence and happy dispositions. They cut to feel sexual pleasure and arousal, rather than to punish themselves or deal with mental illness.

– Kinkly n.d.

Cutting to Bleed

As practitioners, we must discern the line between healthy kink and the physical manifestation of emotional turmoil and self-abuse. This is especially true of cutting, where an individual may actually be attempting to self-treat. From a Chinese Medicine perspective, Bleeding releases Heat or Blood Stasis. Considering the specific areas a client chooses to cut can help pinpoint the location of Heat and/or Stasis. In either condition, the presence of emotional etiology in the form of underlying Desire, Craving, Guilt, Lying, Repression, or Secrecy is extremely likely, and these emotions must be addressed to ensure long-term resolution (see Section IV). The following are some likely diagnostic findings and treatment options based on area of injury:

Sternum-Clavicle or Intrascapular: Blood Stasis in the Chest

- Acupuncture: KI 22–27, Ren 17, PC 1, 6, HT 1, 5, 6, LU 1, 2, UB 14, 15, 17, 18, 43, 44, 46, 48.

- Herbal Formulae: Xue Fu Zhu Yu Wan, Tao Hong Si Wu Wan.

Sternum-Clavicle or Intrascapular: Heart Fire

- Acupuncture: Ren 17, PC 1, 3, 6, 8, HT 1, 3, 5, 6, 8, LU 1, 2, KI 2, LI 11, UB 14, 15, 17, 18, 43, 44, 46, 48.

- Herbal Formulae: Huang Lian Jie Du Wan, Tao Chih Wan, Suan Zao Ren Wan, Tian Wang Bu Xin Wan.

Inner Thigh: Blood Stasis in the Lower Jiao

- Acupuncture: Zigong, SP 10, LV 8 (*all directed toward the genital region*); KI 11–15, Ren 4, 6, ST 31, 32, 36, SP 6, 8, 11, 15, GB 30–34; UB 17, 26–40, 53, 54.

- Herbal Formulae: Shao Fu Zhu Yu Wan, Tong Jing Wan, Tao Hong Si Wu Wan.

Inner Thigh: Liver Fire – Blood Heat

- Acupuncture: SP 10, LV 8 (*both directed toward the genital region*); LV 2, 3, LI 11, UB 17, 18.

- Herbal Formulae: Long Dan Xie Gan Wan.

Diagnosis by Kink

Individuals that consistently yearn for specific BDSM activities may be attempting to self-treat. Blending this information with other Chinese Medicine diagnostics (tongue, pulse, etc.) could formulate a comprehensive treatment plan. When considering this, it is important to note that using kink as a diagnostic tool *does not make kink pathological*. The focus is not to 'cure' a client's kink. Instead, the focus is to address underlying pathology, treat physical damage, and prevent the development of chronic Craving.

Impact play – whether a thud or a sting, mild or extreme – is a dispersive technique. Any bruising that it results in is a clear sign that Blood is 'broken.' This could be an attempt to work on deep-seated Qi Stagnation or Blood Stasis, which may be caused by underlying scar tissue from physical Trauma, or by the emotions of Guilt and Repression (see Section IV). Cupping is the best solution for pulling any deep stagnation to the surface, where it can be more easily processed through the channels.

When someone yearns to be bound on a regular basis, they may be suffering from a Yin Deficient–Yang Rising pattern, or from extreme deficiency of the Vital Substances. Straightjackets and other physical confinements (cages, jail cells, etc.) provide resistance to one's natural physical movement. When consensual, frustrated mobility can force pent-up Yang to transform into a Yin state of softness and pliability. This helps a Yin Deficient–Yang Rising individual feel temporarily more at ease, but will not solve the underlying Yin Deficiency. Herbs, proper Diet, and mental rest should be the primary treatment modalities.

Snug-fitting constraints could indicate an extreme deficiency of Qi, Jing, Blood, or Body Fluids. The emotional and physical desperation that stems from chronic deficiency can be temporarily lessened in intensity by being bound: the same mechanism by which babies are soothed in a snug-fitting swaddle. On an emotional level, this practice could signify lack of love, or the inability to notice love (see Chapter 8). It can also be associated with depletion from chronic Craving or Fear (see Section IV). Regardless of etiology, incorporating Herbal Formulae and Diet suggestions to 'feed' the underlying deficiency is critical to alleviate the need to self-treat.

SEXUAL MANIPULATION AND ABUSE

Power exchange can get ugly fast when consent is not at the forefront. Anytime a relationship enters non-consensual power dynamics, where the recipient has not agreed to be humiliated, degraded, or used, it is abuse. To a distant observer, the power wielded in a non-consensual dynamic may appear similar to the

Yang energy of sadistic topping or Domination, but the critical difference is in lack of consent, mutual respect, and compassion. It is worthy to note that perpetrators under the scrutiny of the public eye often claim they suffer from 'sex addiction,' but, as discussed in Chapter 7, there is no scientific evidence or support from mental health providers, sex educators, or sex therapists of a sex-related addiction model. In other words, *there is no excuse for any person engaging in non-consensual power play.*

Sexual manipulation and abuse come in many forms, so this is a large subject requiring a book of its own to parse out the various and subtle effects on the Three Treasures and one's ability to engage in the Nine Palaces. The following information covers only the basic energetics and a few treatment options.

Manipulation

When sexual activity is at its best, it stimulates the *Ming Men* Fire, the Ren, Chong, and Du Vessels, and the internal flow of the Three Treasures. Orgasm brings the effulgence of the Extraordinary Vessels out into the Primary Channels, which can help rectify the entire Qi Mechanism. When the participants are emotionally and spiritually connected, the Wuji space of one-ness may be entered and a blending of souls might occur (see Chapter 6).

Sexual manipulation, on the other hand, is sexual activity at its worst. The abuser may use Shame and Guilt to curtail their partner's sexuality, with elements of Repression, Frustration, Anger, or Trauma contributing to the victim's pathology. A primary example is when sexual activity is wielded as a system of punishment and reward. This is typically a chronic situation where non-consensual denial of sex is the norm, not the exception. In the 'withholding' phase, Desire for sex is denied by the abuser, causing Heat and stagnation to build up in the suffering individual's Lower Jiao, Ren, Chong, and Du Vessels. In response, the body may break down communication between the Three Treasures in order to protect the Qi-Emotion and Shen-Spirit levels from the unrequited Heat-Stagnation that stirs the Jing-Essence in the Lower Jiao. When this combines with trauma from the ongoing emotional stress (see Chapter 11), the San Jiao and the entire Qi Mechanism will suffer.

During the 'giving' phase, the sufferer is unlikely to allow themselves to fully express their sexuality with the manipulative partner so the pent-up Heat and Stagnation will not be fully released. Instead, it will lead to a state of extreme physical and emotional stress that sexual activity cannot satisfy. The ongoing presence of Heat and Stagnation will eventually create Damp-Heat as well, with physical symptoms of enduring genital area rash, reduced ejaculate, erectile dysfunction, prostatitis, UTI-type symptoms, and various menstrual difficulties (i.e., heavy flow, early flow, severe cramping, bloating, low back pain). In certain Constitutions, the Damp-Heat formed in the Lower Jiao may transfer locally to the Large Intestine (diverticulitis, ulcerative colitis, etc.), or to the Gallbladder (cholecystitis, cholelithiasis, etc.) as the *Ming Men* Fire travels to support digestion.

Emotional impact from the Stagnation and Heat/Damp-Heat in the Lower Jiao includes the development or exacerbation of Shame, Desire, or Craving; this could manifest as Obsession or excessive masturbation, only further exacerbating the condition (see Chapter 7). When treating this condition, exercise caution with Acupuncture and Medical Qigong as the likelihood of transference is higher than usual.

- Treatment Principles: Clear Heat and Stagnation in the Lower Jiao, Rectify the Ren, Du, Chong Vessels (as appropriate); Harmonize the Three Treasures and Three *Dan Tian*.

- Acupuncture: Ren 2, 3, 4, KI 11–15, ST 25–29, LI 4, 11, LV 2, 3, 8, SP 8, 10, ST 30, UB 22, 26–35; Ear: Shenmen, Zero Point, Heart, Kidney. *Note: Do not over-treat the Extraordinary Vessels to rectify this condition – focus on local pelvic points to release Heat and Stagnation from the Lower Jiao first!*

- Herbal Formulae: Huang Lian Jie Du Wan, Long Dan Xie Gan Wan, Bi Xie Sheng Shi Wan, Zhi Bai Di Huang Wan.

- Diet: Cooling and Damp-clearing foods (peppermint tea, watermelon, cranberry juice, etc.); eliminate alcohol, caffeine, spicy foods (chili pepper, clove, etc.), high-fat and fried foods, processed sugar.

- Medical Qigong: Clearing the Lower Jiao:

  – Connect to the Lower *Dan Tian* by placing one hand under the lower abdomen or sacrum, with the opposite hand on the other side

  – Starting at or just above the skin level, slowly circle the top palm counterclockwise while rising up, drawing the Xie/Evil Qi out

  – Repeat until the sensation of excess Heat dissipates from the Lower *Dan Tian*.

- Qigong: Qi Circulation/Tai Yang Circulation (laying), Gathering the Rice.

- Lifestyle: Address relationship issues or terminate relationship; mental health counseling may be necessary to navigate issues of self-acceptance and emotional pathology.

CLIENT EXAMPLE

A heterosexual, polyamorous male in his early 50s presents with ongoing erectile dysfunction and urinary incontinence after treatment for prostate cancer almost five years prior. He has been divorced twice, and admits he is still angry about both marriages: 'With both of them, I felt tricked.' He lives alone, but is sexually involved with five separate women and has sex with each of them typically once a week. He sits a lot for his office job, and has a large lower-middle abdomen with thin arms and legs. He drinks alcohol (3+ shots of hard liquor), coffee (2–4 cups), and exercises daily (swimming and/or biking). His tongue is reddish-pink, dry, swollen on the sides, with no coat, a deep central crack (Stomach position) and dark sublingual veins. His pulse is wiry. He is treated for Damp-Heat in the Lower Jiao, Chong, Ren, Dai, and Du Mai obstructions, and disharmony of the Three Treasures. He is resistant to stopping alcohol and coffee, but can easily reduce casual sex to three to four times a week. He wants to schedule for every other week, so Herbal Formulae will be the primary treatment modality; one to three years is expected for full resolution.

Sexual Abuse

Sexual abuse, including sexual assault and rape, forces the arousal of Heat and internal flowing of Jing-Essence through unwanted sexual contact. When a victim is fully aware of what is happening, counter-flow Qi sets in at every level, causing emotional Shock as well as immediate damage to the flow of Qi, Yang, and Jing-Essence in the Lower Jiao, the Extraordinary Vessels (Chong, Du, and Ren), the Three Treasures, the Qi Mechanism, the *Dan Tian*, and the Taiji pole. Residual, chronic damage is dependent upon multiple factors, including the age and emotional maturity of the survivor, the frequency of the abuse, the specific type of abuse (i.e., oral versus anal or vaginal contact), and the victim's menstrual cycle.

Etiology starts with resistance: the victim is – *quite understandably and naturally* – trying to escape the situation itself and all associated sensations. In order to do so, the body has a few 'safety mechanisms' that can be activated, either individually or simultaneously:

- Disconnect the Three Treasures: Purposefully misalign the Jing-Essence from the Qi-Emotion and Shen-Spirit levels, helping 'protect' these aspects of the self from the impact of Trauma. Genital numbness and inability to orgasm are common chronic symptoms. One might also experience a degree of physical pleasure with future sex partners, but not be able to emotionally or spiritually connect during sex. This will lead to *Ming Men* Fire and Kidney depletion, among other problems.

- Disconnect the San Jiao: Purposefully split the Lower Jiao from the Middle Jiao, helping to 'bind' the counter-flow Qi in the Lower Jiao. Extreme Heat and Qi Stagnation in the Lower Jiao are common, with Fluid Stasis development in both the Middle and Lower Jiao areas. An East–West Axial Trauma pattern affecting the Wood–Earth–Metal dynamic is also likely (see Chapter 11).

- Disconnect the Dai Mai: Purposefully divide the body into 'top' and 'bottom' along the major horizontal axis. In this case, the development of Heat Above–Cold Below conditions are common, with Qi and Fluid Stagnation primarily focused in the Lower Jiao. Other 'horizontal conditions' may present, including jaw tension, TMJ, occipital headaches, and diaphragmatic constriction. Both North–South Axial Trauma patterns affecting the Fire–Earth–Water dynamic and East–West Axial Trauma patterns affecting the Wood–Earth–Metal dynamic are possible (see Chapter 11).

Emotions and Extraordinary Vessels

Damage from unwanted sex is never entirely physical. The emotional complications most commonly seen in survivors are a combination of Shame, Guilt, and Trauma (see Section IV). Shame and Guilt are both associated with Fluid Stasis pathology, making Blood Stasis and Phlegm common. Because the Shame or Guilt are associated with sex, Chronic Fluid Stasis will likely appear in the Lower Jiao – at least initially. Trauma can impact any part of the Qi Mechanism, leading to more system-wide complications.

Other common emotional complications of sexual abuse include Fear and Disgust. Fear will impact the Kidneys and Water Element, and could lead to physical manifestations such as incontinence (urinary or fecal), chronic UTIs, loss of libido, poor posture, bone issues, and memory gaps. Emotionally, fear may manifest as anxiety or panic attacks (Yin Water aspect), distrust or suspicion (Yang Water aspect), or both.

Disgust is a natural feeling of repulsion, similar to that which occurs with rotten food. It is rooted in the Earth Element as it reflects an inability to accept what the external world has offered. Physical manifestations of disgust include food sensitivities, allergies, bloating, and acid reflux/GERD. Disgust can also impact the Liver or Large Intestine Organs, either through redirection of the Qi Mechanism (i.e., get away from the source of disgust) or an inability to determine how to handle the situation (i.e., knowing when to let go or hold on).

In terms of physical damage to the Extraordinary Vessels, stagnation is more likely in acute cases, but mixed Excess–Deficiency concerns are prevalent among childhood survivors that were not able to fully comprehend the Trauma.

Evidence of pathology to any of the three Extraordinary Vessels may appear separate and distinct, or present concurrently. The development of certain emotions is associated with specific EV damage as well. These differences may help pinpoint where the Trauma occurred (see also Chapter 6):

Chong Mai – Blood

- Pathology: Blood Stasis, Blood Deficiency–Stasis.

- Typical Cause: Internal Trauma to the Lower Jiao, i.e., vaginal or anal penetration.

- Symptoms: Menstrual difficulties, combined with digestive symptoms, Heart pathology (anxiety, palpitations), hip and psoas muscle tension, mixed Hot–Cold syndromes, and any condition related to Liver Qi Constraint or Stagnation.

- Associated Emotions: Anxiety, Guilt, Shame, Suicidal Ideation.

- *Note: The Chong is also 'responsible for passing traumas to the next generation,' (Holman 2018, p.299) so if the client has no memories of abuse, the damage may have occurred in an ancestor's life (this is more common with maternal lineage).*

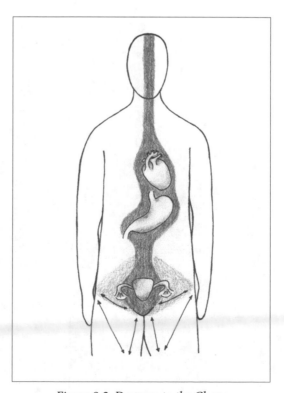

Figure 9.2: Damage to the Chong

Ren Mai – Yin

- Pathology: Yin Deficiency, usually with Dampness or Phlegm (i.e., mixed Excess–Deficiency presentation).

- Typical Cause: Trauma to the oral cavity, which will also impact Earth organs; can also be caused by forced external – clitoral or penile – abuse, especially with orgasm.

- Symptoms: Anorexia, bulimia, acid reflux/GERD, food allergies or intolerances, metabolic syndrome, tonsil stones, sinus congestion, asthma, thyroid conditions, pectoral, scalene/neck/SCM, and occipital tension areas.

- Associated Emotions: Fear, Lying, Secrecy, Shame.

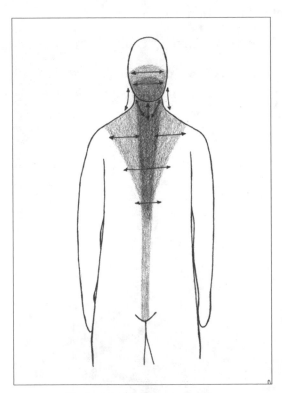

Figure 9.3: Damage to the Ren

Du Mai – Yang

- Pathology: Fire, Yang Rising, Mixed Hot–Cold.

- Typical Cause: Internal Trauma to the Lower Jiao, i.e., anal penetration. Can also be caused by vaginal penetration or forced penile orgasm.

- Symptoms: Headaches, sinus congestion, 'quick temper,' digestive complaints (chronic constipation, diarrhea, IBS, intestinal polyps, inflammatory bowel disorders), issues with the spine and postural alignment, upper back, IT band, and hamstring tension.

- Associated Emotions: Fear, Desire, Craving.

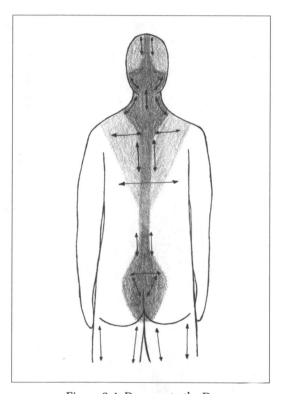

Figure 9.4: Damage to the Du

Dai Mai – Dampness

- Pathology: Dampness /Phlegm, Mixed Hot–Cold.

- Typical Cause: Any type of trauma to the Lower Jiao, especially early childhood abuse.

- Symptoms: Weight accumulation in the lower abdomen and around the waist, heaviness of the legs and abdomen, altered bowel movements, cloudy urine on occasion, delayed orgasm or erectile dysfunction, vaginal discharge/leukorrhea, menstrual cramping, discolored menses (typically brownish), heat in the face and chest with extreme cold below the navel.

- Associated Emotions: Shame, Repression, Secrecy, Self-Loathing.

- *Note: The Trauma event can be 'bound' by pathological Yin to hold it in 'latency' until the conscious mind is able to process the event.*

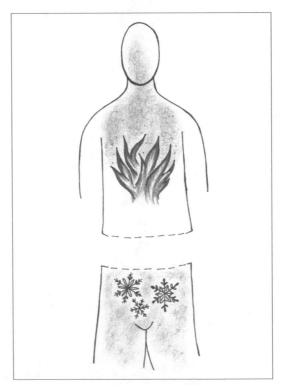

Figure 9.5: Damage to the Dai

Figures 9.2–9.5 provide a visual concept for the impact of sexual abuse on the Extraordinary Vessels. As with any Extraordinary Vessel Trauma, the physical symptoms listed above may also include localized numbness in the genital region, erectile dysfunction, and various menstrual difficulties. Menstrual symptoms can be further differentiated by specific EV based on the Blood, Yin, or Yang pathology. For example, Chong Mai Trauma might present with blood clots, extreme cramping, and amenorrhea, whereas Ren Mai Trauma might present with excessive vaginal discharge, delayed flow, and extreme bloating along the midline.

When approaching a case of sexual abuse, one must simultaneously treat the following:

- Harmonize the Three Treasures, San Jiao, Qi Mechanism, and the appropriate Extraordinary Vessels.

- Clear stagnation in the Lower Jiao.

- Resolve any Fluid Stasis conditions.

- Address impact to the Water and Earth Elements.

- Calm the Shen and treat associated emotions.

To prevent emotional overwhelm from the re-alignment of the internal structures, *always progress slowly* when treating sexual abuse. This is especially important with recent Trauma or when occluded memories are suspected. Another factor is to *not treat the EVs with Acupuncture, as they are already damaged*. Medical Qigong, Essential Oils, and Gemstones will not further damage the EVs; small press beads and gentle acupressure can also be used for short periods. Stress reduction is encouraged for all areas of life while treatment is underway, along with talk therapy or mental health counseling, regular, nutritious meals, and daily light–moderate exercise.

CLIENT EXAMPLE

A 15-year-old female is looking for help with weight loss. She also has anxiety, depression, and occasional heart palpitations and low back pain. She doesn't know when her last period was (menarche at age 12). Two months ago she was caught cutting (inner thigh), and is now seeing a psychiatrist and taking anti-depressants. She is visibly obese, especially around her hips, buttocks, lower abdomen, and thighs. Her cheeks are quite red, but her feet are ice-cold. When asked if there is a reason she cuts, she says: 'I don't even feel the pain, really.' Her flesh feels swollen and tight, except over her abdomen, where the flesh is flaccid and slightly nodular. Her tongue is swollen, tooth-marked, with hardly any coat, a dip at the rear, and pale-thick sublingual veins. Her pulse is slippery, wiry, weak, and thin. She is diagnosed with Kidney Yang Deficiency, Spleen Qi Deficiency, Blood Deficiency, and Damp-Phlegm, with an underlying disharmony of the Three Treasures, San Jiao, and Dai Mai.

To encourage underlying etiology to rise, she is prescribed a six-week course of Herbal Formulae (Liu Jun Zi Wan, Tao Hong Si Wu Wan, and Xiao Yao Wan), with tumbled Gemstones to carry (snowflake obsidian, sunstone), and 10–15 minutes of daily Qigong (Five Animal Frolics–Crane).

Note: It is likely that sexual abuse may be the root of this condition with damage to other Extraordinary Vessels combined with Shame and Secrecy. Weight loss/physical changes will likely occur only after emotional roots are exposed, so the client must be counseled to be patient. It is expected that one to three months of treatment will be required before the EV damage and primary emotional involvement can be fully diagnosed, another three to 12 months of treatment for resolution of Self-Loathing, and she will likely require maintenance treatment for another two to five years.

CLIENT EXAMPLE

A heterosexual female in her mid 20s presents with anxiety, insomnia, headaches (occipital and temporal), digestive upset (nausea, bloating, diarrhea), and menstrual difficulties (delayed, painful, with bloating and back pain). The anxiety and menstrual problems have been present since around age 14–16; her menses never regulated well after menarche. The other problems started in the past six months after a 'bad breakup.' Her tongue is normal color, dry, with thick pale sublingual veins. Her pulse is choppy-thin on the left, and wiry-slippery on the right.

The initial diagnosis is Chong Mai Disharmony and Liver Qi Stagnation, treated with Acupuncture at SP 4–LV 3–PC 6, SP 10, ST 36, LV 8, Ren 6, 12, 17, GB 20, 21, 34, Yintang, Du 24. She bursts into tears after the treatment and shares information about her ex-boyfriend's sexual abuse. Pole Moxa to KI 1, 3, and SP 6 helps her emotions to settle. She is sent home with Chamomile, Lavender, and Peppermint oils applied to PC 6, Ren 17, LV 3, and KI 27, and prescribed Tian Wang Bu Xin Wan to help her sleep. The next treatment incorporates a trauma-release protocol (KI 6–16–26) with focus on integration of Earth Element to 'accept' what has happened (Ren 11, 12, 13, ST 21, 36, 40, 44, SP 3, 6). She is asked to lightly rub SP 4 and KI 1 each night before bed. The nausea, bloating, and diarrhea stop after this treatment, and she is given Xiao Yao Wan, Nu Ke Ba Zhen Wan, and kept on a low dose of Tian Wang Bu Xin Wan for three months to address the remaining Liver Blood Deficiency–Qi Stagnation and North–South Axial Trauma pattern while encouraged to seek out counseling/talk therapy. *Note: This client will likely require maintenance treatment for one year or more, and may require further treatment when she starts dating/trusting again.*

Rough Sex

Internal Trauma can also derive from consensual, enjoyable, sexual activity. Fisting, 'cock-and-ball torture' (CBT), and other forms of 'rough' sex can cause damage to the external genital tissues, but also to the Extraordinary Vessels that run through the 'Room of Essence.' Injury to the anal region is more likely to injure the Du and Chong Mai, while injury to the vaginal/cervical region will likely impact the Ren and Chong Vessels. The Urinary Bladder, Uterus, and Large Intestine are the local organs of concern for treatment, but the Spleen and Liver also deserve attention, for their ability to make and mobilize Blood for healing, but also because of their channel pathways. *The critical difference between rough sex and sexual abuse is that there will be no evidence of San Jiao, Three Treasure, or Qi Mechanism damage, along with no evidence of emotional Shame, Guilt, Trauma, Fear, or Disgust complicating the physical concerns.*

Depending on the type and extent of damage, a blend of the various treatment principles and techniques listed throughout this chapter may prove useful. *Note: Always refer a client out for medical evaluation if tissues are visibly damaged.*

For Women

Urinary Bladder issues are quite common for women after rough sex play, and false UTI symptoms – especially distending pain – may arise in the acute stages of healing. Acupuncture and Herbal Formulae to support Kidney or Spleen energetics and overall healing are more appropriate than UTI-targeting treatments. Kegel exercises and/or Qigong to target pelvic floor muscle strengthening can assist with acute healing and help prevent future damage.

SUMMARY

» Consent is a form of permission granted only between mature adults that have informed knowledge of a situation and its potential consequences.

» 'Safe, Sane, and Consensual' (SSC) describes three aspects of responsible BDSM: identifying and preventing physical or mental health risks (including level of skill, proper equipment use, etc.), mental and physical competency of all parties, and informed consent.

» Individuals that consistently yearn for specific BDSM activities may be attempting to self-treat, *but this does not make kink pathological.*

» Impact play (spanking, cropping, caning, flogging, punching, whipping, etc.) is known for leaving red marks, scrapes, bruises, and welts. It is a dispersive technique that may help treat un-diagnosed, deep-seated Qi Stagnation or Blood Stasis. Acute treatment is focused on accelerating the natural healing process for physical Trauma; pulling out deep stagnation is a secondary priority.

» Bondage involves any act of physical restraint or restriction, either full body or partial; a common problem with lack of training is excessive constriction affecting circulation. Surface wounds and bruises are addressed with Acupuncture and topical Herbs. For deeper tissue damage, internal Herbal Formulae are mandated.

» Consistent use of snug-fitting constraints can signify extreme deficiency of Vital Substances, Yin Deficiency–Yang Rising pathology, lack of love or the ability to experience love, and/or depletion associated with Chronic Fear or Craving.

» Constraint for the purpose of extreme physical transformation, without regard to long-term health consequences, is rooted in issues of self-acceptance and Self-Loathing. Collaboration with a mental health professional is indicated.

» Bleeding releases Heat or Blood Stasis. The areas a client chooses to cut can help pinpoint the location of pathology. The presence of underlying Desire, Craving, Guilt, Lying, Repression, or Secrecy is extremely likely for those that cut to 'feel normal.'

» Anytime a relationship enters non-consensual power dynamics where there is lack of consent, mutual respect, and compassion, it is abuse.

» Perpetrators of sexual manipulation often use Shame or Guilt to curtail a partner's sexuality. The victim will likely experience Repression, Frustration, Anger, or Trauma as well.

» Emotional damage from unwanted sexual contact includes Disgust, Fear, Shame, Guilt, and Trauma.

» Sexual abuse forces the arousal of Heat and internal flowing of Jing-Essence through unwanted sexual contact, causing emotional Shock and damaging the Qi, Yang, and Jing-Essence in the Lower Jiao, the Extraordinary Vessels (Chong, Du, and Ren), the Three Treasures, the Qi Mechanism, the *Dan Tian*, and the Taiji pole.

» Etiology associated with sexual abuse history starts with the activation of 'safety mechanisms' to purposefully disconnect the Three Treasures, the San Jiao, and/or the Dai Mai from the sensations of the assault.

» Residual, chronic damage from sex abuse depends on multiple factors, including the age and emotional maturity of the survivor, the frequency of the abuse, the specific type of abuse (i.e., oral versus anal or vaginal contact), and the victim's menstrual cycle.

» When treating sexual abuse, one must simultaneously Harmonize the Three Treasures, San Jiao, Qi Mechanism, and the Extraordinary Vessels, Clear stagnation in the Lower Jiao, Resolve any Fluid Stasis, address impact to the Water and Earth Elements, Calm the Shen, and treat associated emotional states. Treatment must progress slowly, and Acupuncture to the EVs is generally contraindicated due to the damage caused by physical trauma.

» 'Rough sex' is a consensual, enjoyable, sexual activity that can cause internal Trauma. The critical difference is that there will be no evidence of San Jiao, Three Treasure, or Qi Mechanism damage, along with no evidence of emotional Shame, Guilt, Trauma, Fear, or Disgust complicating the physical concerns.

Section IV

THE EMOTIONAL LANDSCAPE

Too little light, too little water
Too many rocks, too many stones and I've had
Too little light, too little water
But I know the grace
The grace only rough things know

The way we vine,
I won't forget from where I've come

From two little lights with too little water
But I know my way, my way home
When all is done.

                       – Namoli Brennet 2017

Chapter 10

STANDING GUARD
Living in Chronic Fear

- The Illusion of Normal

- Constant Vigilance

- Stages of Concealment

The Master said: Guide them with policies and align them with punishments and the people will evade them and have no shame. Guide them with virtue and align them with li *and the people will have a sense of shame and fulfill their roles.*

– Confucius[1]

The desire to be accepted and embraced by one's community is an innate and natural human need, but 'fitting in' is always based on culture-based beliefs and traditions. For young children, adolescents, teenagers, and young adults experimenting with identity and self-expression, expectations of 'normalcy' and lack of variety in clothing, books, toys/games, advertising, and television programming can pressure them to conform their behavior and language choices to meet cultural expectations. It may even prevent them from consciously recognizing their own gender, sexuality, and relationship style preferences.

In the modern world, the need to maintain social order through strict tradition is quickly losing hold, but backlash from conservative communities can be daunting. Openly DGS individuals can easily find themselves the victim of an attack impacting their employment, housing, child custody rights, or even their physical safety. In some cultures, prejudice against DGS communities is at the

---

1   As translated from Book II of *The Analects of Confucius*, quoted in Eno 2018, p.5.

level of governmental persecution with penalties of imprisonment or execution. Even in close relationships, 'coming out' about one's gender, sexuality, or relationship choices may still result in ostracism from loved ones.

All human beings experience the innate desire for community and authentic connection with others. Although it may still be difficult to freely share one's authentic self in every social circle without repercussions, adults can typically balance their desire for acceptance with appropriate discernment of circumstances: i.e., when and where it is safe for them to be 'out.' Unfortunately, both for younger people and adults, the constant navigation of desire for acceptance and the realities of personal safety can be extremely stressful. For this reason, many DGS individuals live their lives in a state of Chronic Fear.

> *Caring what other people think of you clearly works for some people. For others, it constrains and narrows their lives. If you're surrounded by safe, conservative people – and you care what they think – you are unlikely to move beyond the safe, conservative boundaries that they place on their own lives. No matter how you feel – no matter what your desires – you will feel blind fear at the thought of doing things that upset the people around you.*
>
> – John C. Parkin 2014

THE ILLUSION OF NORMAL

Confucianism prioritizes family and social harmony through cultural traditions and community stability; this is in contradiction to the Buddhist and Daoist emphasis on individual spiritual growth. In their 2016 talk at TCM Kongress – Rothenburg, Nigel Ching commented on the Confucian concept of *Li* 禮, defining it as 'an emphasis on conforming and fitting in to commonly defined norms…[creating] an atmosphere that is inherently prohibitive of gender or sexual deviance.' This Confucian virtue is mirrored in contemporary conservative communities across the planet, a fact that DGS individuals are constantly aware of. In fact, DGS individuals are often hyper-aware of *Li*, with many perpetually performing an elaborate dance between conformity, safety, and the attempt to follow their own path.

Being able to fully express one's self without repercussions is a luxury for most people, which traces back to the concept of *Li*. It is the culture, not the individual, that dictates what 'normal' is, what it isn't, and what the repercussions are. For most people, 'normal' is a simple question of what others might *think* of you: i.e., 'Will my friends like my new haircut?' But for DGS people this question can take on a much more serious tone. Each person must balance the possibility of very real external threats to their personal safety and security against their internal desire for expression. In other words, it may not be a question of 'Is a feather boa too much for this outfit?' but instead, 'Will wearing a feather boa get me killed?'

Being 'outed' remains a tangible and very real fear in DGS communities. In response, many choose to conceal their authentic selves to better align with the *Li* of their culture:

- Bi/Pan/Omnisexuals may choose to only partner with the opposite sex/gender, concealing their real sexual identity.

- Transgender people may focus intensely on 'passing' by spending thousands of dollars on hormone therapy, cosmetics, hair removal, surgeries and implants, as well as moving to a new area and cutting off contact with pre-transition friends and communities.

- Polyamorous people may only have long-distance relationships, or may cheat to keep each relationship secret from their other partner(s).

- Kinksters and swingers may only attend private parties far from their homes, or become obsessed with pornography and rarely attend public events.

Because of the stress involved with constantly analyzing and attempting to conform to other people's rules, Liver Qi Constraint or Stagnation patterns are extremely common in modern culture; DGS individuals are not immune to this issue.

Daoism provides a way to compassionately embrace the spiritual journey our client has embarked upon, without placing blame on the *Li* of the culture or consistently labeling any individual a 'victim' in the events of their lives. As discussed in Chapter 4, the events occurring in each person's life – both good and bad – are meant to assist that individual with the curriculum of the Nine Palaces and the manifestation of Destiny. Without dismissing the very real emotional strain that an individual is experiencing, we can recognize that even this struggle is another aspect of the spiritual journey; another challenge in their life curriculum.

In terms of permanent resolution, only the client knows what the right answer is for them. Should they leave their church or workplace? Should they divorce their unsupportive partner or stop attending large family events? Should they move to a larger city or country with more 'liberal' views? It is not for the practitioner to determine the correct solution; only the client can dive in deeply to their authentic self to know what is right. Unfortunately, the *answer* may also create Fear, Worry, Anxiety or other emotional strain, as the 'right' decision may further contradict with an individual's upbringing, cultural traditions and mores.

As practitioners, we know that choosing to hide the authentic self will continue to create disease. Treatment of Chronic Fear must be focused on helping the client feel safe, so that they might realize and remember their sacred place within the *Dao* and regain the innate ability to determine and follow their own right path.

Fear and the Water Element

From Chapter 4: 'It is the strength and stability of Water and the Lower *Dan Tian* that enables an individual to ignore their Fear in order to manifest and integrate gender and sexuality through the Three Treasures.'

From Chapter 7: 'Fear is the emotion of the Water Element rooted in the *Zhi/Will* to survive of Kidney Yin–Yang in the Lower Jiao. Fear is a binding emotion that forces energy downward and inward, the exact opposite direction of the expansive and upward energy of arousal. Fear...if not properly managed can easily deplete the overall energy of the Kidneys.'

CONSTANT VIGILANCE

Already mentioned are the lack of inclusion, safety concerns, and other consequences that DGS people may face when they share themselves. Fear for one's survival is a natural consequence of living in these conditions, and a state of Chronic Fear and Kidney taxation is prevalent for this reason. For even when an individual enjoys the comfort of a community that fully embraces them, the reality of persecution in other cultures is constant.

Fear has come up a few times in this book. Chapter 4 discussed Fear as an issue of Water Element and Lower *Dan Tian* stability. Chapter 7 discussed Fear in relation to masturbation and sex practices, offering the image of a large knot in the Lower Jiao pulling Qi in and down (see Figure 7.3). When examining the symptoms and impact of Chronic Fear in this chapter, we must first examine hyperarousal, a form of vigilant awareness commonly known as the 'acute stress' or 'fight or flight' response.

In the acute hyperarousal state, adrenaline is released, the heart rate accelerates, breathing becomes shallow and more rapid, sweat may be released, and the muscles tense to prepare for movement (i.e., hit or run), all in response to a perceived threat. Under normal circumstances, this is a short-lived condition that quickly mobilizes the energy of the Heart, Kidneys, and Liver to immediately react to a unique and unfamiliar situation. Once the threat is transformed or eliminated, all systems are allowed to return to a relaxed state.

Chronic hyperarousal also mobilizes the energy of the Heart, Kidneys, and Liver, but the response is being triggered too frequently to allow these systems to return to a state of total rest. A chronic hyperarousal state is often associated with PTSD, but in this case there is no actual trauma, just the constant vigilance of *Li* creating quiet internal whispers of 'Fit in. Be small. Don't be seen.'

Expression of gender, sexuality, and relationship preferences are forms of outward movement that stem from the Qi-Emotions of the Middle *Dan Tian*. Physical and energetic movement through the world is the responsibility of the extremities: the feet and legs set the path and pace of movement, the arms and hands choose what to interact with along the way. Figure 10.1 shows the binds of cultural conformity on the individual: the legs are still free to move at their own pace, but the arms are bound at the side, restricting breath, upper body movement, and external interactions.

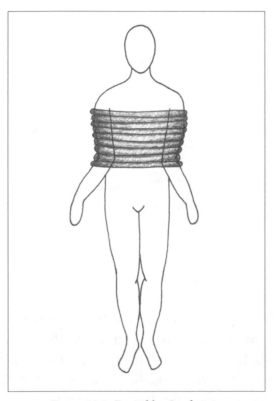

Figure 10.1: Bound by Conformity

Binding the arms clearly impacts the movement of Qi in the arm channels, but it also obstructs the expansion of the diaphragm, affecting the Liver and Lung Qi as well. In an acute situation, tense posture and shallow breathing are the likely symptoms; these can easily readjust after a few stretches, some deep breaths, or a massage. When held on to, the tension of the upper back and arms blocks Qi flow in the local channels. A moderate version of this state can be maintained long-term, but the intrascapular region, jaw, neck, and occipital muscles will likely require regular stretching and massage to avoid pain.

If untreated, the channel obstructions will lead to excess in the Gallbladder, Small Intestine, and Urinary Bladder Channels of the upper back, forcing a 'hunched' posture that encourages the anterior chest at the clavicles, upper sternum, and Lung 1–2 to 'collapse.' There may also be forearm tension or clenched fists because of the 'fight' aspect of hyperarousal. Figure 10.2 shows the long-term tension impact of Chronic Fear in the Primary Channels. Physical complaints may include anxiety, heart palpitations, and asthma, as well as stubborn tension spots (such as already listed) above the diaphragm, and brachial plexus or carpal tunnel syndrome concerns.

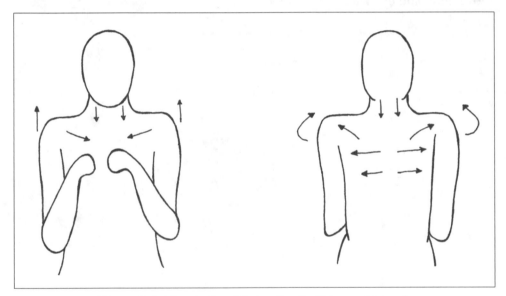

Figure 10.2: Chronic Fear Obstructing the Primary Channels

On an emotional level, outward movement is the responsibility of the Pericardium working to 'relate' to others. Chronic Fear affects this outward movement as well, adversely impacting the Pericardium's ability to relate to others, which will only emphasize the individual's unfulfilled desire for authentic connection. The ensuing combination of loneliness, lack of relationship, and grief will further impact the *Zong*/Chest Qi (Lungs, Heart, Pericardium) and Liver Qi.

If Chronic Fear continues to compound, the excess Qi used to keep the Gallbladder, Small Intestine, and Urinary Bladder Channels 'aroused' will deplete the overall Post-Natal Qi, and impact the respective Yin organs: Liver, Heart, or Kidney. Figures 10.3–10.5 show the corresponding symptom areas for the Yin organs most commonly involved in Chronic Fear. Liver involvement will likely include tension areas in the upper back and occipital region, along with anger, aggression, impulsiveness, anxiety/mania, and depression. Heart symptoms may include intrascapular, sternum, intercostal/pectoral tension areas as well as Deficiency-type insomnia, nightmares, and poor concentration or short-term memory issues. Hyperarousal itself is a sign of Kidney involvement, which will likely impact concentration and memory as well as creating tension anywhere in the back or neck, hamstrings and knee joints, incontinence, chronic UTIs, and low libido.

Specific presentation will naturally depend on the balance of Stagnation–Deficiency, what organs are impacted, and any underlying Constitutional issues. Any combination of these three organ pathologies will eventually affect the overall functioning of the Qi Mechanism and the entire Five Element generating sequence. If Fear remains constant for many years, the person will eventually experience debilitating fatigue (sometimes referred to as 'adrenal exhaustion'), or alternating periods of fatigue and hyperarousal symptoms. If an individual has not been properly evaluated, long-term Chronic Fear can easily be misinterpreted as anxiety, depression, manic-depression, or mild bipolar disorder.

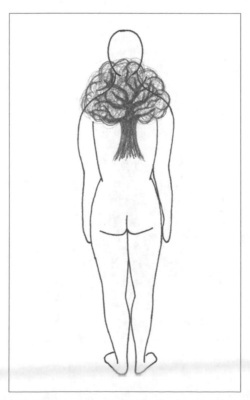

Figure 10.3: Chronic Fear Affecting the Liver

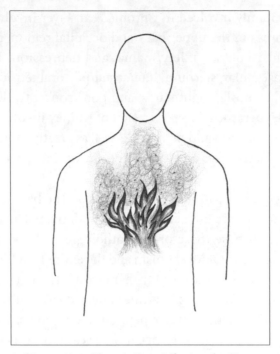

Figure 10.4: Chronic Fear Affecting the Heart

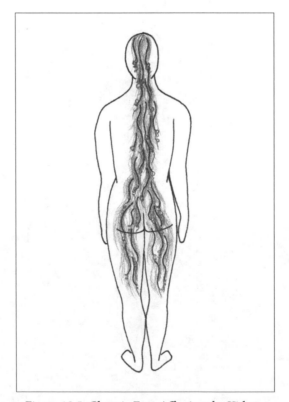

Figure 10.5: Chronic Fear Affecting the Kidneys

STAGES OF CONCEALMENT

Treatment for Chronic Fear falls under three general stages, which can overlap or alternate in presentation depending on external stress factors. As cultural rejection is part of the root etiology for Chronic Fear, it tends to present alongside Trauma, Shame, Guilt, Craving, or Self-Loathing (see Chapters 11–15). Because of this, it is critical that a gentle, compassionate, and non-judgmental approach be integrated at all levels of treatment to ensure the client feels warmly accepted in one's practice, including inter-personal interactions, treatment modality selection, and any take-home suggestions (see Chapter 2).

One general recommendation for Chronic Fear comes from Jeffrey Yuen (2017a), who says the Ren Mai can establish a 'sense of stability and support' in order to counterbalance the emotion of Fear (see Chapter 4). Harmonizing the Ren by treating any concerns found through palpation along Ren 2–22 is particularly useful to re-establish stability, with emphasis on the lower abdomen points Ren 2–8. Utilizing Ren points from all three Jiaos can also help integrate any treatment. For example, using Acupuncture, Moxa, or Essential Oils on Ren 4 or 6 (Lower Jiao) combined with Ren 10 or 12 (Middle Jiao), and Ren 17 or 22 (Upper Jiao).

Stage I: Sitting on the Sidelines

The stagnation present in this condition is primarily emotional, and therefore more an issue of Qi Constraint than Qi Stagnation. There is likely no Kidney impact at this stage, but postural issues are common due to the involvement of the diaphragm (one of the Ancestral Sinews, see Chapter 5).[2] Treatment must be adjusted to an overall gentle technique to focus on the psycho-spiritual level. Any physical complaints will resolve relatively quickly.

- Typical Presentation: Tense posture with arms tight at sides, legs crossed, or otherwise not 'taking up space.' Shallow breathing or mild asthma (especially with exercise) are likely, as is shoulder tension and tenderness at Ren 17. Emotional and spiritual complaints include loneliness, lack of authentic connection with others, sadness, worry (bound Lungs), frustration, PMS (bound Liver), and mild anxiety or an increased startle response (bound Heart/Pericardium).

---

2   The Ancestral Sinews include the following five muscle groups: sterno-cleido-mastoid, diaphragm, paravertebrals, abdominal rectus, psoas. For a more complete explanation of this system, see Franks 2016, p.389.

- Treatment Principles: Open the Chest and Harmonize the *Zong*/Chest Qi (Lungs, Heart, Pericardium), Relax the Diaphragm, Course Qi (and promote outward movement of the Qi Mechanism), Soothe the Liver.

Primary Modalities – Energetic Focus

- Acupuncture – *Note: Distal points must be used to clear stagnation away from the local area and prevent exacerbation*:

  - *Local:* SP 21, Ren 17, KI 22–27, Other sternum points, LU 1, 2, ST 12, 14–16; UB 13, 42, 14, 43, 15, 44, 16, 45, 17, 46, 18, 47, 19, 48

  - *General:* PC 6, LI 4, LV 3, GB 21, 31–34, 40, ST 36, Windows to the Sky, Du 20, 24, Yintang.

- Medical Qigong: Relax and Expand the Diaphragm:

  - Holding the ribcage on opposite sides (front–back or side–side), envision the diaphragm expanding downward as the client inhales (effective without touch as well)

  - Place hands on Lung 1/2 area, envision the expansion happening throughout the entire chest cavity.

- Essential Oils: Angelica, Frankincense, Lavender, Melissa, Rosemary, Sandalwood.

- Qigong: Five Dragons Beat the Drum; Five Animal Frolics–Crane; Butterfly; Gathering the Rice.

Secondary Modalities

- Herbal Formulae: Si Ni Wan, Xiao Yao Wan.

- Cupping: Flash Cupping on sub-clavicular pectoral region, intrascapular, and upper back/shoulders (can be combined with Gua Sha or Tuina).

- Tuina: Rhomboid and scapula release techniques; Grasp and vibrate subscapularis and Spleen 21 area; vibrate the arm channels.

- Gemstones: Blue Tourmaline, Calcite (Green Or White), Carnelian, Green Aventurine, Larimar/Pectolite, Malachite, Peridot, Quartz (Clear, Amethyst, Tangerine, White), Sapphire, Tree Agate-Jasper.

- Lifestyle: 'Doorway stretches' for the pectoral-intrascapular region; cardiovascular activity and deep-breath meditation for *Zong Qi*;

massage/bodywork combined with awareness of etiology can be an effective alternative modality or used for maintenance.

> If we consider cultural oppression as an external threat, like an external pathogen of Wind, Heat or Dampness, then the use of internal Herbal Formulae to support the Wei Qi may be appropriate. If the client suffers from seasonal allergies or other signs of environmental intolerance, consider adding a formula such as Yu Ping Feng Wan or Gui Zhi Wan to the treatment protocol.

Stage II: Tucked Away

Fear has gone beyond the emotional level and settled into the surface layers of the physical body. As the diaphragm remains constricted and Chronic Fear is rooted in external oppression, channels of the upper body are most affected, following either Six Stage Theory (Tai Yang, Yang Ming, Shao Yang) or any pre-existing vulnerability. The most prevalent symptom at this stage is upper body tension and pain that does not improve with massage or bodywork, or is only relieved for a day or two. Channel obstructions are thwarting full range of physical movement at this stage, but the client might not yet realize it. For example, a common UB channel symptom is an inability to bend down to touch the toes combined with reduced mobility of the sacro-iliac joints (but without the pain or extreme limitations of Stage III).

It is also common for people to 'catch a cold' anytime they receive bodywork as trapped Wind is forced from the stagnant channels. *Note: With Chronic Fear as a potential 'hidden pathogen,' make sure the Heart and Kidneys are strong enough to process those experiences before using Gua Sha or Cupping to pull them to the surface!*

- Typical Presentation: Chronic tension or pain (upper back, intrascapular, shoulders, neck, occipital muscles, jaw, head, forearms, hands), with headaches, migraines, TMJD, dizziness/vertigo, chronic sinus or ear congestion. There may also be low back pain, postural problems, shallow breathing, anxiety, asthma, and brachial plexus or carpal tunnel syndrome symptoms. Emotional and spiritual complaints include loneliness, grief, anger, frustration, and lack of relationship.

- Treatment Principles: Clear channel obstructions, Move Qi and Blood, Open the Chest and Harmonize the *Zong*/Chest Qi (Lungs, Heart, Pericardium), Nourish or 'enliven' the channels (especially for menstruating women), Calm the Shen (Pericardium).

Primary Modalities – External/Channel Focus

- Acupuncture: GB 2, 8, 14, 20, 21, 34, Du 14, 13, SI 3, 9–15, UB 12–60, SJ 5, 15, 17, LI 4, 7–11, 20, ST 3–8, LU 1, 2, 5, PC 6, Ren 17, Bafeng, Japanese Arm San Yang Jiao, Jianneiling; *Carpal tunnel*: threaded needle from Pericardium 6–7.

- Cupping: Stationary, flash, and running/moving on upper back, intrascapular, and chest.

- Gua Sha to clear 'diverted pathogens' obstructing the Luo Channels or *Cou Li* spaces.

- Tuina: Pecking, rolling, pressing, and pushing to clear local, stubborn stagnation; vigorous scrubbing with the palm (such as for treating EPFs) on pressure-sensitive areas to avoid the 'guard reflex'; gentle scrubbing with fingertips to 'enliven' under-nourished channels.

- Topical Formulae: Po Sum On (Warming), White Flower Oil (Cooling).

- Lifestyle: Community-building and connection are a must, including online or in-person groups; talk therapy or mental health counseling may help to address Fear from oppression head-on.

Secondary Modalities

- Essential Oils: Lavender, Mimosa, Rose, Rosemary, Vanilla, Vetiver, Ylang Ylang.

- Gemstones: Amethyst, Amazonite, Black Tourmaline, Blue Beryl/Aquamarine, Cat's Eye/Chrysoberyl, Charorite, Garnet, Obsidian (Mahogany, Rainbow), Rhodonite.

- Qigong: Silk-reeling (systemic), Pounding and Scrubbing–Yang Channels (especially upper body), Winding the Silken Thread, Combing the Hair.

Stage III: Immobilized

Fear has fully penetrated both the emotional and external Channel stages, depleting Post-Natal Qi and the Vital Substances of the Liver, Heart, and/or Kidneys. This progression always results in a combined Excess-Deficiency presentation incorporating elements of the two previous stages. Due to the binding nature of Fear, the physical pain will be consistent or constant, with pronounced limitation of movement. As Hicks, Hicks, and Mole eloquently noted:

People can become 'paralyzed' or 'freeze up' when afraid. On the inside they may be a quivering mass of Fear… On the surface, however, they may pretend that everything is all right and appear cool, calm and collected… People who 'freeze' up in the face of Fear may restrict what they do in order to compensate. Sometimes people may find it difficult to go out and are labeled 'agoraphobic.' Others may just find that they are extremely nervous when they go out and have their antennae out waiting for an 'attack' from the outside even if logically they know they are safe. (2011, pp.175–176)

At this stage, the primary treatment focus is to rectify organ and Vital Substance deficiencies. Secondary focus is to repair the overall Qi Mechanism and clear away Channel obstructions. This is typically a long-standing issue related to the life curriculum, and therefore Gemstones are strongly recommended.

- Typical Presentation: Chronic musculoskeletal tension, pain, and physical mobility/range-of-motion limitation primarily located in the upper body, arms or along Yang Channel pathways, back pain, knee or tendon instability, debilitating fatigue, sleep disturbances (insomnia, nightmares, waking early), urinary concerns (incontinence, chronic UTIs), digestive difficulties, poor concentration, low libido. Emotional and spiritual complaints include anxiety, depression, quick-temper (frustration, anger, aggression, impulsiveness), and manic-depression.

- Treatment Principles depend upon the affected Organs (see below).

- Primary Modalities – Internal/Organ focus: Acupuncture, Herbal Formulae, Medical Qigong, Gemstones, Qigong, Meditations/Affirmations/Mindful relaxation techniques.

General Treatments

The following can be used for any condition of compounded Chronic Fear impacting the Liver, Heat, and/or Kidneys:

- Gemstones: Amazonite, Blue Beryl/Aquamarine, Carnelian, Charorite, Garnet (Red, Green), Green Aventurine, Obsidian (Mahogany, Rainbow).

- Qigong: Five Healing Sounds; Five Healing Colors; Wuji Pose – standing or moving; Buddhist Greeting (seated); Qi Circulation/Tai Yang Circulation or Daoist Napping/Shao Yin Circulation (lying).

- Affirmation: 'I am safe and loved and protected by the universe' (Holman 2018, p.196).[3]

---

3   CT Holman's text provides many other affirmations that are useful for Fear and Trauma work.

Liver depleted by Chronic Fear, with Qi obstruction and Yang Rising

- Treatment Principles: Subdue Liver Yang, Clear Heat, Course Qi, Calm the Hun, Nourish Liver Blood/Yin – *see preceding categories for secondary musculoskeletal concerns.*

- Acupuncture: LV 2, 3, 8, GB 20, 21, 31–33 (by palpation), 34, 40, UB 18, 19, 47, 48, Yintang, LV 14 and LU 1 (in combination).

- Herbal Formulae: Zhen Gan Xi Feng Wan, Chai Hu Long Gu Mu Li Wan, Yi Guan Jian, Suan Zao Ren Wan, An Shen Bu Xin Wan, Shao Yao Gan Cao Wan.

- Medical Qigong:

    - Cultivate gemstone-quality blue-green light over the Liver

    - Hold Liver 3 or 8 with Pericardium 8/Lao Gong.

- Gemstones: Amazonite, Malachite, Peridot, Sapphire (Blue), Tangerine Quartz.

- Qigong: Gathering the Rice.

- Lifestyle: Yoga or deep stretching to soften and unbind the tendons.

Heart depleted by Chronic Fear, with Heat due to improper Heart–Kidney communication

- Treatment Principles: Clear Heat (Empty or Full), Calm the Shen, Nourish Heart Blood/Yin – *see preceding categories for secondary musculoskeletal concerns.*

- Acupuncture: Ren 17, HT 5–7, PC 1, 3, 6–8, KI 25–27 (sternum points), KI 6 and 16 and 26 (in combination), LU 1–2, UB 13–17, 42–46, Yintang, Du 24.

- Herbal Formulae: Tian Wang Bu Xin Wan, Suan Zao Ren Wan, An Shen Bu Xin Wan.

- Medical Qigong:

    - Cultivate gemstone-quality pink or ruby-red light over the Heart

    - Hold or circle clockwise above Pericardium 8/Lao Gong

    - Holding Ren 17 and also Ren 17–Ren 4/6.

- Gemstones: Amethyst, Sapphire (Pink/Red), Rose Quartz.

- Qigong: Butterfly, Combing the Hair.

- Lifestyle: Daily cardiovascular exercise to help 'unbind the Heart'; bitter foods (broccoli, dandelion and other greens, dark beer, dark chocolate, etc.).

Kidneys depleted by Chronic Fear: Hot, Cold, or mixed

- Cold due to improper Heart–Kidney communication or Yang Deficiency.

- Hot due to Yin Deficiency–Empty Heat or Lower Jiao stagnation.

- Treatment Principles: Tonify and Nourish Kidneys (Yin, Yang, or both), Anchor the *Ming Men*, Clear Heat (as applicable) – *see preceding categories for secondary musculoskeletal concerns*.

- Acupuncture: KI 1–3, 6, 10, Ren 3, 4, 6, UB 23, 52, Du 4 – *Moxa is applicable*.

- Herbal Formulae: Zuo Gui Wan, You Gui Wan, Er Xian Wan, Ba Ji Yin Yang Wan, Liu Wei Di Huang Wan, Zhi Bai Di Huang Wan, Da Bu Yin Wan, Jin Gui Shen Qi Wan.

- Medical Qigong:

  – Hold Kidney 1 with Pericardium 8/Lao Gong

  – Cultivate gemstone-quality indigo light while circling clockwise over the lower abdomen (especially Ren 4–6) and/or the sacrum

  – Course the leg channels (by leading energy up the Yin leg aspect, and down the Yang leg aspect).

- Gemstones: Tourmaline (Black, Blue), Quartz (Tourmalinated, Yellow).

- Lifestyle: Physical and mental rest.

CLIENT EXAMPLE

A lesbian female in her early 30s presents with carpal tunnel syndrome that developed six months ago. She also has shoulder–neck–upper back tension, mild headaches (two to three times per week), chronic sinusitis, allergies (environmental, animals), asthma (childhood onset), and menstrual irregularities (delayed, bloating, light flow, small clots, low back pain). She sits with her legs tightly crossed, leaning forward, with crossed arms and hunched shoulders.

Range of motion tests show limitations with the Lung/LI and Heart/SI Channels, and she can barely touch her knees when bending down. She winces upon palpation of Lung 1, 2, GB 20, 21, Ren 17, San Jiao 5–6, and Pericardium 1, 6, 7. Her tongue is pale, tooth-marked, swollen, with a thin yellow coat. Her pulse is present in all positions, wiry on the surface, weak underneath. She is diagnosed with channel obstructions (LI, SI, UB, GB, Lung, Heart, Pericardium), Liver Qi Stagnation, and Spleen, Heart, and Liver Blood Deficiency. She is prescribed Gui Pi Wan, Jia Wei Xiao Yao Wan, and Pe Min Kan Wan, and instructed to do daily stretching/Yoga. Weekly Acupuncture treatment alternates front and back treatment, including points such as GB 20, 21, 32, 34, LI 4, 10, 11, 20, SI 3, 9, 10, 11, 14, 15, LU 1, 2, 7, Jianneiling, ST 36; UB 13, 14, 15, 17–19, 26–37, 40, 43, 44, 46–48, 60. Essential Oils (Angelica, Chamomile, Jasmine, Pine, and Spruce) are frequently used. Her posture gradually changes over the course of 12 weeks, sitting up straighter and more relaxed. Her wrist pain, upper-body tension, and headaches are noticeably lessened in intensity and frequency, and her last menstrual cycle arrived on time, with minimal bloating and no pain for the past two cycles. At almost three months of weekly treatment she divulges the emotional abuse she suffered in her relationship with her ex-wife, which she never told her family about because of their homophobia. Treatment principles change to help boost the Wei Qi using a low dose of Yu Ping Feng Wan, and release underlying emotions of Shame, Trauma, and Guilt through Cupping and Tuina. *Note: Although the client's Chronic Fear has been lifted, she will likely remain a long-term client (one to three years) to address the other emotions present.*

SUMMARY

» Confucianism prioritizes family and social harmony through cultural traditions and community stability. These cultural expectations are called *Li*.

» Individuals experience pressure to conform their behavior and language choices to the *Li* of their culture at any age. Between lack of inclusion and perceived safety threats, these pressures may prevent people from consciously recognizing their own gender, sexuality, or relationship preferences.

» Being 'outed' remains a very real fear in DGS communities, and many choose to conceal their gender, sexuality, or relationship choices. Fear of expressing one's self in an authentic way creates Qi Constraint or Stagnation affecting the Liver and *Zong*/Chest Qi (Lungs, Heart/Pericardium).

» Chronic Fear mobilizes the energy of the Heart, Kidneys, and Liver too frequently to allow these systems to return to a state of total rest. It also tends to present alongside Trauma, Shame, Guilt, Craving, or Self-Loathing.

» The initial stage of Chronic Fear is primarily emotional, with Qi Constraint and postural issues, but minimal-to-no Kidney impact.

» In the second stage, Chronic Fear has penetrated the physical level and is obstructing energetic and physical movement in the channels. The most prevalent symptom is upper body tension and pain that does not improve with massage or bodywork, or is only relieved for a day or two.

» The third stage of Chronic Fear is always a mixed Excess–Deficiency presentation involving the emotions (1st stage), channel obstructions (2nd stage), and depletion of Qi, Vital Substances, and the Liver, Heart, and/or Kidney organs. Pain is consistent or constant, with pronounced limitation of movement.

» One Extraordinary Vessel, the Ren Mai (Ren 2–22, especially Ren 2–8) provides stability to counterbalance Fear.

» Treatment of Chronic Fear must focus on client safety and regaining the ability to determine and follow their right path. It is critical that a gentle, compassionate, and non-judgmental approach be integrated at all levels of treatment to ensure the client feels warmly accepted.

Chapter 11

DISINTEGRATION
The Impact of Emotional Trauma

- Yin Substances and the Heart

- Vertical and Horizontal Axes

- Navigating the External World

Emotional or psychological Trauma is the result of witnessing or experiencing an extremely upsetting event, where one's ability to integrate the various emotions involved becomes compromised. Emotional trauma is a large subject that deserves a book of its own, but some of the basics are covered here under three distinct types: direct, indirect, and complex.

Direct exposure includes a specific 'triggering' event that is experienced or witnessed first-hand (i.e., physical or sexual abuse, violence, persecution, rejection, etc.). Clients are typically able to self-report a direct trauma, and may already have a diagnosis of PTS/PTSD. Those who are subject to indirect or complex Trauma may have no specific incident to report, and likely have no knowledge that they are suffering from Trauma. Indirect exposure includes learning about events second-hand, through narrative accounts, media reports, and other external influences. Complex Trauma is based on cumulative exposure over a period of time, such as with ongoing verbal abuse, Chronic Fear, or multiple indirect exposures. As Brené Brown notes, both indirect and complex Trauma have become unfortunately commonplace:

> From 9/11, multiple wars, and the recession, to catastrophic natural disasters and the increase in random violence and school shootings, we've survived and are surviving events that have torn at our sense of safety with such force that we've experienced them as trauma even if we weren't directly involved. (2012a, p.27)

Regardless of type, the first step in treatment is to identify it. One method to gather information is through health history intake forms. This can be as simple as 'list any surgeries, major accidents, or other traumatic incidents (abuse, etc.) that may have impacted your overall health.' Compassionate and uninterrupted listening to a client's verbal description of any event is necessary to establish trust, and a sincere, forward-looking response can demonstrate hope: 'I am so sorry this happened and would be happy to help lessen the burden for you.'

Complicating a complete diagnosis will be clients that do not accurately report emotions, or who mislabel trauma-level stress as anxiety or depression, which is incredibly common. DGS individuals have often spent extensive periods of time hiding their authentic selves, which can distort a client's perspective regarding 'normal' emotions or events. In such situations, observational diagnosis holds more importance:

- Can the client breathe slowly, relaxedly, and fully into their abdomen?

- Can the client allow their body to be moved – without providing physical assistance?

- Can the client close their eyes, stop speaking, and truly rest during a treatment?

If the answer to these questions is no, and this persists beyond the trust-building of the first two or three visits, it is reasonable to conclude that the client is suffering from emotional Trauma. Fortunately, confirmation via tongue, pulse, and pattern diagnosis is relatively easy, as extreme emotional stress – even if short-lived – will always affect the Yin Substances and the Heart. As Giovanni Maciocia described, 'All emotions…affect the Heart indirectly because the Heart houses the Mind. It alone, being responsible for consciousness and cognition, can recognize and feel the effect of emotional tension' (2005, p.246).

Both indirect and complex exposure Trauma consistently impact Heart-Blood, as it is Blood that assists the Heart in processing emotional experience into memories. If the event was mild or short-lived, an acute and easily resolved Heart-Blood pattern may be the only pathology that ever develops. DGS individuals, however, face regular traumatic exposure in their daily lives through the ever-present threat of physical violence, or the Chronic Fear of being 'outed' without adequate legal protection. In addition to this, tragic events such as the 2016 Orlando, Florida, nightclub massacre, the state-sponsored Chechnyan 'purge' of 2017, or the 2018 interment of Matthew Shepard in Washington, DC, serve as reminders of compromised safety. This combination of enduring indirect and complex exposure Trauma will always engender deeper pathology.

When left untreated, constant re-triggering of Trauma can actually 'break' the axes of internal organ communication and alter overall Qi Mechanism functioning. Depending on the client's age or level of emotional maturity, the San Jiao and the Wei Qi may also be affected, impacting a person's psychological development and their ability to properly interact with others. Those subject to direct Trauma can show immediate impact at this profound level, especially when the event(s) occurred in early childhood.

Notes on Trauma Treatment

Each client must be in an emotionally safe and supportive environment – including intimate relationship(s), home, work, social and spiritual connections – *prior to starting* Trauma resolution work. Clients may experience post-treatment emotional upheaval anytime during the Primary Channels' 24–48 hour Qi cycle as trauma is released. Encouraging a client to *allow* this release is a critical component to processing the event(s) without inducing more fear and resistance.

YIN SUBSTANCES AND THE HEART

The Heart 'Governs the Blood,' making it responsible for Blood's production and circulation. When mild emotional stress becomes chronic, these Heart functions will suffer. In short-term cases (one to six months) the quality of Blood is depleted by the over-processing of emotional strain. This will most likely present as Heart Blood Deficiency, an extremely common pattern associated with elevated stress and anxiety. Concurrent Spleen Qi Deficiency often goes hand in hand with Heart Blood Deficiency as the Spleen attempts to rectify the Blood by overproducing Gu Qi. The typical symptoms that present are a perfect depiction of acute stress affecting the Shen-Spirit: increased worry or anxiety, inability to fall asleep easily and/or restless sleep, being easily startled, and poor concentration, with a pale-dry, possibly thin tongue, and a thin, weak pulse. As the Heart has a direct link to the Uterus through the *Bao Mai,* women may also experience lighter menstrual flow or early menses. Intense sweet cravings are also possible as this flavor tonifies the Spleen and is found in many Blood-nourishing foods, such as meats, dates, and cherries. Figure 11.1 shows the organs (Heart, Kidneys, and Pancreas/Spleen) involved in Heart Blood Deficiency, the most common pattern caused by the emotional stress of indirect Trauma.

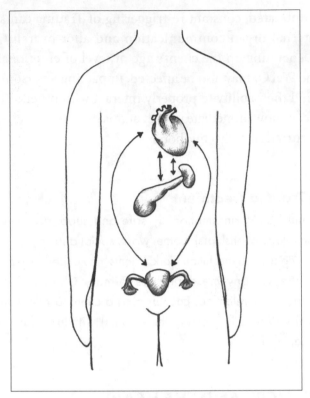

Figure 11.1: Indirect Trauma – Heart Blood Deficiency Impact

Although the quality of the Blood may be affected, increased Blood circulation can usually manage the ebb and flow of indirect Trauma. Complex emotional Trauma, however, involves regularly occurring emotional stress over the course of many months, or even years. This is more likely to present as Blood Stasis because the Heart's relentless attempts to process intense emotions energetically 'churns' the Blood. As Qi is the 'Commander of Blood,' the extra demand on Qi to keep Blood flowing and prevent Stasis will likely create Qi Stagnation and/or Deficiency as well. Body Fluids may also be used to 'thin' the Blood to prevent stasis, so these may also be depleted to keep Blood flowing properly. Heart Blood Stasis can therefore appear concurrently with Heart Blood Deficiency, Heart Yin Deficiency, Qi Stagnation (Liver, Lung, or *Zong*/Chest), and Phlegm conditions.

Symptoms will remain Heart and Uterus focused, but as Blood Stasis is involved, pain will present. Whereas Blood Stasis in the Uterus will clearly present with menstrual cramping and clotted menstrual flow, Blood Stasis around the Heart is more likely to present as chronic upper back, intrascapular, chest, pectoralis, intercostal, or sternal attachment tension that does not improve with massage. There may also be heart palpitations or extreme tenderness at Ren 17. Cupping on the upper back and intrascapular region will likely confirm the diagnosis with the presence of dark, purplish *Sha* that appears quickly and leaves bruises.

Blood and Yin Deficiency issues will also present in the Heart and Uterus; the symptoms discussed earlier for Blood Deficiency alone will worsen and include dryness of the mouth, tongue, or vagina. Any concurrent Phlegm may 'Mist the Mind,' obstructing clarity of thought. This lack of clarity may make the client emotionally overwhelmed by situations that any other person would easily dismiss, creating an even larger burden of emotional Trauma for the Heart to process.

Figure 11.2 shows the psychological 'churning' of emotions and Yin Substances that originate from the Heart. The most common patterns that result are Heart Blood Stasis, *Zong*/Chest Qi Stagnation, and Phlegm Misting the Mind, along with issues related to physical pain (i.e., channel obstructions, etc.). Clearly these patterns are more likely to show up as Heart/Pericardium Organ problems, but as the entire Kingdom serves to protect the Emperor, there can always be concurrent Fluid damage elsewhere.

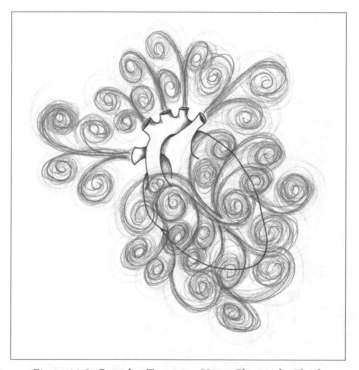

Figure 11.2: Complex Trauma – Heart Churns the Fluids

Treatment Options: Heart Blood Deficiency

Physical substances are required to nourish Blood adequately, so Herbal Formulae and Diet are the primary treatment modalities, with either meditation or mental rest to ensure the emotions have 'quiet time' to reset. Acupuncture and Essential

Oils are good secondary approaches. This pattern can resolve in two to 12 weeks if the source of extreme stress is properly managed along with treatment.

- Typical Presentation: Chronic Worry/Anxiety, inability to fall asleep easily and/or restless sleep, being easily startled, poor concentration, sweet cravings, menstrual irregularities (light flow, early menses). Pulse: tight, thin, choppy, or weak. Tongue: thin, dry and/or fine red dots at the tip.

- Treatment Principles: Nourish Blood and Heart; Calm the Shen.

Primary Modalities

- Herbal Formulae: Si Wu Wan, Nu Ke Ba Zhen Wan, Gui Pi Wan.

- Diet: Blood-nourishing foods (meats/high protein intake, soups, whole grains, etc.); bitter foods (broccoli, dandelion and other greens, dark beer, dark chocolate, etc.).

- Lifestyle: Meditation or mental rest; short, daily exercise in nature.

Secondary Modalities

- Acupuncture: ST 36, SP 6, HT 6, 7, PC 6, LV 8, Yintang, Du 20, Ren 6, 12, 14, 17, UB 13, 14, 17, 18, 43, 44.

- Essential Oils: Angelica, Chamomile, Lavender.

- Gemstones: Amethyst, Bloodstone, Garnet, Hematite, Rose Quartz.

- Qigong: Five Animal Frolics–Crane.

CT Holman recommends points along the Ren vessel, especially Ren 4, 6, 9, and Ren 11–13, for anytime 'Emotional trauma unsettles the yin and blood' (2018, p.89).

Treatment Options: Fluid Stasis – Blood and Phlegm

Fluid Stasis issues make complex trauma more difficult to treat than indirect. Herbal Formulae, Acupuncture, and any 'vibrational' techniques that help break the stasis will be the primary treatment modalities. Cardiovascular exercise is another critical component to support quick resolution (estimation: one to six months).

- Typical Presentation: Chronic pain and tension not improving with massage (upper back, intrascapular, chest, pectoralis, intercostal, sternal attachment, etc.), heart palpitations, sternal tenderness (Ren 17 area), menstrual irregularities (cramping, clots, dark-thick flow), confusion or emotional overwhelm. Pulse: wiry, slippery, choppy. Tongue: purple tone, dark or distended sublingual veins, thick coat (may only be present at rear).

- Treatment Principles – *chosen from the following as applicable*: Move Blood and Clear Stasis; Clear Phlegm and Open the Orifices; Regulate *Zong*/Chest Qi and Open the Chest; Nourish Fluids; Calm the Shen.

Primary Modalities

- Herbal Formulae: Xue Fu Zhu Yu Wan, Tao Hong Si Wu Wan, Dan Shen Yin Wan, Tian Wang Bu Xin Wan, An Shen Ding Zhi Wan, Bu Nao Wan, Yan Hu Suo Zhi Tong Wan.

- Acupuncture: HT 1, 3, 5, 6, Ren 17, PC 1, 5, 6, SP 6, 9, 10, 21, ST 36, 40, GB 34, 40, LI 4, Chong Mai (LV 3–SP 4–PC 6), Windows of the Sky.

- Tuina: Arm and leg channel vibrations or shaking; vibration over any pain areas.

Secondary Modalities

- Cupping: Flash Cupping to break stasis; running Cupping to dredge stasis to the surface.

- Qigong:

  - General: Five Animal Frolics–Crane

  - To increase cardiovascular activity: Butterfly, Gathering the Rice

  - To disperse stagnations: Golden Rooster Shakes his Feathers; Sheng Zhen Qigong: Releasing the Heart/Mohammed Standing – Pure Heart Descends.

- Gemstones: Amethyst, Amber, Garnet, Lapis Lazuli, Meteorite, Ruby, Sapphire.

- Lifestyle: Cardiovascular activity (biking, walking, light running, Qigong, etc.) and any form of 'vibration'/'shaking' therapy (dance, chanting, Shamanic drumming, etc.).

CLIENT EXAMPLE

A mid 20s female presents with constant anxiety, difficulty concentrating, and difficulty sleeping (hard to fall asleep, vivid dreams). The main source of her anxiety is from graduate school tests and papers; she is in her second semester, hates taking tests, and has never been out of school. Her other concerns are excess weight (about 30 pounds), sugar cravings (donuts, candy, chocolate, etc.), and shoulder–neck–jaw tension. Her menstrual flow is typically light for one to two days, with dark blood and a few small clots; she also experiences bloating at ovulation. Her pulse is wiry-slippery in the right middle and front positions, and thin in the left middle and front positions. Her tongue is pale, swollen, tooth-marked, with reddish tip, peeled sides, a thin coat at the rear only, and thick-pale sublingual veins. She is diagnosed with Heart Blood Deficiency–Empty Heat, Liver Blood Deficiency–Qi Stagnation, Blood Stasis, and Spleen Qi Deficiency–Dampness due to indirect and complex emotional Trauma. She is initially treated with Acupuncture (points include SP 6, 9, 10, LV 3, 8, PC 6, Ren 6, 12, 17, HT 5, 6, 7, GB 21, 34, Taiyang, Yintang), Herbal Formulae (Nu Ke Ba Zhen Wan, Xiao Yao Wan, and An Shen Bu Xin Wan), and she is also instructed to eat Blood-nourishing foods for meals and frequent snacks. She is diligent with herbs and diet and notices a 50 percent reduction in anxiety, insomnia, and sugar cravings within two weeks of treatment. After one month of treatment her menstrual cycle is much heavier, with larger clots and increased cramps, and a new pre-menstrual headache. She is given Yan Hu Suo Zhi Tong Wan to maintain at a low dose until the next cycle. Her next menstrual cycle is greatly improved with no headache, hardly any cramps and only a few small clots, but the dark color remains. She only gets anxiety, insomnia, and sugar cravings at the end of her menses now, and her tension is only apparent while studying and taking tests. As she is still in school, she is put on a maintenance dose of all formulas to continue for three to six months, with treatment recommended every two to four weeks for prevention and monitoring. After another month of treatment she confides that she is openly bisexual to her friends, but has never come out to her family for fear of ostracism. She is given Bloodstone, Tiger Eye, and Hematite to place together on her bedside table overnight, with instructions to carry one of them each day. During her next treatment she says, 'I wonder if I would still be in school if I wasn't trying to please my parents all the time.' Rose Quartz is added to her gemstone options. Before her next visit, she joins a Yoga class and has found a classmate to take 15–30-minute walks with between classes a few days each week. *Note: This client's pathology shows elements of cultural conformity and Chronic Fear, but clearly exhibits the Blood and Fluid pathologies of Trauma without the channel stagnations, Kidney depletion, or 'living small' that are common in chronic fear. Her remaining symptoms will likely disappear once she graduates and stays away from the ongoing source of emotional stress. Resolving the issue of sexuality disclosure ('coming out' or not) to her family will ensure full pattern resolution and the ability to pursue her right path.*

THE VERTICAL AND HORIZONTAL AXES

Whenever there is a single and extreme incident of direct emotional Trauma to the system, or even a small event occurring on top of years of complex Trauma, the Yin Substances will not be strong enough to buffer the impact of the event. This is when damage to the energetic alignment of the internal organs and the Qi Mechanism will occur. Frequently seen is the type of client that has been managing indirect or complex emotional Trauma for some time, with both deficiencies and stagnations leaving them fewer reserves and less emotional flexibility. When a new and particularly stressful event occurs, there can be an immediate axial 'break.' Because this occurred well after the psychological fabric of the individual was fully developed, proper and immediate treatment of this single event will promote quick and full resolution of any acute symptoms (usually within two to four treatments). Long-term maintenance (one to 12 months, depending on the chronicity of symptoms) can heal the underlying Fluid concerns and prevent the impact from any future minor events.

Organ alignment is more easily damaged by traumatic events that occur in childhood or adolescence. The first two 'Cycles of Seven and Eight' are when psychological development is still fragile and easily disrupted, so this is a particularly vulnerable time. For young DGS children already under heightened stress from constantly navigating terrain that does not fully embrace them, even a small Trauma – one which may seem trivial to an adult mind – can be all it takes to damage an axis.

Adults that have experienced emotional Trauma are typically able to report the incident on their health history, or may say something like, 'I have never been the same since "this" happened.' If a person has taken advantage of mindfulness training or mental health treatment (Yoga, talk therapy, etc.), they may even be able to indicate physical symptoms that are linked to their Trauma history. Emotional Trauma from early childhood however, may not be recognized by an adult client. This can be diagnosed by mindful listening and careful observation as the client shares their early life experiences, paying close attention to changes in breath, pulse, and speech that may indicate unprocessed distress. For example, a rapid or irregular pace can show up in the breath, pulse, or the pattern of speech. The breath may become very shallow, or even disappear for periods of time. They may suddenly have an inability to find the right words or become 'tongue-tied.' They may consistently close their eyes or look away when talking about a particular subject. All of these indicate difficulty in emotional processing.

Regardless of the age of the client, there are two major types of misalignment which occur along the Yin–Yang poles of the Taiji. This is shown in Figure 11.3, where the Elements and internal organs are arranged in polar pairs: these are the North–South and East–West axes.

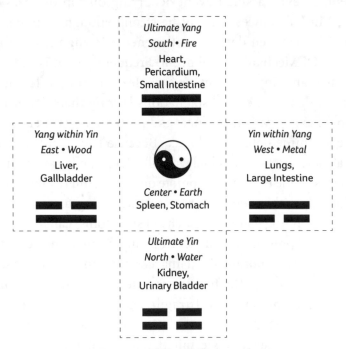

Figure 11.3: Axial Alignment

It is important to note that Earth sits directly at the center of the Taiji, reflecting one's ability to remain calm and stable in the midst of change. Due to this central position, the Earth organs are involved in any disruption of either axis. The Stomach and Spleen are also responsible for 'accepting' one's life experiences, the first to decide what experiences are 'clear' or 'turbid' (just as with food and drink). It is for these reasons that digestive symptoms are likely to appear in any case of axial disruption. Figure 11.4 shows the Earth organ process of emotional acceptance, sending 'clear' emotions and experiences we are ready to feel up to the Heart and chest, and pushing the 'turbid' that we are not yet ready to face down to the Small Intestine for storage in the abdominal cavity.

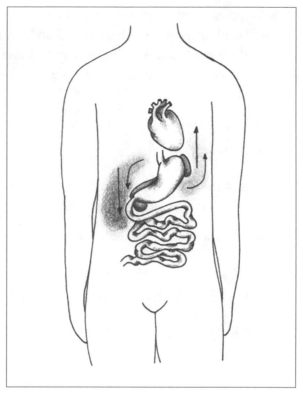

Figure 11.4: Earth at the Center

Table 11.1: Basic Axial Pathology

Axis	Elements	Yin Organs	Yang Organs	Emotions	Likely event	Possible symptoms
North South	Fire Earth Water	Heart Spleen Kidney	Small Intestine Stomach Bladder	*Anxiety* Worry Fear	Young child Safety threat Sexual Abuse	Nightmares Bedwetting Constipation Sexual shyness/lack of libido
East West	Wood Earth Metal	Liver Spleen Lungs	Gallbladder Stomach Large Intestine	*Anger* Worry Sadness	Teen/Young Adult Abusive/ restrictive environment	Distant/ Unresponsive Self-abuse (cutting, smoking, etc.) IBS/diarrhea or constipation

Which axis has been damaged and where that break occurred are the most important things to identify when approaching this depth of emotional Trauma. Table 11.1 shows the basics of North–South and East–West Axial pathology, including likely examples of triggering event(s). This table is a mere sampling, and *is not meant to fully represent all possible events and symptoms associated with Axial Trauma patterns*. Fortunately, the 'dis-harmonic' combinations created by axial damage are some of the most common patterns in Chinese Medicine, and traditional Zang Fu diagnosis may pinpoint areas where emotional Trauma has settled in.

North–South Axis Patterns

- Spleen Qi and Heart Blood Deficiency – *a more enduring version than that caused by indirect Trauma, usually in combination with another pattern.*

- Spleen and Kidney Yang Deficiency with Dampness.

- Heart–Kidney Disharmony.

- Heart, Spleen, and Kidney Yang Deficiency.

- Heart and Kidney Yin Deficiency with Empty-Heat and Dampness/Phlegm.

East–West Axis Patterns

- Lung and Spleen Qi Deficiency with Dampness.

- Liver and Lung Qi Stagnation with Dampness and/or Spleen Qi Deficiency.

- Liver Qi Stagnation and Spleen Qi Deficiency with Dampness/Phlegm.

- Damp-Heat in the Large Intestine with Spleen Qi Deficiency.

These patterns will be mixed with others that are related to the specifics of the client's emotional stress history (i.e., Fear with Kidney Depletion, Secrecy with Binding Depression of Qi, etc.).

Both North–South and East–West Axial disruptions can, of course, co-exist – a complication commonly brought on by multiple emotional traumas, usually in both childhood and adulthood. This is extremely common in DGS individuals who spend a childhood in fearful isolation and an adulthood fighting for civil rights. The overall Qi Mechanism can be righted by proper treatment of the affected axis, its associated organs/channels, Fluid concerns, and any underlying emotions, but if the patterns were established in childhood or have been ongoing for some time, the San Jiao and Wei Qi may require special attention (see below).

When these patterns have been present for some time, full resolution may take 6 to 18 months or more. There are too many axial patterns to address each one individually here, but some general options are:

- Treatment Principles: Rectify Fluid Deficiencies and Stagnations, Harmonize the affected Axis, Rectify the Qi Mechanism, Calm the Shen-Spirit.

- Acupuncture – general suggestions:

  - North–South – *use vertical combinations across all three Jiaos*: Ren 4 or 6 and 12 and 17 or 22; KI 6 and 16 and 26; KI 1 and Ren 8 (Moxa) and Du 20; Ankle–Navel–Wrist combinations such as KI 3 with Four Doors (Ren 12, ST 25, Ren 4 or 6) and PC 6

  - East–West – *use horizontal and centralized combinations, especially in the Middle Jiao*: LV 13 and Ren 12; Four Doors (Ren 12, ST 25, Ren 4 or 6); Four Flowers (Ren 13, 12, 11, ST 21)

  - Ren Mai to counteract Fear, and nourish or stabilize the resources of Yin and Blood

  - Chong Mai to 'reset the blueprint, re-enliven the spirit and one's nature, and align it back with one's curriculum' and to 'bring us back in touch with intuition, trust, faith, and an overall sense of comfort' (Rosen 2018, p.349).

- Gemstones: Apophyllite, Calcite (Orange/Yellow), Carnelian, Coral, Lepidolite, Peridot, Rhodonite, Sugilite, Tangerine Quartz.

- Qigong – *whole body integration:* Gathering the Rice; Taiyang/Qi Circulation, Daoist Napping (laying postures); Hun Yuan Gong–Grinding the Corn; Qi Pouring/Pouring Qi.

- Lifestyle: Talk therapy or mental health counseling; friendship/ community-building to transform isolation (online, local, etc.); mental rest, cardiovascular exercise, and 'vibration' therapy (as mentioned above).

- *Medical Qigong, Essential Oils, and Herbal Formulae are determined by the appropriate pattern.*

CLIENT EXAMPLE

A gay, polyamorous male in his early 50s presents with acute insomnia, anxiety, and indigestion (bloating, easily full, no appetite) since an unexpected diagnosis of HIV+ ten days prior. He is in otherwise good health with no major concerns, exercises regularly, and does not know how he contracted HIV. He has disclosed the diagnosis to his two partners (a closed triad; both are HIV-) and a few close friends, but not yet to his adult children or other family. His tongue is dry at the front half with a moderately thick white coat at the rear. His pulse is vibrating in the middle and front positions on both sides, and weak-deep in both rear positions. He is diagnosed with North–South Axial damage (Heart–Kidney Disharmony, Damp Obstruction in the Middle Jiao). He is treated with Acupuncture (Yintang, Du 20, 24, Sishencong, KI 6, 16, 26, Ren 4, 6, 11, 12, 13, ST 21, 25, 36), Herbal Formulae (Tian Wang Bu Xin Wan), Essential Oils (Angelica, Chamomile, Frankincense, Lavender, Sandalwood, Vanilla), and given temporary Diet recommendations (snacks instead of meals, reduce stress while eating, etc.). He is treated twice a week for two weeks. Digestion and insomnia are reduced after the first treatment, and resolved after the second. Herbs are switched to Gui Pi Wan for the second week. The anxiety is greatly reduced by the end of the two weeks, and he is able to tell his family. Treatment focus switches to nourishing Yin and regulating the Dai Mai to help induce latency, and he returns for four more weekly sessions to accept and integrate his new life.

CLIENT EXAMPLE

A gay male in his mid 40s presents with headaches, chronic shoulder–neck–intrascapular tension, daily digestive upsets (bloating after meals, foul-smelling diarrhea), fatigue, and a desire to quit smoking (currently one pack per day). He is overall thin, his complexion is reddish, skin is warm to the touch, and he has a few extra pounds in his middle and lower abdomen. He is extremely sarcastic in conversation. His diet 'isn't great' and he tends to binge drink (more than four mixed drinks per night) on the weekends to manage work stress. His pulse is wiry, rapid, and slippery overall. His tongue is reddish overall with large red dots on the sides and rear, a thin brown-yellow-greasy coat, and swollen-curled sides ('taco' shape). He is diagnosed with an East–West Axial obstruction (Liver Qi Stagnation-Heat, Spleen Qi Deficiency, and Damp-Heat in the Large Intestine). Weekly Acupuncture sessions (alternating front-and-back treatments including: LI 4, 10, 11, LV 2, 3, 5, 13, GB 20, 21, 34, 40, 43, Four Doors (Ren 4 or 6, 12, Stomach 25), Four Flowers (Ren 13, 12, 11, ST 21), ST 36, SP 6, Ren Mai (LU 7–KI 6), Yintang, UB 14, 15, 18, 19, 20, 21, 22, 23, 25, 27, 28, 43, 44, 46, 47, 48, 51, 52, and Herbal Formulae (including Long Dan Xie Gan Wan, Chai Hu Long Gu Mu Li Wan, Huang Lian Jie Du Wan, Mu Xiang Shun Qi Wan) are the primary treatment modalities, with both flash and running Cupping to clear channel obstructions in the upper back and neck. After the first treatment he notices a substantial difference in digestive distress, tension, and fatigue. Energy improves over the next four weeks of treatment, and he reports clothes fit better, less overall stress, fewer cigarettes each day, and fewer drinks on the weekend. After three months of consistent, slow symptom reduction, he divulges that he has been extremely lonely since his former partner died of cancer five years prior, and that watching his partner die was exhausting and painful: 'Life has just never been the same since then.' After a lengthy conversation about mindfulness and self-care, he commits to reducing smoking to less than half a pack daily and only two drinks per night, as well as figuring out how to cultivate contentment and joy in his life. He continues weekly treatment for six more months, during which time he quits his job, reduces smoking to two cigarettes per day, takes dance classes, and starts dating again. *Note: Although not divulged, it was assumed from the start that this client had emotional Trauma due to the combination of patterns and regular use of 'numbing' behaviors (alcohol, cigarettes, poor diet choices).*

NAVIGATING THE EXTERNAL WORLD

Axial breaks in either direction will clearly impact the Qi Mechanism, which affects the overall functioning of the San Jiao. When the San Jiao is compromised it becomes difficult to fully integrate new thoughts and emotions; in terms of an individual's psychological growth and development, this translates into *an inability to evaluate and learn from new experiences.* As the San Jiao is intimately related to the 'spreading' of Wei Qi throughout the body, San Jiao damage impacts the ability to defend the system from external insult, making a person even more vulnerable to emotional Trauma.

Together, the San Jiao and the Wei Qi support the ability to relate with others and to properly function in the world. If left untreated, long-term impact to these systems can have lasting repercussions on an individual's personality and the ability to manifest their Destiny. There are two ways the San Jiao can be impacted through a traumatic axial break: deficiency with accumulation, and stagnation with inflammation.

Deficiency and Accumulation in the San Jiao

A North–South Axis disruption makes the San Jiao overwork to ascend and descend Fluids between the three body cavities. This causes the San Jiao to draw more heavily on the *Yuan*/Source Qi, which will impact both the Kidneys and the client's overall Constitution. If the San Jiao's ability to move Fluids continues to disintegrate, the *Zheng*/Upright Qi is compromised and gravity will allow Fluids to accumulate in the Lower Burner.

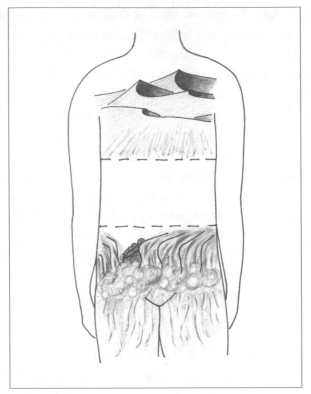

Figure 11.5: Deficiency and Accumulation in the San Jiao

Initial symptoms of Lower Burner Fluid accumulation will be Dampness or Damp-Cold (due to the Kidney Deficiency), but over time this condition will transform to Damp-Heat or Phlegm because of the failure of the San Jiao to 'spread' the *Ming Men* Fire. Eventually, the Upper Jiao will also display clear symptoms of Dryness from the failure of the San Jiao to 'mist' the Upper Jiao; the Dryness symptoms will likely be more subtle than the Lower Jiao Dampness, Damp-Heat, or Phlegm symptomology. Figure 11.5 uses an overflowing river and a sandy desert to help visualize the combination of wetness and dryness.

North–South Axial Trauma is more likely to have occurred in early childhood, and sexual abuse is one of the primary causes. If this type of assault is involved, the Extraordinary Vessels may also show signs of damage (see Chapter 9).

Stagnation and Inflammation in the San Jiao

In an East–West Axis pattern, the stirring and spreading function of the Middle Jiao will fail, preventing the proper separation of 'Clear' and 'Turbid' while allowing the Gallbladder's digestive Fire to 'brew'. This leads to the San Jiao holding on to fluids the body no longer needs, creating Qi Stagnation and Dampness/Damp-Phlegm in the Middle Jiao, evidenced by abdominal weight gain, the 'love handles' that sit lateral to the outer UB line above the waistline, or gallstones. Without proper circulation in the Middle Jiao, the Gallbladder's warmth (which should have been spread to support the other digestive Organs) will transform the Middle Jiao Dampness/Damp-Phlegm into a Hot condition (i.e., Damp-Heat or Phlegm-Heat). As Heat will always rise, it will eventually create a Dry-Heat in the Upper Jiao as well.

The balance of Damp versus Heat in depends on the individual's Constitution, Diet, level of exercise (and purgative sweating), environmental factors, and accompanying emotions. Regardless, an enduring stagnant Dampness and Heat in the Middle Jiao will form the basis for inflammation. If the Heat becomes intensified by other factors, it could easily brew into a Phlegm-Fire condition.

The various 'spaces' of the *San Jiao* will become easily affected by this inflammation. *Cou Li* impact can be seen in hypertonicity of the flesh, especially near the San Jiao Channel on the forearms: skin will feel objectively tight, bony markers are less distinct (even if the patient is thin or average-sized), and Acupuncture points (especially on the San Jiao Channel) become difficult to locate. Figure 11.6 shows the condensing of excessive fluids by Heat, sending an overabundance of warmth to the Upper Jiao.

Middle Jiao Stagnation and systemic inflammation more likely occur with East–West Axial patterns that impact older teenagers and adults. When this trauma is rooted in restrictive home/family environments, there is typically a combination of Chronic Fear, Secrecy, and Repression at the root.

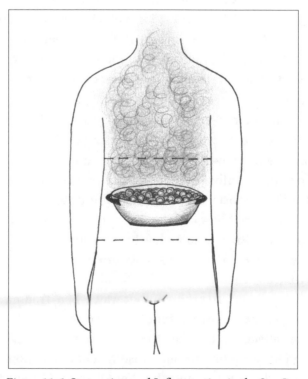

Figure 11.6: Stagnation and Inflammation in the San Jiao

A combination of:

- Upper Jiao Dryness or Yin Deficiency–Heat, with

- Dampness, Damp-Heat, or Phlegm in the Middle or Lower Jiao

is a good indicator that the integrity of the San Jiao was compromised by Trauma.

Wei Qi Involvement

Wei/Defensive Qi defends the skin and surface channels against attack by External Wind by forming a defensive 'net' around and inside the body. In daytime, it circulates primarily in the *Cou Li*, the space of the San Jiao, helping warm and enliven the flesh while protecting the body from pathogenic factors. At night, Wei Qi retreats inward to circulate among the organs, helping warm and protect the deepest layers of the body from pathological factors. By its inward and outward movement, Wei Qi contributes to our ability to engage with the world while awake, and to retreat inwardly for 'down time.' When Wei Qi is strong, one can move about the world with a sense of safety; but when it is weak, one needs to be cautious about how much to engage.

In Medical Qigong theory, Wei Qi also circulates just outside the physical body, forming the energetic aura that extends into and beyond a person's physical body (Johnson 2000, pp.284–285). Wei Qi therefore helps protect from both physical (i.e., Wind or EPF invasion) and energetic (i.e., emotional or spiritual) attack, enabling the individual to move out into the world *believing that they are safe* in whatever situation they might encounter.

On an emotional level, External Wind is another person's feelings, circulating and extending from their own Qi field. If an individual has healthy Wei Qi maintaining a strong emotional border, that person will have healthy boundaries that clearly delineate their own emotional state from another person's, even in intimate relationship (family, lovers, etc.). By preserving healthy emotional boundaries, Wei Qi supports an individual's ability to take responsibility for their own actions and emotions, without taking on responsibility for the actions or emotions of others. When Trauma has broken down the Wei Qi, however, a person may experience emotional sensitivity or empathy to the needs of others that goes far beyond any concept of 'health,' including co-dependent entwinement with an inadequate partner. To say it another way, when Trauma strikes the Wei Qi a person may lose their sense of 'mine versus yours.'

When Trauma affects the San Jiao, the circulation of Wei Qi within the *Cou Li* space is compromised, either through insufficient circulation or obstruction. If Trauma impacts the San Jiao and the Wei Qi in childhood, teenage years, or any time before the psychological fabric is solidified, it is highly likely that long-lasting patterns of emotional immaturity and unhealthy boundaries will be established. The following are just a few examples of this complication:

As the San Jiao is affected...

- Trust no one/stranger danger: Limited social circle, phobias, limited work possibilities and ability to make money, fear of sex or intimacy.

- Letting everyone in: Inability to distinguish between friend and acquaintance or appropriate partners/relationship styles, sexual promiscuity or infidelity.

- Learning and growing from life's experiences: Child-like behavior/extended reliance on parents (financial, emotional, etc.), complete avoidance of responsibility, martyr complex (i.e., Why is this always happening to me?).

As the Wei Qi is damaged...

- When to extend and when to retreat: Anxiety, depression, inability to motivate/leave their home, phobias, fear of crowds/new places, inability to maintain work or relationship.

- Emotional boundaries: Extreme empathy for others' feelings, repeated engagement in abusive/co-dependent relationships, inability to maintain self-care practices.

- Acceptance/Fear of change: Inappropriate dress, inability to apply for work or take on new responsibilities, living in a child-like state.

Treatment of emotional Trauma at this level requires everything already mentioned under axial alignment, as well as special attention to Fluid Stasis in the San Jiao and the inability of the Wei Qi to properly function. Acute-onset symptoms from recent Trauma may be managed within two to four months, but repairing long-standing damage at this level typically takes over a year of treatment. Modalities must be varied and treatment principles will change frequently during this time in order to address holistic re-integration. Talk therapy and long-term maintenance with Chinese Medicine are strongly recommended for all cases of childhood-onset emotional Trauma, along with Tuina, Shiatsu, Massage, or other bodywork to address the San Jiao, *Cou Li*, and Wei Qi circulation.

- Typical Presentation: Regularly-occurring 'fear of wind' (air conditioning, fan breezes) with shivers, skin numbness or varied surface temperatures, emotional immaturity, frequent colds and flus, atopic asthma or eczema, environmental allergies, food allergies/sensitivities, and various other immune system/auto-immune conditions. *Note: Other symptoms will be based on the location of the axial break and the type of San Jiao impact.*

- Treatment Principles: Clear Dampness, Damp-Heat, and/or Phlegm, Tonify Wei Qi (through the Lung–Spleen–Kidney axis), Harmonize the San Jiao (and Axial Patterns).

- Acupuncture – general suggestions:

    - ST 8, 36, 40, GB 34, 38, 40, LV 3, 5, SP 3, 6, 9, Ren 4, 6, 10–13, LU 1, 2, 5, 7, KI 1 (Moxa), 3, 7, 10, Du 4, 14, 20, SJ 5, 6, 14, 17, UB 13, 14, 13, 42, 20, 23 (with Heat: LI 11, ST 44, GB 43, LV 2)

    - Du Mai to regulate the senses (hypersensitivity or dulled senses) and one's ability to engage with or disengage from external stimuli

    - Dai Mai to clear the 'latency' of unprocessed Trauma, as well as release the suppression of one's natural power reservoir (Jing-Essence)

    - Combination: Yintang with Du 20 and/or 24 to soothe the Sea of Marrow, reduce 'psychological disruptions,' and improve concentration/memory.

- Herbal Formulae: Xiao Chai Hu Wan, Yu Ping Feng San Wan, Er Chen Wan, Bu Nao Wan (with Nu Ke Ba Zhen Wan, Si Jun Zi Wan).

- Gua Sha for upper body channels to 'raise' Wei Qi.

- Tuina (or other bodywork) to clear the *Cou Li* spaces and address whole-body integration.

- Gemstones: Azurite, Azurite-Malachite, Black Jade, Obsidian (Apache Tears, Mahogany), Yellow Tourmaline, Zircon.

- Lifestyle: Talk therapy or mental health counseling; Tuina, Shiatsu, massage or other bodywork; avoidance of situations and people that cause emotional stress; warm clothing to protect the Wei Qi.

- Self-treatment for 'checking out,' numbing, or flashbacks: tapping on Du 26 to awaken the conscious mind.

Emotional Trauma – especially occurring in the formative years – molds a person's beliefs and ideas about the external environment... The challenging nature of breaking these patterns requires the combination of multiple treatment methods to 'keep the body guessing,' which ultimately shifts the ingrained nature of a Trauma.

– CT Holman 2018, p.126

The Psychological Impact of Trauma

Trauma impacts the *Wu Shen* through axial damage, the accompanying breakdown of the Qi Mechanism, and by striking the psycho-emotional aspects of the San Jiao and the Wei Qi. In early childhood-onset, Trauma can enter directly into the psychological fabric, with significant repercussions on the individual's ability to properly perceive the world, integrate and learn from their experiences, and form or maintain healthy relationships. Personal and emotional growth can be effectively frozen at the age the trauma took place, disabling a person's ability to address their life curriculum and manifest their Destiny. Figure 11.7 shows the three types of emotional Trauma and their most common associated pathologies.

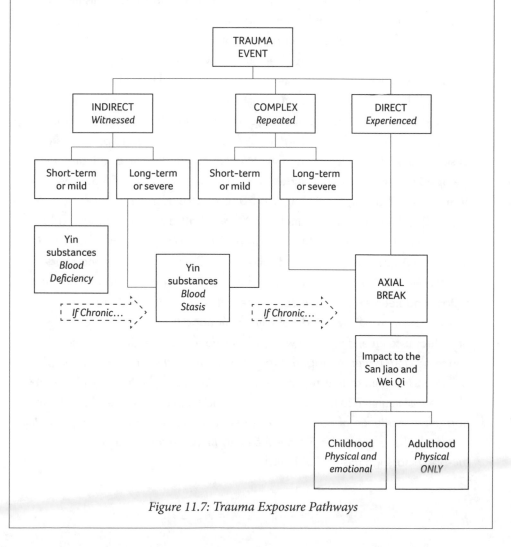

Figure 11.7: Trauma Exposure Pathways

CLIENT EXAMPLE

A heterosexual female in her early 50s presents with obesity (her estimated weight is 300–325 pounds), bipolar disorder (she loves the mania phase – 'I get so much done!' – but wants help with the depression phase), fibromyalgia, and chronic fatigue syndrome. She also reports ongoing agoraphobia, claustrophobia, food and environmental sensitivities, and memory concerns. She grew up in a rural area and was repeatedly molested and raped by older siblings and cousins as a child, which was ignored by her drug-addicted parents. She ran away at age 17 after her second abortion, and currently lives in a gated community that she leaves only for medical appointments (she even gets groceries delivered). She sees a therapist twice weekly, and a psychiatrist once a month for medication management (Lithium). She is showered and clean, with polished nails, but her clothing is stained, unfashionable, and mismatched. She talks loudly and is unable to maintain eye contact or linear conversation. Her tongue is pale, wet, swollen-puffy, tooth-marked, with a dip at the rear, peeled sides, and a red-thin tip. Her pulse is wiry, tight, and slippery prior to needling; with needles it switches to slippery, weak, and thin. She is diagnosed with both North–South and East–West axial breaks and failure of the San Jiao and the Wei Qi due to trauma (Heart–Kidney Disharmony, Liver–Spleen Disharmony, Phlegm Obstructing the Orifices). Initial treatment principles are to stabilize the Earth Element and the Wei Qi, Clear Phlegm, and Harmonize the San Jiao. Acupuncture includes ST 8, 36 (with Moxa), 40, SP 3, 6, 9, Ren Mai (LU 7–KI 6), SJ 17, GB 40, UB 60, and Moxa on Four Doors (Ren 6, 12, ST 25). Herbal Formulae includes Xiang Sha Liu Jun Zi Wan with a low dose of Chai Hu Long Gu Mu Li Wan and Tian Wang Bu Xin Wan. She is also given Amazonite, Amber, and Yellow Jade Gemstones. She is encouraged to take two 10–20 minute walks per day, eat smaller meals up to five times a day, and keep external stressors limited. It is recommended that she return weekly for an indefinite period of time to manage the bipolar, fibromyalgia, and chronic fatigue, and to not worry about the excess weight until these other concerns were better managed. *Note: It is assumed that Treatment Principles will change within one to two months of treatment, and that she will require lifetime maintenance to manage symptoms and maintain a sense of emotional normalcy. Incidence of transference is heightened in this case, so she would eventually be referred to a massage center/therapist for San Jiao integration full-body massage (instead of Tuina).*

SUMMARY

» Emotional or psychological Trauma results from witnessing or experiencing an extremely upsetting event, where one's ability to integrate the various emotions is compromised.

» Indirect trauma is emotional stress from a second-hand event (i.e., narrative accounts, media reports, other external influences). When chronic, it impacts the Heart Yin Substances; the most common Zang Fu pattern is Heart Blood and Spleen Qi Deficiency.

» Complex trauma is emotional stress from cumulative exposure (i.e., ongoing verbal abuse, Chronic Fear, multiple indirect exposures). As the Heart attempts to process the relentless distress, it 'churns' the Blood. The most common Zang Fu pattern is Heart Blood Stasis, which commonly presents with Heart Blood or Yin Deficiency, Qi Stagnation (Liver, Lung, or Chest Qi), or Phlegm.

» Direct trauma includes a specific event that is experienced or witnessed first-hand (i.e., physical/sexual abuse, violence, persecution, rejection, etc.). The Heart and its Yin Substances are not strong enough to buffer these events, so damage to the internal organ alignment and Qi Mechanism occurs.

» A single incident of direct Trauma, especially occurring in childhood or adolescence, can cause an axial 'break' that permanently damages internal organ communication and Qi Mechanism functioning. Chronic re-triggering of indirect and complex trauma can also lead to such 'breaks.'

» North–South and East–West Axial disruptions can co-exist, more commonly found in those with a history of multiple traumatic events in both childhood and adulthood (e.g., DGS individuals in fearful isolation as kids, then fighting for civil rights as adults).

» Earth reflects stability in the midst of change, and acceptance of one's life experiences. It sits directly at the center of the Taiji, so it is involved in disruption of either axis.

» Axial breaks in either direction impact the Qi Mechanism, which affects the functioning of the San Jiao. When the San Jiao is compromised, it becomes difficult to fully integrate new thoughts and emotions, leading to an inability to evaluate or learn from new experiences.

» There are two ways the San Jiao can be impacted through a traumatic axial break: deficiency with accumulation (limited Heat), and stagnation with inflammation (intense Heat).

» A North–South Axis disruption makes the San Jiao overwork to ascend and descend Fluids between the three body cavities. If the San Jiao's ability to move Fluids continues to disintegrate, the *Zheng*/Upright Qi is compromised and gravity will allow Fluids to accumulate in the Lower Burner.

» In an East–West Axis pattern, the stirring and spreading function of the Middle Jiao will fail, preventing proper separation of 'Clear' and 'Turbid' while allowing the Gallbladder's digestive Fire to 'brew'. This leads to the San Jiao holding on to fluids the body no longer needs, creating Qi Stagnation and Damp-Heat/Phlegm-Heat in the Middle Jiao. As Heat always rises, Dry- or Damp-Heat will eventually present in the Upper Jiao as well.

» Wei/Defensive Qi contributes to our ability to engage with the world while awake, and to retreat inwardly for 'down time'. If an individual has healthy Wei Qi maintaining a strong emotional border, that person will have healthy boundaries that clearly delineate their own emotional state from another person's, even in intimate relationship (family, lovers, etc.).

» If Trauma impacts the San Jiao and the Wei Qi in childhood, teenage years, or any time before the psychological fabric is solidified, it is highly likely that long-lasting patterns of emotional immaturity and unhealthy boundaries will be established.

» Make sure that a client is in an emotionally safe and supportive environment *prior to starting* emotional Trauma resolution. Talk therapy and long-term maintenance with Chinese Medicine are strongly recommended for all cases of childhood-onset emotional Trauma, along with Tuina, Shiatsu, Massage, or other bodywork to address the San Jiao, Cou Li, and Wei Qi circulation.

Chapter 12

BEING JUDGED
Guilt and Shame

- Heavy and Ephemeral Fluids

- The Chains of Guilt

- The Swamp of Shame

Shame and Guilt are both aspects of moral judgment about what is right and what is wrong. Starting at a very early age, these emotions are taught as ways to reinforce *Li*, the Confucian concept of conforming to social expectations that are dictated by family and culture (see Chapter 10). Those in the psychology field often refer to the *usefulness* of Guilt as a motivational tool. According to Brené Brown, 'We feel guilty when we hold up something we've done or failed to do against our values and find they don't match up. It's an uncomfortable feeling, but one that's helpful. The psychological discomfort…is what motivates meaningful change' (2012a, p.72). But like all emotions, too much of a good thing is *never* a good thing: when Guilt and Shame are chronic and unprocessed, pathology ensues.

The two emotions have strong similarities, but also a few differences. Both are related to moral principles, with deep association to conservative or religious traditions. Guilt is a value judgment of one's *behavior*: 'I *did* something – or want to *do* something – that is bad.' Unprocessed Guilt results from the inability to admit a *potential* wrong-doing, either because of emotional maturity or anticipation of rejection. Guilt is always in reaction to an external response or perception of the individual's behavior – either real or imagined – which typically manifests along with Fear and Secrecy (see Chapters 10, 13).

Shame, on the other hand, is a judgment on one's very *existence*: 'I *am* bad.' Shame is not reliant upon other people's perceptions, nor is it dependent on any actual behavior or Desire. As Brown states, 'Shame is the intensely painful feeling or experience of believing that we are flawed and therefore unworthy of love and belonging' (2012a, p.69). Brown has also described Shame as 'highly, highly correlated with addiction, depression, violence, aggression, bullying, suicide, eating disorders' (2012b, @14.25), while noting that Guilt is inversely related to those very same behaviors. This evidence demonstrates how much easier it is to say, 'I *did* that, and I'm sorry,' than to say, 'I *am* that, and I'm sorry.'

Because of ongoing cultural reinforcement, Shame and Guilt are among the most difficult emotions to treat, requiring dismantling and re-wiring of deep, subconscious-level belief structures that undermine the individual's ability to truly experience self-worth. As Shame is directly linked to self-worth and frequently presents with Self-Loathing (see Chapter 15), it is considered more difficult to treat than Guilt.

HEAVY AND EPHEMERAL FLUIDS

There are three similarities between Shame and unprocessed Guilt: they both create Fluid Stasis, are both heavy and descending in nature, and may only present on the emotional or ephemeral level (ephemeral being defined as non-physical, fleeting, or come-and-go in nature).

The Fluid Stasis of Shame or Guilt is engendered by extreme Qi Stagnation affecting either the Liver or Spleen. Guilt is associated with action, either by total prevention of movement or by forced, undesirable action. Any frustrated action or inaction impacts the tendons, so acute Guilt corresponds to the Liver organ and Liver Qi Stagnation. As Qi is the 'Commander of Blood' this Qi Stagnation will inevitably lead to Blood Stasis, the primary pathological pattern associated with chronic, unprocessed Guilt.

Shame is related to self-worth and self-acceptance, the spiritual lessons of the Spleen and Earth Elements. When the proper functioning of Earth is obstructed, the separation of 'Clear' and 'Turbid' and the transportation and transformation functions will falter. Dampness and eventually Phlegm will form, obstructing the Qi Mechanism leading to Qi Stagnation. As Stagnation-Heat will cook the Damp fluids, Phlegm is the primary pathological pattern associated with chronic shame.

Fluid Stasis itself is heavy and tends to sink. When gender and sexuality issues are at the root, these conditions easily settle into the Lower Jiao and the Jing-Essence, and are likely to impact the reproductive organs. As there is an ephemeral quality even with physical presentation, the presence of pathology is likely to have remained hidden for years, such as with primary amenorrhea, polycystic ovarian disease, infertility, etc. Symptoms are also likely to be extremely responsive to the environment, diet, menstrual cycle, and current stress levels.

For example, pathology may appear more dramatic in humid environments or seasons where excess fluids become apparent, but be difficult to discern in dry, desert climates. Excessive dairy, wheat, soy, and processed foods in the diet as well as lack of exercise or movement will exacerbate either condition, as can the effulgence of body fluids that occurs at ovulation and pre-menstruation. Conversely, a diet free of Damp/Phlegm-engendering foods can dramatically lessen the presence of fluid pathology, and regular cardiovascular exercise can also reduce symptoms, especially for Blood Stasis. Finally, emotional worry or stress can deplete the Spleen Qi and lead to an increase in Dampness, or it can stagnate the Liver Qi and aggravate Blood Stasis. Again due to the ephemeral nature, once the trigger (environmental, dietary, emotional, etc.) is relieved, symptoms related to Shame or Guilt may completely disappear between these acute episodes.

When Shame or Guilt has been present for some time, the ephemeral quality will wane, and both Fluid Stasis and Qi Stagnation will eventually present systemically. On a general physical level, Fluid Stasis conditions that obstruct movement include Bi/Obstruction syndrome, arthritis, fibromyalgia, and chronic fatigue. Giovanni Maciocia wrote that both Shame and Guilt affect the Heart: 'Guilt affects the Kidneys and Heart. Shame affects the Heart and Spleen' (2013, p.299). Between the emotional root and the *Bao Mai* that connects the 'Room of Essence' to the Heart, the ephemeral Fluid Stasis can easily impact the Heart as well. When Shame and its corresponding Phlegm are involved, this commonly results in clouded thinking or poor memory, making it difficult to get accurate health history; other emotional conditions may include a general lack of inspiration, depression, anxiety, manic-depressive cycles, or even bipolar disorders. If Shame or Guilt is experienced as long-term emotional stress, either of them can also develop into Trauma. Both Shame and Guilt can damage the North–South Axis of Water–Earth–Fire elements, but Guilt is more likely to damage the East–West Axis of Wood–Earth–Metal due to its correspondence with actions, tendons, and the Liver. In any case, there will always be Lower Jiao and reproductive organ involvement with Shame or Guilt related to gender or sexuality.

In terms of diagnosis, both Shame and Guilt can present with a wiry middle pulse due to obstruction affecting the Liver or Spleen. The specific location – left or right – may help point toward the underlying emotion in an early presentation, but it is important to remember that Shame and Guilt can easily appear together or be masked by other factors such as Constitution and diet. Another diagnostic similarity comes from Jeffrey Yuen (2017a), who has described a visible vein between the eyes at Yintang when long-standing Shame or Guilt are present. Both Shame and Guilt may also present concurrently with Lying, which is associated with pathology in the throat including thyroid issues or goiter, strep throat, tonsillitis, and plum pit Qi (see Chapter 13). For treatment, Yuen (2017a) recommends Windows of the Sky Acupuncture points to address throat concerns associated with Lying, and points of the Chong Mai pathway (Spleen 4, 12, etc.) to 'rectify' the Qi flow that was damaged by excessive adherence to *Li*.

Table 12.1 shows the general similarities of Shame and Guilt as well as the critical differences that distinguish them. Because Shame and Guilt can be ephemeral in presentation, are often subconscious, and are culturally enforced from childhood, they are among the most difficult emotions to treat. If Shame and Guilt are the underlying root of any condition, expectations of cure must be properly managed.

Table 12.1: Guilt and Shame Basics

Both	Fluid Stasis, Heavy, Descending, Ephemeral
	Gender & Sexuality: Lower Jiao and Reproductive Organs, Heart
	Systemic: Arthritis, fibromyalgia, chronic fatigue
	Emotional: Lack of motivation, anxiety, depression, bipolar
	Wiry Pulse
	Difficult to treat
Guilt	Blood Stasis and Qi Stagnation
	Liver, Tendons (secondary: Heart, Kidneys)
	East–West Trauma (secondary: North–South)
Shame	Dampness, Phlegm, Qi Deficiency
	Spleen (secondary: Heart)
	North–South Trauma

THE CHAINS OF GUILT

Guilt stems from internalized cultural judgment of one's past, current, or antici-pated behaviors. Examples of this in relation to gender and sexuality include the LGBTQ+ child that doesn't 'come out' because their parents or friends may reject them, or the polyamorist that repeatedly attempts (and fails at) monogamous relationships. As denial of self becomes chronic, Fear (see Chapter 11), Lying, and Secrecy (see Chapter 13) often present alongside unprocessed Guilt.

Guilt prevents action and obstructs the movements of tendons, creating Qi Stagnation in the Liver. Whereas Anger invokes the outward and upward movement traditionally associated with Wood energy, Guilt does the opposite. Instead of Qi being directed toward the Upper Jiao and Head, Guilt directs Qi inward and downward, anchoring into the Middle and Lower Jiaos to bind the authentic self. Figures 12.1 and 12.2 show the difference between the up-out movement of Anger and the in-down, heavy nature of Guilt.

Maciocia described Guilt as a 'dark emotion with no redemption' (2013, p.296). The combination of darkness with Qi Stagnation and inward-downward movement explains how unprocessed Guilt quickly transforms into Blood Stasis. The Blood Stasis of Guilt will primarily impact the Liver organ, but may also affect other systems through various relationships:

- Lungs or Large Intestine: Metal controls Wood and is easily injured by Wood Excess.

- Heart: Experiences and processes all emotions, as well as 'governs' the Blood.

- Spleen or Stomach: Earth is easily injured by Wood Excess, and Spleen 'controls' the Blood.

- Kidneys: The 'mother' of Wood and 'ruler' of the Lower Jiao.

As tension created by the thwarted movements of the tendons easily depletes Liver Blood, Blood Deficiency may co-exist with the Blood Stasis of Guilt (see a discussion on Blood Deficiency at the end of this chapter). It is also possible for Heat to arise from stasis, but it will not be a primary presentation without other co-factors such as environment, diet, Constitution, Desire or Craving.

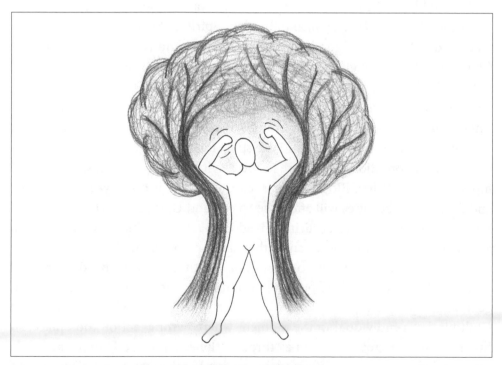

Figure 12.1: The Shape of Anger

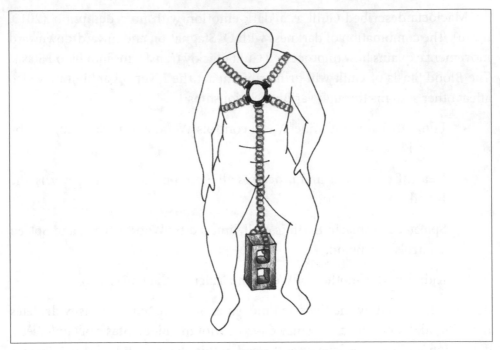

Figure 12.2: The Shape of Guilt

Figure 12.2 depicts the heavy and descending nature of Guilt as chains that anchor and bind the body. This inward-downward weight limits the free flow of the Heart, Upper *Dan Tian*, and the Shen-Spirit that support self-knowledge and the development of gender identity, sexuality, and relationship needs (see Chapters 4, 6). Although the stagnation of unprocessed Guilt will always begin in the Middle Jiao and Liver organ, Blood Stasis related to gender and sexuality will eventually settle into the Lower Jiao as well. There it can affect the uterus (menstrual irregularities – clots, cramps, dark/heavy flow, amenorrhea, etc.), prostate, urinary bladder (interstitial cystitis, incontinence, etc.), or create pain and arthritic conditions anywhere in the pelvic region (sacrum, sacro-iliac or hip joints, etc.). When Blood Stasis is left untreated for many years, the heavy and descending qualities will affect the Spleen and Upright Qi; this may lead to Lower Jiao prolapses (uterus, urinary bladder, haemorrhoids, miscarriage, etc.), although these are more prevalent with pathology rooted in Shame.

As the cultural backdrop to feelings of Guilt typically begins during early childhood or adolescence, patterns of emotional immaturity, naiveté, and generalized 'people-pleasing' behaviors are extremely likely. On a spiritual level Guilt binds an individual in the moment where 'wrong' action took place, so further spiritual growth – such as through the steps of the Nine Palaces – is very unlikely. The lessons offered by the Travel and Adventure Palace are the most commonly rejected as these relate to seeing new ways of doing things and re-evaluating familial or cultural traditions. So instead of the individual embarking on a self-determined pursuit of Destiny based in self-knowledge and self-acceptance, *Li* will overrule their major life choices. If Guilt combines with Trauma during early childhood, the San Jiao and Wei Qi impact can be extremely difficult to unwind (see Chapter 11). Because of the emotional and spiritual blocks caused by Guilt, individuals working toward healing this emotional state typically have a lot of personal growth to accomplish. As healing progresses, it is common for major life transformations to occur, including career choice, geographic relocation, and divorce.

- Typical Presentation: Extreme tendon tension (especially IT band, jaw/scalp, occipital – shoulder along the GB Channel, inner knee along Liver Channel – *all unrelieved by massage*); varicosities (especially thighs, IT band, middle Jiao/hypochondriac ribcage); focused and non-moving pain; menstrual irregularities (clots, cramps, dark, heavy/flooding, early, delayed); digestive complaints (bloating, constipation or mixed bowel movements); moderate Middle Jiao weight gain; pulses: wiry, choppy, firm, overflowing; tongue: purple spots or distended and dark sub-lingual veins.

- Treatment Principles: Move and course Qi, Move or 'break' Blood, Clear Stagnation from the Middle and/or Lower Jiao, Soothe Tendons (*and nourish Liver Blood and Kidney Yin as applicable*).

Primary Modalities

- Acupuncture: Ren 4, 6, 12 (Moxa applicable); SP 8, 10, LV 3, 8, LI 4, PC 6, GB 34, Yintang:

  - Combinations: Du 20 with Sishencong – the 'Princess Crown' at the 7th Chakra to help remember one's Divine place in the world; GB 40 with UB 60 – to 'rectify movement' by aligning the feet

  - Local points for pain: ST 7, 25–30, Zigong, GB 2, 20, 21, 26–28, 31–33, SI 16, SJ 21, etc.

  - Points along the Chong to rectify *Li*, and Windows of the Sky for throat symptoms.

- Herbal Formulae: Xue Fu Zhu Yu Tang, Tao Hong Si Wu Wan, Tong Jing Wan, Yan Hu Suo Zhi Tong Wan, Jin Gu Die Sheng Wan, Huo Luo Xiao Ling Wan, Ge Xia Zhu Yu Wan, Shao Fu Zhu Yu Wan.

- Cupping: Flash to break up stagnation – especially useful for tendons (hamstrings and IT band), and upper chest or intrascapular areas.

- Tuina: Vibrational techniques to break up stasis.

- Gemstones: Amethyst, Rose Quartz, Bloodstone, Carnelian, Garnet, Hematite, Lapis Lazuli, Red Jasper, Sodalite, Sunstone.

Secondary Modalities

- Medical Qigong: Counterclockwise circling and gentle 'thumping' against the physical energetic field to disperse stagnations, then lead the Excess out through the closest extremities. *Note: Blood Stasis typically reads as a black-purple color.*

- Essential Oils: Cinnamon, Cumin, Frankincense, Ginger, Myrrh, Onion, Parsley, Tarragon.

- Qigong: Hun Yuan Gong – Opening and Closing the Three *Dan Tian*, Rotating Qi in the Lower *Dan Tian*; Butterfly Qigong; Silk-Reeling; Pounding and Scrubbing the Channels.

- Lifestyle: Blood-moving foods; cardiovascular exercise and healthy sexual activity; living one's life 'without limits.'

- Affirmation: 'My body and spirit are free.'

THE SWAMP OF SHAME

As discussed, Shame is an internal value judgment placed upon one's self, irrespective of actual behaviors or external perspective. Shame is predominantly based in childhood lessons of morality, and often presents alongside Self-Loathing (see Chapter 15). Lying and Secrecy also frequently appear with Shame, but are not always present or apparent (see Chapter 13). As an internal form of judgment, Shame can completely overwhelm the individual with periods of intense and endless self-criticism. A shamed individual is being judged at all times in the courtroom of their own mind, even when they are alone.

When an individual suffers from Shame, they will likely be putting effort into staying small, 'flying under the radar,' and remaining hidden from the view of others. This will play out across all major life decisions, including career and relationship choices. Shame pulls a person inward and downward, just like Blood Stasis, but the heaviness is more intense, preventing movement of the feet, lifting of the head, or even looking out to see reality reflected back. In this way, Shame is the opposite of self-less pride, which is an outward expression of self-worth that radiates from within like a golden star. Figures 12.3 and 12.4 show the difference between pride and Shame, with pride unburdened by the heavy weight of Shame, able to stand tall, chin up, with springs under the feet to easily bounce forward into life's adventures. On the other hand, Shame has overburdened the Middle Jiao, making it impossible to maintain an erect spine. The person has collapsed from the weight of their own self-deprecation, and now sits with feet of concrete, unable to get up, move forward, or look at anything other than their own puddle of Shame.

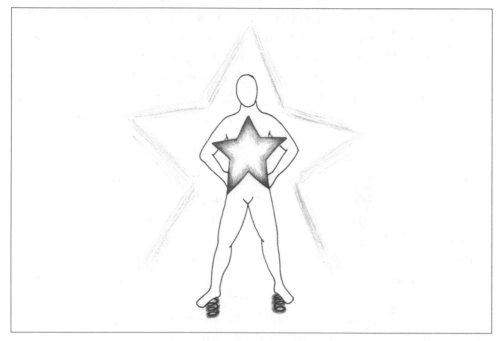

Figure 12.3: The Shape of Pride

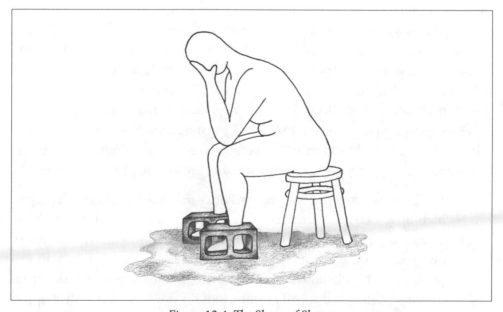

Figure 12.4: The Shape of Shame

Shame completely obstructs self-acceptance and self-forgiveness, creating Qi Stagnation in the Earth Element organs (Stomach, Spleen, Pancreas) on a spiritual level. Just as the 'Turbid' is separated from the 'Clear,' the belief that one's very existence is wrong is a belief that deserves to be discarded. This lack of compassion toward the self thwarts the spiritual aspect of the Spleen and Earth Element, leading to enduring Dampness or Phlegm. The weight of Shame creates a sense of helpless impotence that can psycho-spiritually 'freeze' a person at a moment in time and space, leading to an inability to 'move forward' either emotionally or physically. Limitation of movement from Shame will be rooted in either Yang Deficiency or Cold, not in Qi Stagnation (as with Guilt). The ongoing presence of Deficient or Excess Cold along with Dampness or Phlegm will quickly overburden both the *Zheng*/Upright Qi and the San Jiao, making mixed Qi Deficiency–Stagnation a more prevalent presentation in Shame than a purely excess Qi Stagnation condition.

Depletion of the Spleen, San Jiao, and Upright Qi will not be able to stop the forces of gravity, so the Dampness or Phlegm will settle into the Lower Jiao and impact the Kidneys almost immediately. Dampness and Phlegm are also self-engendering: as they continue to obstruct the Spleen, San Jiao, and Kidneys, more Dampness and Phlegm will be allowed to collect. This is further exacerbated by Shame related to sex or sexuality, which focuses in the Lower *Dan Tian*. Extreme weight gain can be expected to develop in the pelvic region, lower abdomen, hips, and upper thighs, with moderate weight gain in the Middle Jiao as well. 'Leakage' from the Lower Yin Orifices is likely, along with pelvic tension to 'stop' the leakage of Qi/Fluids, especially with issues of sexual abuse.

The self-engendering Dampness and Phlegm of Shame makes it extremely difficult to fully resolve the root emotion. Obstacles may include an inability to recognize abusive self-talk, along with inability to cultivate empathy or forgiveness of the self for having allowed Shame to dictate their life choices. Creating authentic and supportive friendships that allow honest dialogue to expose areas of Shame, as well as crafting a daily program of physical self-care and emotional self-affirmations, are a critical part of the long journey away from this emotion. To ensure lasting progress, the individual must address their own ingrained, self-demeaning thought patterns: talk therapy, compassion/mindfulness training practices, Yoga, Qigong, and prayer/meditation are all strongly recommended.

- Typical Presentation: Lower Jiao/pelvic region weight gain and 'leakages,' including diarrhea, urinary incontinence, chronic UTI symptoms, menstrual irregularities (leukorrhea, spotting, miscarriage); areas of numbness in the Lower Jiao, especially feet, legs (or inability to feel sex/genital stimulation/very slow to orgasm); heavy legs/feet, slow gait, trips easily, slouched spinal posture, looking downward; digestive upsets (indigestion, bloating, nausea, hiccups after eating); frequent colds/not feeling well, chronic sinus congestion; heavy weight gain around the pelvis/hips/buttock/thighs, moderate in the Middle Jiao; pelvic/sacrum/hip/IT band/hamstring tension. Pulse: wiry, slippery. Tongue: swollen.

- Treatment Principles: Drain Dampness, Clear Phlegm, Tonify Spleen, Kidneys, and the Upright Qi, Harmonize the San Jiao, Tonify and warm Qi/Yang (clear Cold *as appropriate*). *Note: Qi Stagnation is secondary to Qi Deficiency; once the Deficiency resolves, Stagnation may become more apparent.*

Primary Modalities

- Herbal Formulae: Bi Xie Sheng Shi Wan, Er Chen Wan, Xiang Sha Liu Jun Zi Wan, Liu Jun Zi Wan, Bu Zhong Yi Qi Wan.

- Massage/Gua Sha/Tuina: Vibration and shaking techniques to break up Phlegm deposits; pushing and pressing to address whole-body integration.

- Diet: Foods to clear Dampness and Phlegm (i.e., almonds, celery, garlic, mustard greens, jasmine green tea, onion, parsley, pear, scallions, thyme, walnuts, etc.); avoidance of grains, wheat, dairy, beer, high-fat, processed, and 'sticky foods'; eating small meals without stress.

- Lifestyle: Mindfulness training around self-critical thought patterns, empathy, and forgiveness of self; open, honest, authentic friendships; talk therapy or mental health counseling for further support; walking, biking, or any form of smooth, self-paced movement to promote freedom of internal movement. *Note: If Stagnation is predominant, movement should include short bursts of more vigorous 'bounce' to break up Phlegm without further depleting the Qi (dance, running, etc.).*

Secondary Modalities

- Acupuncture: SP 3, 6, 9, ST 8, 25, 36, 40, GB 40, KI 3, Yintang, Ren 4 (Moxa), 6 (Moxa), 12 (Moxa), UB 14, 15, 20, 21, 22, 23, 28, 43, 44, 49, 50, 51, 52, DU 4 (Moxa):

  - Combinations: Du 20 with Sishencong – the 'Princess Crown' at the 7th Chakra to help remember one's Divine place in the world; Four Flowers (Ren 11, 12, 13, ST 21); Four Doors (ST 25, Ren 12, Ren 6 – all with Moxa)

  - Local points for Lower Jiao: UB 31–36, 40, GB 26–28, 30–32, Dai Mai (GB 41–SJ 5), etc.

- – Points along the Chong to rectify *Li*, and Windows of the Sky for throat symptoms.

- Essential Oils: Birch, Caraway, Cardamom, Cedar, Fir, Ginger, Grapefruit, Neroli, Onion, Parsley, Sandalwood.

- Qigong: Healing Sounds and Colors – Earth Element; Abdominal Round-Rubbing; Butterfly Qigong; Silk-Reeling Qigong; Sheng Zhen Qigong: Heaven Nature/Kuan Yin Standing – Boat Rowing in the Stream of Air; Hun Yuan Gong–Grinding the Corn; Sinking the Turbid and Washing the Organs. (*Note: 'Sinking the Turbid and Washing the Organs' may increase Damp–Turbidity if not done properly*.)

- Gemstones: Agate (Green, Moss), Alexandrite, Amber, Beryl (Yellow, Golden), Peridot, Phrenite, Spinel (Yellow, Clear), Sodalite, Sunstone, Yellow Jade, Yellow Jasper, Zircon.

- Affirmation: 'I accept myself completely.'

Guilt, Shame, and Blood Deficiency

As Blood passes through the Heart, it helps process sensation and experience while nourishing the tissue to help with verbal expression of emotion. When Blood is stored in the Liver, it simultaneously detoxifies and nourishes the organ, soothing frustrations and stagnations while supporting decision making, imagination, and courage. When Guilt or Shame constantly thwart the ability to express one's self (tongue, Heart) or be one's authentic self (movement, Liver), this will always affect the proper production, storage, or circulation of Blood.

As already mentioned, Guilt prevents freedom of movement which depletes Blood from the tendons. In simple, acute cases this may present only as tendon tension (calf cramps, restless legs, jaw tension, etc.). When severe or chronic, more systemic Liver Blood Deficiency conditions (including delayed or scanty menses, amenorrhea, eye floaters, and headaches) will appear alongside the classic Blood Stasis of Guilt.

Shame's obstruction of Pride thwarts the ability to compassionately understand and love one's self, primarily impacting the Earth organs. Alongside the development of Dampness, this will affect the quality of Gu Qi that supports the creation of Blood, leading to acute symptoms of Spleen–Heart Blood Deficiency (anxiety, worry, insomnia, palpitations, etc.). In more severe conditions, the ongoing Deficiency will eventually 'dry out' the Spleen, Stomach, and Pancreas, leading to malabsorption or auto-immune conditions such as anemia, pancreatitis, diabetes, Celiac, and Crohn's disease.

CLIENT EXAMPLE

A bisexual-queer female in her mid 30s presents with uterine fibroids, ovarian cysts, and a history of pelvic pain starting in her late teens. The current pain is near right Zigong, sometimes bilateral. She has already had the left ovary removed, and is considering a full hysterectomy to address the pain. She exercises regularly, is average weight, and there are visible veins along her right hypochondriac region and both inner knees (near Liver 8–Spleen 10). She gets migraines at the start of her menstrual cycle, which is dark and clotted. Her pulse is slightly wiry, tongue is unremarkable. Overall complexion and skin tone are slightly pale. Japanese Acupuncture *Hara* (abdominal) palpation reveals a 'Cross Pattern' with tension and reaction along the right ribs, the left pelvis/ASIS area, and Stomach 25–27, especially on the right side where the pain is located. Ion cords are attached to needles at PC 6–SP 4 on the right, and SJ 5–GB 41 on the left. After five minutes, *Hara* symptoms are reduced by 10–20 percent. Needles are removed, and cords are taped to the skin on the opposite sides: SJ 5–GB 41 on the right, PC 6–SP 4 on the left. After another five minutes, there is no abdominal pain remaining, except for the right Zigong area, which is reduced by over 50 percent. After a month of weekly treatment, pain is consistently at 25 percent or less than before the first treatment; she also divulges the conservative religious upbringing that created extreme internal conflict for her as a child and teenager. Treatment shifts focus to the emotional root of Guilt and Repression related to gender and sexuality using a two-month course of Herbal Formulae (Shao Fu Zhu Yu Wan, Huo Luo Xiao Ling Wan), and Gemstone therapy (Amethyst, Hematite, Red Jasper, Sodalite, Sunstone). She is encouraged to get weekly massages during this time to continue unwinding physical stagnation, and seek talk therapy to determine areas of self-limitation. *Note: As this condition has been developing for well over a decade and Guilt and Repression are both present, symptoms are expected to recur during periods of stress.*

CLIENT EXAMPLE

Female in her mid-teens presents with anxiety and panic attacks that occur one to three times per week; they started six months ago. She is also obese (Middle and Lower Jiao focused), with secondary amenorrhea for the past eight months. The panic attacks happen in the afternoon and evening (not while at school); she is woken by her heart 'racing' occasionally. When asked about any stressors or life changes that occurred prior to onset of amenorrhea or panic attacks, the client looks down, shuffles her feet, gets red in the face, and says, 'No. Not really,' without looking up. She has no appetite for breakfast, doesn't eat much at school, but then snacks a lot at home before and after dinner. She has 'always been heavy and lazy,' reports her mother, but also divulges that her sister, mother, grandmother, and female cousins are all overweight. Her menstrual cycle started at age 12, after a short transition was regular for about two years, but had gotten irregular in timing (every 32–40 days) and color (brown mixed with red), with fatigue and extreme sugar cravings for about six months prior to stopping. She has thick vaginal discharge, slightly yellow but without odor. Her bowels are always loose, and sometimes urgent. Her complexion is pale, with rosy red cheeks. She complains of feeling very hot all the time, but her skin feels overall cool, and her legs below the knee are very cold with cold-sweaty feet. Pulse is slippery, weak, and thin; completely hidden in the right-rear position. Tongue is pale, swollen, tooth-marked, and slightly wet, with pale-thick-distended sublingual veins. She is diagnosed with Heart–Spleen–Kidney Yang Deficiency, Damp-Heat in the Lower and Middle Burners, and Heart and Liver Blood Deficiency–Stasis. She is treated weekly for two months using Acupuncture (SP 3, 6, 9, ST 36, 40, KI 3, Ren 4, 6, 12, 17, Du 20, Yintang) and Herbal Formulae (Bu Zhong Yi Qi Wan, Tao Hong Si Wu Wan, Tong Jing Wan) along with diet and exercise recommendations (eat breakfast, small meals, no dairy or processed foods, increased protein – especially red meat and beans; short walks or other easy, daily exercise). She is able to take the herbs and goes for a few walks, but she has been unable to make any diet changes that go against the family's eating habits. Instead of acknowledging the family's struggle to honor their daughter's needs, the mother comments, 'I just don't know what to do with her. She has to figure this out for herself.' The client's menses came for one day (brown, clotted, painful), but there was no change to the panic attacks. Acupuncture protocol changes to include the Ren (to nurture, stabilize, and combat Fear) and Chong Mai (to counteract *Li*). Herbs are switched to Liu Jun Zi Wan, Tao Hong Si Wu Wan, and Tian Wang Bu Xin Wan, with a Gemstone recommendation of Yellow Jade and Sunstone, and a diet recommendation of cooked oatmeal or rice with cinnamon and cardamom in the morning (instead of toast, butter, and cold orange juice). Her next menses is on time (28 days) with brighter red color and two solid days of flow, and her panic attacks were reduced to only two that month. *Note: Between her mother's derogatory comments and the client's posture (looking down, feet shuffling), it is assumed that this client's pathology contains a combination of Shame with Secrecy and/or Repression. Her symptoms may recur until she leaves her parent's home and finds self-acceptance.*

SUMMARY

» Starting at a very early age, Guilt and Shame are taught to reinforce *Li*, the Confucian concept of conforming to social expectations that are dictated by family and culture.

» Guilt is a value judgment of one's behavior: 'I did something – or want to do something – that is bad.' Shame, on the other hand, is a judgment on one's very existence: 'I am bad.' Shame is not reliant upon other people's perceptions or any actual behavior or Desire.

» Shame and Guilt are among the most difficult emotions to treat, requiring the dismantling and re-wiring of deep, subconscious-level belief structures that undermine the individual's ability to truly experience self-worth.

» There are three similarities between Shame and unprocessed Guilt: they both create Fluid Stasis, are both heavy and descending in nature, and may only present on the emotional or ephemeral level (ephemeral being defined as non-physical, fleeting, or come-and-go in nature). They can also appear together, or be masked by other factors like Constitution or Diet.

» Fluid Stasis itself is heavy and tends to sink. With gender and sexuality issues at the root, these conditions easily settle into the Lower Jiao and the *Jing*-Essence, and will likely impact the reproductive organs.

» Guilt impacts the Liver, Kidneys, and Heart, stemming from internalized cultural judgment of one's past, current, or anticipated behaviors. Guilt is like heavy chains that anchor and bind the body, limiting the free flow of the Heart, Upper *Dan Tian*, and the Shen-Spirit that supports self-knowledge.

» On a spiritual level Guilt 'binds' an individual at the moment where 'wrong' action took place, so patterns of emotional immaturity, naiveté, and generalized 'people-pleasing' behaviors are extremely likely. Further spiritual growth – such as through the steps of the Nine Palaces – is very unlikely, as *Li* will likely overrule any major life choices.

» Guilt prevents action and obstructs the movements of tendons, creating Qi Stagnation in the Liver. Chronic, unprocessed Guilt leads to Blood Stasis; when related to gender and sexuality issues, it will settle into the Lower Jiao. Blood Deficiency may co-exist with Blood Stasis, as Guilt's inability to move forward depletes Blood from the tendons, causing calf cramps, restless legs, jaw tension, etc.

» Shame is an internal form of judgment predominantly based in childhood lessons of morality. When an individual suffers from Shame, they will likely be putting effort into staying small, 'flying under the radar,' and remaining hidden from the view of others. Shame impacts the Heart and the Spleen, and is consistently paired with Self-Loathing, Secrecy or Lying, and periods of endless self-criticism. Phlegm is the primary Zang Fu pattern associated with chronic Shame.

» Shame creates a sense of helpless impotence that can psycho-spiritually 'freeze' a person at a moment in time and space, leading to an inability to 'move forward' either emotionally or physically, rooted in either Yang Deficiency or Cold.

» Shame's obstruction depletes the quality of Gu Qi and Heart Blood, leading to acute symptoms of Spleen–Heart Blood Deficiency. In severe, ongoing conditions, the Stomach, Pancreas, and immune system may also become involved, leading to malabsorption or auto-immune conditions such as anemia, pancreatitis, diabetes, Celiac, and Crohn's disease.

Chapter 13

TIED IN KNOTS
Secrecy and Repression

- Binding the Qi

- Living in Secrecy

- Locked by Repression

Secrecy is the purposeful withholding or concealment of information from others, typically done as a form of self-protection. A certain degree of secrecy in a person's life is actually healthy, such as with information regarding one's personal or sexual life. For anyone that must completely hide their authentic self in order to survive, however, Secrecy can easily become pathological. Secret-keeping is always associated with the emotion of Fear – fear of being discovered or 'found out' (see Chapter 10). Because of Fear, chronic Secrecy tends to impact the Kidneys and Lower Jiao; this is only emphasized in conditions related to gender or sexuality. Secrecy typically involves the act of Lying; i.e., telling others intentionally false information in order to protect the secret. Lying has strong correspondence to one's spoken and unspoken words, so there will likely be Heart, tongue, throat, and/or thyroid pathology combined with the Lower Jiao impact of Secrecy.

Repression is the act of subduing, inhibiting, or suppressing information. Whereas Secrecy involves 'external' dishonesty, Repression is a form of 'internal' dishonesty, where there is a purposeful disconnect between the unconscious, subconscious, and conscious states. As a Freudian ego-defense mechanism, Repression is used to cover up ideas, emotions, and memories by pushing them into the deep unconscious; it is a subconscious yet purposeful decision to 'never think of this again.' Repression operates without the individual's awareness to prevent thought, memory, and emotion from surfacing. By thwarting knowledge

267

of self and psycho-spiritual growth, Repression frequently incorporates aspects of Self-Loathing (see Chapter 15).

A repressed individual typically has no conscious awareness of holding back truth, so Repression does not necessarily involve the Lying and throat pathology so common in Secrecy. Instead, Repression impacts deeper 'necks' of the body, including the vaginal canal and cervix, the anus and prostate, and the cavities of the spine. In both Secrecy and Repression there is a personal quality or event that must be kept hidden, so it is expected that another emotion – i.e., Trauma, Shame, Guilt, Desire, or Craving – will be at the root of either presentation.

A life spent living in Secrecy or hiding in Repression is a life spent 'holding back,' which is an obvious reference to lack of free flow and the development of Qi Stagnation. The constant friction from Qi Stagnation strongly alters the overall Qi Mechanism, the Wood Element, and the San Jiao. The predominant pattern created by this triumvirate in the acute phase is Qi Stagnation-Heat. Due to the Wood Element, Secrecy or Repression will always include expression of Anger or Frustration: most commonly this presents as passive-aggressive behavior, especially for females or those with middle- or upper-class backgrounds where Anger is considered 'unacceptable' and therefore always subdued.

Physically, an individual suffering from Secrecy or Repression will be unable to move in some way. Extreme physical tension is common in the early phases, with Fluid Stasis and structural obstructions occurring in later stages. A lifetime of Secrecy and Repression will eventually manifest with one or more of the aptly named 'knotty' diseases of Chinese Medicine, deriving from extreme binding of Qi, Heat, and Fluids.

Marijuana for Secrecy and Repression

The Qi Stagnation of Secrecy or Repression responds well to small, regularly administered amounts of CBD oils (topical for musculoskeletal tension, internal for emotional pathology) and/or medical marijuana (such as THC micro-dosing). Administration methods should be cool or neutral in nature to avoid engendering more Heat, and dosage must be kept to a minimum effective level in order to prevent Phlegm accumulation or 'misting' the Mind.

BINDING THE QI

In the acute phase of either Secrecy or Repression, Qi becomes temporarily 'bound' in the Middle *Dan Tian* at the Qi-Emotion level of the Three Treasures. Primary initial impact is to the Stomach and Earth Element that are attempting to process and integrate the information, with secondary effects in the Heart, as it experiences all emotion. If a secret is kept or a thought repressed for a brief period of time, there will be only a mild impact from the flash of Fear, Anxiety, or Worry that accompanies the act of holding back. Any immediate physical sensations (such as palpitations, hiccups, belching, or 'butterflies in the stomach') will quickly resolve on their own, especially if the act of hiding is justified, such as when concealing information about a surprise birthday party or holding back a thought until a more appropriate social situation.

When a thought or emotion is hidden for a longer period of time, or in the case of a constitutional Fire or Earth weakness, the Stomach and Heart become 'knotted' by the unprocessed thought or emotion. In this situation, indigestion and palpitations will likely come and go whenever the topic arises to conscious level; for most people this resolves once the secret is told. The heavy knots around the Stomach and Heart are shown in Figure 13.1, but this is only the acute phase of Secrecy or Repression.

If Secrecy and Repression become chronic, knotting will transform the entire Middle Jiao, impacting the Qi Mechanism, the San Jiao, and the Wood Element organs. As the Earth Element is already struggling to process – i.e., transform and transport – the idea or event, the first consequence will likely be a Wood–Earth Disharmony. The phrases 'I cannot accept this' or 'sick to my stomach' both apply to the symptoms that can arise, including general indigestion, bloating, nausea, loss of appetite, and bowel disorders. Depending on Constitution and other emotional factors (especially Trauma and Self-Loathing), the pathology of Secrecy and Repression may stay focused in the Earth Element, manifesting in a variety of eating disorders that attempt to keep the hidden information 'stuffed down.'

The next phase of injury focuses on the Liver Excess that develops from Qi Stagnation. As the Liver corresponds to the tendons, symptoms of Secrecy and Repression will expand beyond the digestion, settling into the musculoskeletal channels associated with Wood Element pathology: Liver, Gallbladder, and San Jiao. For many individuals, acute digestive or heart palpitation symptoms cease as secrets are moved into these 'storage zones.' In the Gallbladder Channel, Secrecy tends to settle into the muscle groups around the neck and throat (jaw, occiput, sternocleidomastoid, trapezius, etc.), whereas Repression will present with tension in deeper and larger muscle groups such as the subscapularis, paraspinals, quadratus lumborum, or the IT band. In the Liver Channel along the inner aspect of the leg, Secrecy or Repression might cause calf cramps, restless legs, knee ligament pulls, and ilio-psoas tension. Regardless of location, any areas of musculoskeletal tension will require excessive nourishment to avoid injury, placing more demand on the supply of Liver Blood. Very quickly the combination of inhibited Qi flow, physical tension, Anger or frustration, and Liver Blood Deficiency will lead to pain, decreased movement, and increasing Excess and Empty Heat levels.

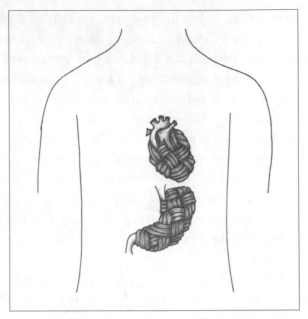

Figure 13.1: Bound Qi – Middle Dan Tian

Because of pain and decreased movement, stagnation will eventually spread throughout the body, but the primary pattern of Qi Stagnation-Heat will predominate in all conditions. William Maclean (2017) has established a 'Primary Pathological Triad' (PPT) theory that describes a 'catch-22' phenomenon of Liver Qi Stagnation, Spleen Yang/Qi Deficiency, and Heat from constraint, which Maclean describes as 'three patterns of pathology that frequently occur simultaneously, are tightly interlinked and mutually engendering.' Secrecy or Repression involves Earth Deficiency, Wood Excess, Qi Stagnation, and Heat pathology just like in Maclean's PPT diagram, shown here as Figure 13.2.

Maclean's theory demonstrates how Fluid Stasis and/or Deficiency patterns arise from Qi Stagnation-Heat and Earth dysfunction. In conditions related to Secrecy and Repression, fluid pathology will strongly impact the Liver and Gallbladder first, and through their channels affect the San Jiao and the Dai Mai. In an attempt to rectify the Qi Mechanism, Qi will be diverted from other organs, leading to multiple organ deficiency patterns before manifesting mixed Excess–Deficiency patterns. It is extremely common in Secrecy or Repression to also find an East–West Trauma pattern due to the Middle Jiao stagnation and San Jiao involvement. Figure 13.3 shows the results of long-term Secrecy or Repression, where the entire body becomes energetically bound by inward-pulling obstruction, leading to an inability to 'move' physically, emotionally, or spiritually.

Inability to move will allow the internal 'knotting' to fester. Because of the Heat and Fluid impact from Qi Stagnation, toxic levels of internal Damp-Heat can form, leading to chronic inflammatory conditions and some of the 'knottiest' contemporary medical conditions. In cases of long-term Secrecy and Repression, one might see fibromyalgia, chronic fatigue, rheumatoid arthritis, Graves' disease, scleroderma, or various cancers.

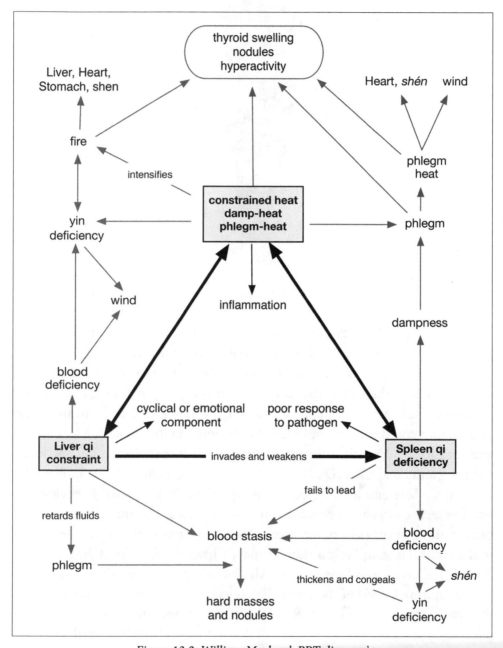

Figure 13.2: William Maclean's PPT diagram[1]

---

1   Reproduced from Maclean and Taylor (2016) with permission of Eastland Press.

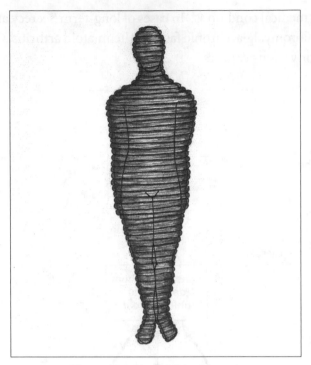

Figure 13.3: Bound Qi – Systemic

For most people, Secrecy and Repression are used as coping mechanisms in reaction to the *Li* of one's culture (the only common exception is with early childhood Trauma). As the Liver Channel moves internally from the base of the ribcage into the Upper Jiao cavity, it can easily deposit the Qi Stagnation of unprocessed Secrecy or Repression among the Lung, Pericardium, and Heart organs. Intercostal and/or diaphragmatic tension, shallow breathing tendencies, and occasional heart palpitations are indicative of Liver Qi Stagnation impacting the Lung and *Zong*/Chest Qi. For those coming from conservative families with conditional love and high expectations regarding duty, 'proper' behavior, and obedience, Secrecy and Repression can also manifest as childhood or early-adult onset asthma or other respiratory conditions. Any physical obstructions found in the Heart, Lung, or Pericardium Primary Channels may reflect the long-term presence of Secrecy and Repression, which could also impact the emotional or psycho-spiritual levels of the Upper Jiao organs. This is shown in Table 13.1 by the traditional levels of external disease penetration, but any organ could be affected by the penetration of Liver Qi depending on Constitutional weakness or other factors.

Table 13.1: Psycho-spiritual Impact to the Upper Jiao

Channel	Action	Consequence	Likely pathology
Lung	Release *'I will let go of this, slowly.'*	Leaking Qi	*Lung*: All respiratory *LI*: IBS (diarrhea or constipation type), ulcerative colitis
Pericardium	Adaptation *'I will learn to live with it.'*	Enemy within	Auto-immune conditions, cancer
Heart	Change, Metamorphosis *'I will become someone else.'*	Denial of Shen-Spirit and Destiny	'Numbing'/escapist behavior Psychiatric: Bipolar, dissociative identity disorder (multiple personality), etc.

Because of the innate human desire to 'fit in' with one's culture, resistance to root treatment is commonplace. Rather than attempting aggressive Acupuncture or Herbal Formulae that could break up stagnation before a client is emotionally ready, Qigong, Essential Oils, and Gemstone therapy are encouraged to help memories, thoughts, or ideas 'come out of latency' to the conscious state at the client's own pace. Individuals will likely experience waves of Grief and Sadness as Secrecy and Repression are cleared; clinical experience thus far indicates this is associated with the 'lost time' to live authentically. Talk therapy with a licensed professional is strongly recommended for additional support. The following are basic treatment suggestions for Secrecy or Repression in their acute phase, or when it is difficult to discern the two aspects.

- Treatment Principles: Harmonize Wood–Earth (i.e., Course Liver Qi, Tonify Spleen Qi), Clear Channel obstructions (i.e., Gallbladder, Liver, Lung, Heart, and/or Pericardium – *as applicable*), Clear Heat, Nourish Blood, Harmonize the San Jiao.

Primary Modalities

- Acupuncture: LV 2, 3, 8, 13, 14, LI 4, 11, ST 36, Ren 6, 12, SP 3, 6, GB 21, 34, 38, Du 20, UB 17, 18, 19, 20, 21, 22, 60:

  – Combinations: Four Gates (LV 3–LI 4); utilize points in all three Jiao

  – Ahsi channel points with 'Above and Below' technique for full resolution (see Figure 5.6)

– Points along the Chong Mai (Spleen 4, Spleen 12, etc.) for any issue related to *Li* (Yuen 2017a).

- Herbal Formulae: Jia Wei Xiao Yao Wan, Chai Hu Long Gu Mu Li Wan, Xiao Chai Hu Wan.

- Cupping: Flash to break up stagnation – *especially useful for large tendons (hamstrings and IT band), chest, and intrascapular areas.*

- Medical Qigong: Counterclockwise outward circling over applicable areas to disperse Heat and Stagnation. *Note of caution: Extreme Heat can increase likelihood of transference.*

Secondary Modalities

- Tuina: Vibrations to break up deep stagnations; Pressing, rolling, or other applicable technique for tension areas (often best combined with Cupping).

- Essential Oils: Chamomile, Lavender, Lemon, Peppermint, Rose, Vetiver.

- Gemstones: Blue Calcite, Blue Lace Agate, Chrysoprase, Rainforest Jasper, Malachite, Obsidian (Black, Rainbow), Phrenite, Seraphinite, Tourmaline.

- Qigong: Gathering the Rice; Five Animal Frolics–Crane; Sheng Zhen Qigong: Heaven Nature/Kuan Yin Standing–Traveling Eastward Across the Ocean; Butterfly.

- Lifestyle: Regular, full body exercise to move Qi (walking, running, dancing, Yoga, etc.); Cooling Foods, small meals, eating without stress; talk therapy or mental health counseling.

Secrecy and Repression create Qi Stagnation-Heat that impacts the Qi Mechanism, the Wood and Earth Elements, and the San Jiao. Initial symptoms include digestive issues and mild eating disorders, musculoskeletal tension, pain, and decreasing capacity for physical movement. Long-term complications include respiratory conditions, auto-immune conditions, mental illness, cancer, and various 'knotty diseases.'

LIVING IN SECRECY

Examples of long-term patterns of Secrecy are found in young queer people that hide their gender identity and sexuality, polyamorous adults with lovers in distant places so the 'neighbors don't find out,' and sex abuse survivors that never tell a soul what happened. On top of the impact from the acute stages discussed above, Secrecy relates to Water and the emotion of Fear (see Chapter 10), to the Fire Element through spoken (or unspoken) words and desires, and to Earth with issues of self-acceptance. When Fear impacts the ability to breathe deeply through the Lung–Kidney Axis, there may be evidence of more extreme and long-standing Liver and Lung Qi Stagnation-Heat patterns as well.

Throat obstruction occurs more often in individuals that must frequently lie, without any safe space (community, friends, etc.) in which they can ever be truthful. Constant 'twisting' of truth creates other twisted shapes in the energetic field, easily altering the flow of Qi and Fluids. Counter-flow Qi or insubstantial Phlegm conditions result from this perversity; these most commonly affect the throat but could also settle into the Heart, Jing-Essence, or Sea of Marrow. Figure 13.4 shows the binding of Qi Stagnation-Heat affecting the throat area, creating shoulder and neck tension, occipital headaches, thyroid concerns, and improper flow to and from the head channels and the Sea of Marrow. It is important to note that the binds of Figure 13.3 still exist, but the constant lies create more pronounced Qi Stagnation and Phlegm at this juncture of the Upper Jiao.

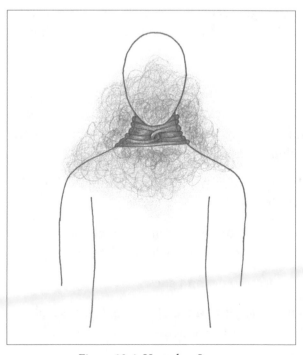

Figure 13.4: Unspoken Issues

The person suffering from Secrecy is subconsciously terrified to move lest their secrets be freed. Fear always 'holds' more tightly than patterns of Qi Stagnation or Qi Stagnation-Heat, so a physical pain condition is inevitable. Because of the intense Heat, pain may still be able to move or come-and-go, such as with menstrual cramps, IBS, or arthritis. Fear can easily contribute to counter-flow Qi patterns as well, causing belching, hiccups, nausea/vomiting, anxiety/panic attacks. Fear tends to affect the Lower Jiao, so the counter-flow Qi and insubstantial Phlegm could impact both proper flow and 'shape' of Jing-Essence. Altering the course of Jing may cause changes in the overall libido (affecting arousal and orgasm), but the alteration of shape can actually transform the specifics of a person's sexual desires. Examples of libido 'twists' stemming from internalized Secrecy and Repression include female bi/pansexual survivors of sexual assault that choose only some-sex relationships, as well as gay men or lesbians that had once spent years in 'happy' heterosexual marriages before freeing themselves.

Any counter-flow Qi or Phlegm condition will reinforce Secrecy by creating more Qi obstruction and Heat, leading to increasing Yin Deficiency and Stasis. Dampness and Phlegm will obstruct the Earth Element even further, easily twisting self-acceptance issues into forms of self-abuse through food and drink, such as over-eating, binging, and excessive alcohol intake to help 'stuff' one's secrets. Secrecy and Lying are not easily admitted to by clients, but unlike Repression *the client is aware of their secrets*. Resistance to the truth is likely, so a cautious approach is mandated. Talk therapy with a licensed professional combined with daily Qigong exercises and Essential Oil or Gemstone application to 'come out' is strongly recommended. Treatment suggestions listed under 'Bound Qi' should be combined with some of the following suggestions.

- Typical Presentation:
  - Upper Jiao: Shortness of breath/inability to breathe deeply without concentration, neck/shoulder/jaw tension, headaches, throat/thyroid, 'plum pit qi,' anxiety, insomnia, mental confusion/'brain fog'/mild dementia states, sinus congestion

  - Middle Jiao: Digestive upsets, bloating, nausea, IBS, 'stuffing' food and/or drink

  - Lower Jiao: Strong/poor libido, changing sexual desires, cramps or bloating with menstruation or ovulation

  - Pain: Moves, comes and goes.

- Treatment Principles: Move Qi, Clear Heat, Resolve Phlegm, Support Water, Fire, and Earth Elements.

- Acupuncture:

  - Water: KI 3, 10, Du 4, 20, 24, UB 23, 52

  - Fire: Ren 17, HT 5, 6, 7, PC 6, Yintang, Du 24, UB 14, 15, 43, 44

  - Earth: ST 8, 36, SP3, 6, 9, Ren 12, UB 20, 21, 49, 50

  - Windows of the Sky for issues related to Lying (Yuen 2017a).

- Herbal Formulae: Ban Xia Hou Po Wan, Er Chen Wan, Bu Nao Wan, Pe Min Kan Wan.

- Medical Qigong: Counterclockwise outward circling targeting the throat area.

- Gemstones: Amber, Amethyst, Blue Beryl/Aquamarine, Blue Aventurine, Blue Chalcedony, Blue Tiger Eye, Blue Topaz, Cavansite, Lapis Lazuli, Larimar/Pectolite, Sodalite, Sunstone, Zircon.

- Qigong: Passing Clouds.

- Lifestyle: Client must be advised to start speaking their truth, even if this is painful. Journaling and talk therapy are both useful tools.

Secrecy and Lying – the Basics

Five Elements: Water, Fire, Earth

Emotions: Fear, self-acceptance

Pathology: 'Twisting' of truth – Counter-flow Qi, Phlegm

Primary impact: Upper Jiao – Throat, Diaphragm; Lower Jiao – Libido, Menses

Pain: Moves, comes and goes

LOCKED BY REPRESSION

The Qi Stagnation-Heat of Repression is internally bound at the deepest levels, where Heat thickens fluids and purposefully stagnates Yin to 'lock' memories, thoughts, or desires at the subconscious level. The 'stuffing' of food and drink that was mentioned under Secrecy is even more likely in Repression, along with more serious eating disorders (obesity, bulimia, anorexia, etc.). When Repression combines with this type of Earth Element dysfunction, bigger issues of self-worth, self-acceptance, and Self-Loathing are usually at play (see Chapter 15). As the body is constantly 'full' from Repression, poor digestion and difficulty accepting new circumstances, environments, or people are likely to coincide with other symptoms.

Unlike Secrecy, the pain found with Repression will not be able to move or come and go. Because of the Fluid Stasis, pain will be fixed and may feel swollen or distended (subjective or objective). The combination of Fluid Stasis and Heat can cause poor circulation, extreme temperature fluctuations, and Desire for Cold with avoidance of Heat (environmental, food and drink, etc.). As Repression is a subconscious level activity, it affects the deepest regions, including the lymphatic system, bones, and cellular structures. It also creates 'hidden' illnesses – those that are not easy to identify in the early stages without advanced medical testing – including diabetes, cholesterol plaques, auto-immune conditions, and cancer. As Repression involves complete obstruction of thought patterns and memories, it is also a contributor to many mental health concerns, including bipolar disorder, schizophrenia, Alzheimer's and other forms of dementia. Figure 13.5 shows the deeply bound nature of Repression, where the binds have sunken inward, creating stagnation at the core of the body. This does not negate the more external binds found in Figure 13.3, as the chronically Repressed individual typically has both internal and external bindings.

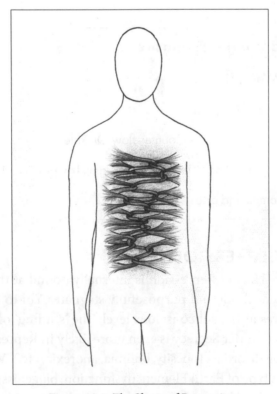

Figure 13.5: The Shape of Repression

At an emotional level, Repression is often at the root of Depressive conditions. As Leon Hammer wrote, Depression is 'a form of mourning throughout the life cycle for part of the self which is spiritually and physically dying from repression' (2005, p.292). It takes energy to maintain the internal binds of Repression, thereby depleting the individual's overall capacity for excitement and curiosity.

When Repression is connected to both Self-Loathing (see Chapter 15) and Craving (see Chapter 14), the deep Qi Stagnation-Heat can also transform into Toxic Fire. This Fire will more quickly deplete and stagnate fluids, likely forming both extreme Blood Stasis and Phlegm. The combination of internal Toxic Fire, Yin Deficiency–Empty Heat, Qi and Blood Stagnation, and Phlegm can create some major health concerns, including malignant and quickly metastasizing cancers. Because of Repression's deeply subconscious nature, any cancerous development would arise at the deepest level: the Bone. The Bone level includes the potential for lymphatic, skeletal, blood, or bone marrow involvement, but when associated with gender and sexuality it could also settle into the Curious Organs of the uterus, cervix, ovaries or prostate. Figure 13.6 shows the burning flames of Craving bound up in the knot of Repression, keeping their combined Heat firmly tucked into the Lower Jiao. Clearly the Middle and Upper Jiao may also show signs of Heat due to 'steam' rising upward, but these will be mild in comparison to the Heat in the Lower Jiao.

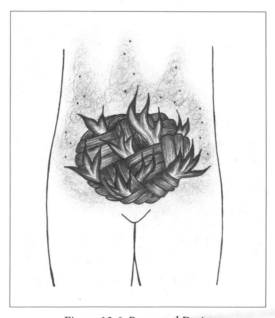

Figure 13.6: Repressed Desire

Repression is hidden from the client experiencing it, so by its very nature it will be resistant to treatment. The first obstacle is to help release the Repression so that the client can recognize their own self-imposed etiology and work together with the practitioner as a team. As already discussed, at-home treatment (Qigong exercises, Essential Oils, Gemstone therapy) to help bring memories and desires 'out of latency' to the conscious state are highly recommended. Herbal Formulae and Medical Qigong are typically better than Acupuncture to penetrate the deep layers and assist with release. As Repression is released, other emotions are likely to unexpectedly rise to the surface, so root treatment must be approached slowly and talk therapy with a licensed professional is strongly recommended to prevent transference. Treatment principles are also likely to dramatically change as treatment progresses, so any course of treatment must be re-evaluated frequently (once a month or more). Treatment suggestions listed in the first section of this chapter can be combined with the following suggestions.

- Typical Presentation: Poor digestion (easily full, bloating) excess weight, eating disorders, difficulty with new situations, physical pain (swollen, fixed), poor circulation or temperature issues (unusual hot flashes, night sweats); may also present with diabetes, elevated cholesterol, inflammatory or auto-immune conditions, Alzheimer's/dementia, bi-polar, schizophrenia, cancer.

- Treatment Principles: Move Qi, Clear Heat (Disperse and Cool Toxic Fire *as applicable*), Break Blood Stasis, Resolve Phlegm.

Primary Modalities

- Herbal Formulae: Si Ni Wan, Jia Wei Xiao Yao Wan, Xue Fu Zhu Yu Wan, Huang Lian Jie Du Wan, Long Dan Xie Gan Wan, Bi Xie Sheng Shi Wan.

- Medical Qigong: Holding (hands on or off) to access deep levels; counterclockwise outward circling to disperse Heat and Stagnation. *Note: Extreme Heat can increase likelihood of transference.*

- Qigong, Gemstones – *see earlier suggestions under 'Binding the Qi' and 'Living in Secrecy.'*

Secondary Modalities

- Acupuncture: LV 2, 3, LI 4, 11, PC 8, HT 8, UB 17, 18, 43, SP 10, ST 36, 40, 44.

- Cupping, Tuina, Essential Oils – *see earlier suggestions under 'Binding the Qi' and 'Living in Secrecy.'*

- Lifestyle: Referral to a mental health professional is likely necessary once the 'binds' start to release; cardiovascular exercise to help increase circulation and disperse Heat; cooling, Blood-moving, or Phlegm-clearing foods *as applicable*.

Repression – The Basics

Five Elements: Wood, Earth

Emotions: Self-Loathing, Desire/Craving, difficulty accepting 'new'

Pathology: 'Stuffing' memory, thought, or Desire; Internally bound Heat

Primary Impact: Deep level: bone; Risk of 'hidden' disease

Pain: Fixed, swollen

CLIENT EXAMPLE

An asexual queer female in her mid 20s was diagnosed with precancerous cervical cell abnormalities via PAP smear and tissue sampling (CIN 3). She also complains of neck and shoulder tension, stress headaches, teeth grinding, depression stemming from seasonal affective disorder, and general inflexibility (she recently started Yoga classes for stress). Her periods are dark, clotted, and painful. She is also vegetarian and admits she drinks 'a lot' of coffee. Pulses are wiry overall, slightly thin on the left. Tongue is swollen and curled on the sides ('taco' shape) with a thin yellow, greasy coat overall, large red dots on the sides, and pale-distended sublingual veins. She is diagnosed with Liver Qi Stagnation-Heat, Blood Deficiency–Stasis, and Damp-Heat in the Lower Jiao with probable stagnation of Jing-Essence due to Repression. She is treated with both Acupuncture (Ren 2, 3, ST 26–28, LV 2, 3, 8, SP 9, 10, ST 40, GB 21, 34, 40, Du Mai, Dai Mai) and Herbal Formulae (Jia Wei Xiao Yao Wan, Tao Hong Si Wu Wan, Yu Dai Wan). She is also given recommendations to stop or reduce coffee and caffeine intake due to Heat, and to replace it with peppermint or jasmine green tea to clear Heat and Dampness. Qigong exercises (Hun Yuan Gong–Grinding the Corn; Sinking the Turbid and Washing the Organs; Gathering the Rice) and Gemstone therapy (Rainbow Obsidian, Hematite) are prescribed at the second appointment. *Note: Pre-cancerous state at this age with no family history indicates probable stagnation of Jing-Essence due to Repression. Based on the patterns and symptoms, there are likely elements of Guilt and Self-Loathing in her etiology; any deeper emotions will naturally clarify once Repression begins to lift.*

CLIENT EXAMPLE

A lesbian female in her late 40s presents with a 10+ year history of irregular PAP smears and an acute, fluid-filled cervical cyst. The cyst was recently drained but is still causing pain with sex and orgasm. She also has yellow, mild-odorous vaginal secretions (for over one year), and menstrual irregularities (light color and flow, mild abdominal bloating immediately prior, and mild cramping). She also has carpal tunnel and brachial plexus concerns due to excessive computer use (numbness of arms and fingers that comes and goes). She clears her throat many times during the interview, and when asked about her personal/sex life she purses her lips, talks slowly, and crosses her arms. She confides that she is not 'out' at work, her female partner is polyamorous and dating other people. Pulse is wiry, slippery, and rapid. Tongue is pink-red, peeled overall with a thin yellow coat at the rear. She is diagnosed with Toxic Damp-Heat in the Lower Jiao, Liver Qi Stagnation, and Yin Deficiency–Empty Heat due to Secrecy. She is treated primarily with Herbal Formulae for almost three months: Long Dan Xie Gan Wan, Bi Xie Sheng Shi Wan, Zhi Bai Di Huang Wan, and Yin Care (vaginal douche). Symptoms improve dramatically in two weeks, continuing to slowly improve over the next two months. She abruptly stops treatment because she says she no longer 'feels right' after taking herbs. *Note: Chronic and extreme Repression are involved in this case, so other emotions are likely to unexpectedly rise to the surface (especially Shame, Fear, and the Emotional Stress of pre-Trauma). Increased incidence of projection and/or sudden termination of treatment is always possible.*

SUMMARY

»   Secrecy and Repression are commonly used to cope with the *Li* of culture, such as with hidden gender identity, abuse history, relationship or sexual preferences. As there is always a personal quality or incident to be concealed, another emotion – such as Trauma, Shame, Guilt, Desire, or Craving – will be revealed through treatment.

»   In the acute phase of Secrecy or Repression, Qi becomes temporarily 'bound' in the Middle *Dan Tian* at the Qi-Emotion level of the Three Treasures. Primary initial impact is to the Stomach and Earth Element that are attempting to process and integrate the information, with secondary effects in the Heart as it experiences all emotion. Because of the impact on Earth organs, both Secrecy and Repression are associated with digestive complaints, eating disorders, and 'hidden' diseases.

» Secrecy and Repression both inhibit energetic and emotional movement, and can result in physical pain conditions. Pain associated with Secrecy is able to move, or come and go. Repression pain will be fixed, and may feel subjectively swollen.

» Secrecy relates to Water and the emotion of Chronic Fear (see Chapter 10), to the Fire Element through spoken (or unspoken) words and desires, and to Earth with issues of self-acceptance. Secrecy commonly presents with Lying and its associated throat pathology.

» Repression is the act of subduing, inhibiting, or suppressing information. It is an 'internal' dishonesty, with purposeful disconnect between the unconscious, subconscious, and conscious states in order to 'never think of this again.'

» Repression can easily manifest as Depression. It takes energy to maintain Repression's internal binds, which depletes overall capacity for excitement and curiosity.

» The Qi Stagnation-Heat of Repression is internally bound at the deepest levels, where Heat thickens fluids and purposefully stagnates Yin to 'lock' memories, thoughts, or desires into the subconscious. Repression can manifest as a 'hidden' or 'knotty' disease at the Bone level or in the deep 'necks' of the body.

Chapter 14

SCORCHING THE SELF
Desire and Craving

- Five Elements of Desire

- Heat and Wind

- Cooling the Flames

What is the Noble Truth of Suffering? Birth is suffering, aging is suffering, sickness is suffering, dissociation from the loved [one] is suffering, not to get what one wants is suffering: in short the five categories affected by clinging are suffering.

– The First Noble Truth of Buddhism[1]

Desire, at its most basic, is an attraction to an experience or thing that is stimulated through touch, sight, sound, or emotion. As all emotions are a fast-moving form of Qi, Desire can easily transform from 'Oh, isn't that interesting?' into 'I want it right now!' Any form of Desire is healthy and natural when it is allowed to arise, be satisfied, and resolve. Examples of the healthy flow of Desire include eating foods that entice with their aroma, feeling the cool ocean waters on a hot day, or kissing a beloved out of joyous connection.

Desire and Craving share the same root, and are the same in many aspects. They are both forms of the Buddhist concept of 'clinging,' the action of tightly holding on to something with persistence, stubbornness, or unhealthy dependence. Craving is a more intense – *and always pathological* – version of Desire. Craving is a chronically unresolved, unsatisfied Desire that an individual

---

1   As quoted in Sumedho 2011, p.12.

maintains well beyond any reasonable period of time. By their relation to clinging, Desire and Craving are warned against by the three major philosophies that have contributed to Chinese Medicine: Buddhism, Confucianism, and Daoism all consider clinging to be the root of human suffering.

As Thich Nhat Hanh wrote:

> The first step in the art of transforming suffering is to come home to our suffering and recognize it… If we try to use consumption to ignore or distract ourselves from our suffering, we end up making the suffering worse. We turn on the television. We talk or text or gossip on the phone. We get on the Internet. We find ourselves in front of the refrigerator over and over again… [D]istractions not only fail to help heal the underlying suffering, they may contain stories or images that feed our craving, jealousy, anger, or despair. Instead of making us feel better, they numb us only briefly, then make us feel worse. To consume in order to cover up our suffering doesn't work. We need a spiritual practice to have the strength and skill to look deeply into our suffering, to get insight into it and make a breakthrough. (2014, pp.22–23)

Both frustrated Desire and Craving run rampant internationally, but they seem most pervasive in capitalist countries where intensive advertising *purposefully stimulates* Desire. Desire or Craving can be oriented toward many things, including sex, material objects, and achievement of status or relationship. Within the DGS communities, pathological Desire or Craving is often found in intense desperation for acceptance, or the unsatisfied yearnings of the Shen-Spirit. Fear, Shame, Guilt, Repression, Secrecy (with Lying), and/or Self-Loathing are other emotions that commonly present alongside Craving.

In any healthy state of sexual, intellectual, or spiritual Desire, the *Ming Men* Fire stirs the Jing-Essence and Yang aspect of Kidney energy. This Water Yang activity stimulates the direction, focus, imagination, and courage of the Wood Element to go after and satisfy the attraction. The Heat from *Ming Men* Fire will also follow the mind's intention to the source of attraction. For example, in a case of sexual Desire, the flow of *Ming Men* Fire will stimulate the Jing-Essence, Kidney Yang, and the Wood Element, but will also flow strongly into the genital region and the Liver Channel (see Chapter 6). With intellectual or spiritual Desire, the *Ming Men* Fire will more strongly stimulate the Sea of Marrow through the Du Mai.

When Desire is frustrated, *Ming Men* Fire continues to stir the Lower Jiao, but it is thwarted from proper movement and instead must 'brew' there. In a temporary situation, Desire is eventually satisfied and the excess Heat is released or dispersed. When Desire remains chronically unsatisfied, Heat continues to build, congealing fluids in the Lower Jiao until some of the Heat 'escapes' through the *Bao Mai* to the Heart and Pericardium. In the Upper Jiao, the excess Heat scatters[2] the Qi of the Heart and harasses the Shen-Spirit. Signs and symptoms associated with chronically frustrated Desire reflect the impact of *Ming Men* Fire on the Heart and Pericardium: palpitations, reddish face, insomnia, dry mouth/thirst, and mental-emotional restlessness (irritability, anxiety, mild mania), with a reddish tongue – especially at the tip. This is where Desire has begun to transform into the state of Craving. The most common Zang Fu patterns associated with this are Heart Fire or Heart Yin Deficiency–Empty Heat.

Chronic states of Desire or Craving can arise on their own through lack of mindful self-control, or they can be created by other chronic states that obstruct Qi movement and increase Heat in the Lower Jiao, including Extraordinary Vessel damage (from premature sex, sexual assault, etc.), Fear, Shame, Guilt, Secrecy, and Repression. The extreme Heat of chronic Craving will eventually unsettle the *Wu Shen* of both Wood and Fire Elements, stir up internal Wind, and can impact the overall alignment of the Qi Mechanism and the Five Elements if not properly managed. This disharmony can even become self-engendering when the stagnant Heat in the Lower Jiao is *never* fulfilled or resolved; instead it continues to stir the *Ming Men* Fire, building more and more Heat, resulting in further dissatisfaction and Craving.

To resolve chronic tendencies toward Craving, the most important treatment modality is mental restraint: the client must be encouraged to take charge of their own thought patterns on a daily basis through mindful and forgiving re-direction away from the intense feeling, while steadily cultivating a more calm and peaceful existence away from attraction triggers. As the Buddhist monk Ajahn Sumedho wrote, 'Desire has power over us and deludes us only as long as we grasp it, believe in it and react to it' (2011, p.30).

Notes on the *Tongue*

The reddish tongue tip found in states of Desire and Craving is actually quite common. It can reflect a Desire for more love among those looking for relationships (see Chapter 8), a consensual delay in sexual satisfaction such as found in long-distance relationships or BDSM dynamics, or it may reflect exposure to intensive advertising and material-wealth-based consumerism. The reddish color and any fine or large red dots may also come and go depending on ever-changing levels of frustration and satisfaction.

---

2   Giovanni Maciocia (2013, p.294) used the term 'scatter' instead of 'disperse' to describe the effect on Heart Qi. Desire and Craving are both Heat conditions that affect the Fire Organs, so the Heart Qi can dissipate extremely quickly and even mimic a mild form of emotional Shock. I agree that 'scatter' seems more appropriate due to the speed of action implied.

> **Notes on the *Pulse***
>
> The pulse of Desire or Craving is traditionally thought of as excess – large, rapid, tight, wiry – in the right-rear position. This aligns well with the theory of *Ming Men* Fire being stirred to vex the Pericardium. In clinical practice, however, the Heat from any ongoing Desire or Craving easily depletes the fluids, creating a mixed presentation of Yin or Blood Deficiency with Excess and Empty Heat. Evidence of this can be found anywhere in the pulse, but especially in the middle and front-left positions due to simultaneous involvement of Wood and Fire Elements. It may also present in the left-rear position if Kidney Yin is being used to balance Wood or Fire.

FIVE ELEMENTS OF DESIRE

The focus of this chapter is the pathology of unresolved or unfettered Desire and Craving, but what about when Desire is *lacking*? Each of the Five Elements interact in the development of *healthy* sexual Desire and deserve recognition for their contributions. Two of the Elements have the greatest impact on sexual Desire: Fire and Water.

Without a healthy presence of Fire (i.e., general Yang energy, including *Ming Men* Fire), it will be very difficult for any Heat to build: any sexual Desire is likely to be fleeting or wane very easily. A client suffering from lack of Fire may even identify as Asexual (see Chapter 7). When Fire is lacking, Desire can be supported through the use of warming foods (shrimp, lamb, walnuts, red wine, etc.) and mild substance use (see text box). On the other hand, excessive Fire (i.e., general Yang energy) can lead to intensified or unfettered Desire, an overall tendency toward Craving, and little to no regard for social norms: a clear example of Fire 'melting' Metal (see 'Cooling the Flames' for treatment options).

Without a healthy presence of Water (i.e., overall Kidney energy, including *Ming Men* Fire), it will be difficult for Heat to stir or impact other systems. Again, sexual Desire may be present, but likely to easily wane. In this case Desire is best supported through rest and self-care routines to rebuild Water energetics. Excess Water Yang can promote a very strong sex drive; this creates pathology and symptoms when there is too much sexual activity for the person's current state of health (see Chapter 6). Excess Yin, however, can dampen the flames of Desire, requiring warming practices like cardiovascular exercise or Moxa therapy to help counteract these effects.

Two other Elements are responsible for ensuring the strength of one's personal boundaries during sexual exploration: Metal and Earth. Any attempt by the Metal Element to temper Desire with reason and sound judgment reflects the Confucian ideal of order and ritual, *Li*. But these choices must also be based in self-knowledge and self-acceptance, the products of healthy Earth. Both Metal and Earth need to be relaxed enough to allow for experimentation and growth, yet strong enough to identify areas of social or personal hazard before engaging in any specific activity.

The Earth Element sits at the center of the two axes, in charge of integrating Desire, mitigating emotion and cultural mores, and making sure that sexual activity is in alignment with one's capacity for self-acceptance. When Earth is strong, self-acceptance will be too, so Metal will allow the individual to choose sexual activity in relation to *their own* rules of conduct. When Earth is weak however, self-acceptance will be diminished and Metal unsupported, so Metal will act from either deficiency or stagnation.

In a deficient state, Metal will not be able to maintain healthy boundaries, so attention to social rules and concern for personal safety may wane, allowing boundaries to be violated. Metal is also easily injured by the Grief and Sadness of not getting what one wants, so this is a common complication of chronic Craving. If Metal stagnates because of weakened Earth, Metal will prioritize the rules of culture over one's own preferences, putting stricter limits on sexual exploration that may increase internal frustration and contribute to Self-Loathing, Shame, or Repression. If Metal stagnates for another reason, such as Liver Qi Stagnation with Wood insulting Metal, healthy Fire is critical to help soften Metal through the control cycle. When Metal is chronically stagnant, however, Desire has to burn intensely to overcome the extreme rigidity. As noted, mild substance use can help soften the obstacles brought on by stagnant Metal in these situations.

It is worthy to also take note of the Wood Element, which is stimulated by the Heat of sexual Desire through the genitals and Liver Channel. The Heat of Desire spurs the Wood Element to engage in sexual activity with direction and courage. If Wood becomes deficient, Desire may still be present, but there may not be enough courage to pursue it. When sexual activity is consistently thwarted – by *Li*, stagnant Metal, or by any deficiency of Fire, Water, or Wood – the Heat stirred by Desire will settle into the Liver or Gallbladder creating enduring stagnation, Fire, and Damp-Heat conditions. For this reason, frustrated Desire and Craving are consistently associated with stubborn Wood pathology, such as frequent herpes outbreaks and gallstones.

Figure 14.1 shows the interaction of Five Elements in supporting healthy sexual Desire. Wood is the element of *action*, providing direction and courage to engage and initiate. Fire is the element of *stability* in maintaining focused Desire over a period of time. Metal is the element of *guidance*, helping align Desire with reason, self-knowledge, and *Li*. Water is the element of *engagement*, providing the foundation for Desire and sexual energy. Earth is again shown at the center, as it is the element of *integration*, including acceptance of one's Desires (physical, emotional, and spiritual). It is also the element in charge of creating Post-Natal Qi, which provides the day-to-day energy that dictates one's ability to form Desire or to participate in sex.

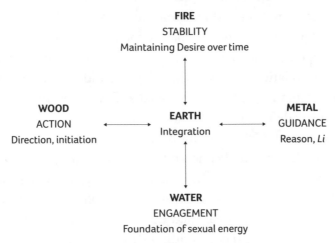

Figure 14.1: Five Elements of Sexual Desire

Desire, Craving and Substance Use

Alcohol and other mind-altering substances have a warming nature that stimulates internal Heat. Increase in internal Fire will warm and soften the cool nature of Metal so that reason, judgment, or rigid belief structures (i.e., the *Li* of culture) become more flexible. Substance-derived Heat also directly warms the Liver Organ and its channel that 'winds' the genitals, stirring the *Ming Men* Fire and stimulating sexual Desire. Warming Metal and Wood is one reason that casual 'hook-ups' and sexual exploration with one's partner are sometimes more easily engaged in when substances are involved. Substance use may even be a subconscious attempt at self-treatment in lieu of therapeutic counseling or other management strategies. Clients must be warned that although minimal substance use can be beneficial for relaxing the Metal Element, excessive use increases Heat and may lead to a combination of Craving and Shame.

HEAT AND WIND

As stated above, Desire is a healthy and natural emotional state when it is able to rise and easily move through the system, either through satisfaction of the act or by letting go of the feeling itself. Ongoing Desire for what one does not have or cannot attain creates a high degree of internalized Frustration. This Frustration is caused by that which is obstructing Desire's proper flow: in regards to gender and sexuality it is the *Li* of culture and any associated emotions of Fear, Trauma, Shame, Guilt, Secrecy, or Repression. Heat from Craving will rise along the *Bao Mai* to harass the Shen-Spirit, Heart, and Pericardium, with symptoms of Heart Fire or Heart Yin Deficiency–Empty Heat. Frustration of any type of movement, including Desire, will always impact the Wood Element and its associated organs, so symptoms of Liver Qi Constraint or Stagnation are commonplace even in acute conditions.

In chronic situations, the Wood system will certainly suffer because:

- Water Yin is injured by excessive Lower Jiao Heat and unable to nourish Wood

- excess Kidney Yang from the Lower Jiao (*Ming Men* Fire) brings excess Heat into the Wood system through both the Five Phase Cycle as well as the Liver Channel, and

- the frustration of overall movement impedes the Qi Mechanism and the capacity of the *Hun* to travel unencumbered.

Patterns of Liver Yang Rising and Liver Fire Blazing will easily develop, with increased libido, headaches and upper body tension (jaw, shoulders, temporal, etc.), red eyes, and mental unrest (irritability, outbursts of rage, etc.).

Once Craving is involved, *Ming Men* Fire will brew in the Lower Jiao and impact the Wood and Fire Elements just like in ongoing Desire, but it will also settle into the Stomach and other digestive organs as it tries – in vain – to 'satisfy' itself. The Stomach is especially vulnerable as the *Bao Mai* brings Heat directly past the Stomach on its way to the Heart and Pericardium. Symptoms of Craving include Heart and Liver patterns, along with mild to severe symptoms of Stomach Heat or Stomach Fire: excessive food cravings, excessive appetite, stomach ulcers, acid reflux, etc. Figure 14.2 shows the Heat of *Ming Men* Fire stirring in the Lower Jiao and flowing into these three primary target areas: the Liver, Heart, and Stomach.

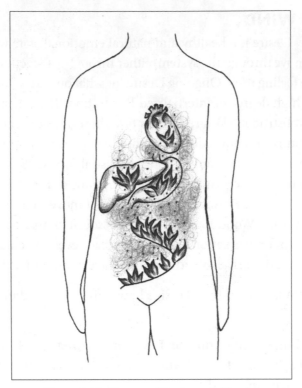

Figure 14.2: Flames of Desire and Craving

When Craving is allowed to 'run amok,' the *Ming Men* Fire will no longer be contained in the Lower *Dan Tian*. As Heat is merely another form of Qi, an uncontained *Ming Men* Fire will follow the mind's intention, increasing temperature in whatever system Desire is grasping at. For example, when Desire is related to sex or sexuality, the Heat in the Lower Jiao and genitals will become much more intense than when focused on material accumulations or career aspirations. In this case, Liver Yang Rising and Liver Fire Blazing symptoms from sexual Craving would be genital focused, with extreme libido, genital rashes or cysts, and increased incidence of herpes or other STI outbreaks. Kidney–Liver Yin (and Blood) Deficiency and Empty-Heat conditions are also expected as the excess Heat 'cooks' fluids in this area: symptoms of low back pain, insomnia, vaginal dryness or irritation, and early, scant menses are likely.

Excess Heat from an uncontained *Ming Men* Fire will deplete the general Yin Substances of the body, which in turn allows the Heat even greater and quicker movement throughout the system. The speed of movement will thwart the Mind's ability to focus and concentrate, allowing Craving to flit between various sources of attraction with little to no focus. The intensity of this unfocused movement combined with Craving's Heat easily stirs up Internal Wind. Manic emotional states, tics, tremors, dizziness/vertigo, and shaking with emotional release are some of the more common symptoms, all of which are likely to come and go with any associated increase or decrease in Desire. Figure 14.3 shows the flames of unanchored Heat whipping upwards to create Internal Wind.

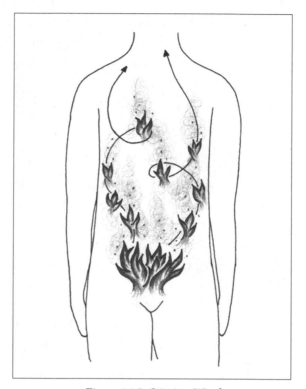

Figure 14.3: Stirring Wind

The Heat from chronically frustrated Desire or Craving settles into the 'area of attraction,' stirs up Internal Wind, and impacts all three Jiaos as follows:

- Lower – Kidneys, Liver Channel, genitals

- Middle – Liver, Gallbladder, Stomach

- Upper – Heart, Pericardium

COOLING THE FLAMES

One of the greatest challenges in treating Desire or Craving is that Heat easily feeds itself. Heat 'cooks' the Yin Substances, leading to Yin or Blood Deficiency, Blood Stasis, and Phlegm, which create Empty-Heat or Stagnation patterns that can promote the development of more Heat. Excess Heat conditions are more common in those with pre-existing Qi Stagnation, commonly due to underlying Repression, Secrecy, Shame, or Guilt. Deficient and Empty-Heat conditions are more common in individuals with pre-existing Yin or Blood Deficiency concerns due to overwork, Chronic Fear, extreme emotional stress, or a North–South Trauma pattern. Yin or Blood Deficiency may also develop in chronic states due to the depletion of fluids by Heat, because as with any disease, the more long-standing the condition the more likely it is to present as a mixed Excess–Deficiency pattern.

Mental rest is a critical component to repairing the Yin Substances, along with Herbs and Diet therapy. This includes the mental restraint already mentioned, as well as general stress reduction and the cultivation of a calm and peaceful existence away from personal and cultural triggers (i.e., advertising, capitalist-consumerism, pornography, etc.).

One potential obstacle, especially in colder climates, is that the Heat arising from *Ming Men* Fire makes many people feel 'more alive', which can contribute to resistance in changing one's underlying thoughts. Another obstacle is Shame (see Chapter 12), which often coincides with Desire or Craving either at the root of *Yuan*/Source Qi displacement (see 'The Creation of Yin Fire' box) or created by Phlegm obstruction as a result of Heat 'scorching' the fluids. Regardless of which emotion presented first, Craving and Shame will easily engender each other because of their interactions with Heat, Fluids, and Qi Stagnation. The TCM patterns commonly associated with Desire and Craving include:

- Heart: Fire, Yin Deficiency–Empty Heat

- Kidney: Yin Deficiency (with or without Empty Heat)

- Liver: Qi Constraint/Stagnation, Yang Rising, Fire Blazing, Damp-Heat, Yin or Blood Deficiency (with or without Empty Heat)

- Stomach: Heat/Fire

- Wind: Internal

- Yin Fire (see text box).

No matter where *Ming Men* Fire has spread, Herbal Formulae and Diet therapy are important to counteract the effects of Heat. Acupuncture can be extremely effective to anchor and contain the *Ming Men*, as well as move stagnation, disperse Wind, and clear Heat. As previously stated, Jeffrey Yuen (2017a) suggests Chong Mai points (Spleen 4, Spleen 12, etc.) to help rectify conditions related to *Li*.

The impact of *Li* upon one's Desires may also be reflected in the obstruction of sensory orifices, especially those that can visualize one's Desires (eyes, eyesight) or ask for them (throat, tongue, voice). Window to the Sky points may prove helpful in such cases. Acupuncture point selection, Herbal Formulae, and Diet recommendations must be customized for the unique presentation of organ involvement, the degree of Heat and Wind, and the depletion of Yin Substances. Some general suggestions are provided below.

- Treatment Principles: Clear Heat and Stagnation, Nourish Yin Substances, Subdue Wind, Anchor and contain *Ming Men* Fire.

Primary Modalities

- Acupuncture: HT 3, 6, 8, KI 1, 2, 10, LIV 2, 3, 8, GB 20, 21, 34, PC 6, 8, SP 10, ST 44, Ren 12, 15, 17, UB 14, 18, 19, 43, 47, 48, Du 14, 20 (directed inferiorly):

  - Du (SI 3–UB 62) and Ren Mai (LU 7–KI 6) to rectify Yin–Yang balance

  - Chong Mai points for conditions related to *Li*

  - Window to the Sky points for visual or throat obstruction.

- Herbal Formulae: Er Xian Wan, Huang Lian Jie Du Wan, Liu Wei Di Huang Wan, Long Dan Xie Gan Wan, Suan Zao Ren Wan, Tian Wang Bu Xin Wan, Yu Quan Wan, Zhen Gan Xi Feng Wan. *Note: These are just a few options; more than one formula is typically required.*

- Diet: Cooling (cucumber, lettuce, melon, peppermint, etc.) and Yin- or Blood-nourishing foods (asparagus, lemon, pear, pork, etc.); soups, steaming, and slow-cooking to preserve or enhance moisture.

- Lifestyle: Mental restraint, including reduction of triggers and cultivation of calmness; working toward realistic goals.

Secondary Modalities

- Essential Oils: Chamomile, Jasmine, Lavender, Lemon, Marjoram, Melissa, Orange, Rose, Sage, Valerian.

- Gemstones: Chrysocolla, Jet, Pearl, Spinel, Zircon.

- Affirmation: 'I am enough.'

Creation of Yin Fire

The traditional development of Yin Fire assumes a preceding condition of Kidney *Yuan*/Source Qi Deficiency brought on by a combination of improper diet, overwork, and lack of mental and physical rest. When *Ming Men* Fire is then stirred by Desire, it 'displaces' and further weakens the Yuan Qi to support itself, creating symptoms of Heat Above–Cold Below (red face, thirst, mouth ulcers, warmth in the chest or face, cold feet or below the waist, fatigue). Treatment of Yin Fire is counterintuitive to its name: the principles of draining Fire and nourishing Yin are inappropriate. Instead, one warms Yuan Qi while gently clearing Heat from *only* the Upper Jiao. Lifestyle changes to rebuild Kidney energy are combined with Acupuncture, Moxa, and Herbal Formulae as the primary treatment modalities. Giovanni Maciocia (2013, p.306) recommended the following Acupuncture treatment:

- Tonify the Original Qi: Ren 4.

- Lift Qi: Du 20, Ren 6.

- Clear Heat in the Upper part of the Body: PC 8, 7, LI 4, LU 7, Ren 15.

- Calm the Mind: Du 24, Du 19, HT 5.

- Regulate the San Jiao: SJ 5, 6.

Further, I personally recommend moxibustion or other Heat therapy on Ren 4, 6, Du 3, 4, and UB 31–43. Any Herbal Formulae must primarily support the Kidney energetics, with a secondary, symptom-based approach to clear Heat and regulate Qi. For example, using You Gui Wan or Jin Gui Shen Qi Wan with Jiao Wei Xiao Yao Wan or Tian Wang Bu Xin Wan.

Although a combination of improper diet, overwork, and lack of mental and physical rest continues to be a significant cause for Yuan Qi Deficiency and the subsequent development of Yin Fire from Desire, another important etiology to be aware of is Shame. In chronic Shame, Damp-Phlegm 'swamps' the entire Lower Jiao, *displacing – but not depleting –* the Yuan Qi. In this case there will be pronounced fatigue, but little-to-none of the constant cold that indicates Yuan Qi Deficiency or a true Heat Above–Cold Below pattern. Resolution of concurrent Shame and Desire is based on clearing Damp-Phlegm, moving Qi, and clearing stagnant Heat, while rectifying the San Jiao and the systemic balance of Fluids. The primary modalities include Acupuncture, Diet, and Herbal Formulae (which must again be used in combination; for example, Liu Jun Zi Wan or Bu Zhong Yi Qi Wan with Zhi Bai Di Huang Wan). Acupuncture may be able to rectify the Yuan Qi alone, but it is more likely that Medical Qigong will be required to properly address this aspect.

CLIENT EXAMPLE

A homosexual Latino male in his mid 50s presents with recurring genital HSV-1 lesions since his relocation to a rural, predominantly white, area over six months prior. The original HSV outbreak was over 20 years ago, and he'd only had one or two outbreaks annually for the past 15+ years. He also has neck and shoulder tension, vivid dreams, and a strong libido. He is a visual artist and former drag queen that is frustrated in his pursuit of a relationship. He admits to extreme loneliness, but talks loudly, rapidly, and laughs frequently. He is very thin and muscular. Pulse is tight, slightly rapid. Tongue is very long, dark red, and completely dry. He is diagnosed with Damp-Heat brewing in the Liver Channel, Liver and Heart Fire, and Heart–Liver–Kidney Yin Deficiency due to Craving. He is afraid of needles, and due to the presence of extreme Heat there is an increased risk of transference from Tuina or Medical Qigong. Therefore, (to clear patterns and manage latency) combined with flash and running Cupping (to clear away musculoskeletal tension) are the primary treatment modalities. The first course of herbs is two weeks on Huang Lian Jie Du Wan, Long Dan Xie Gan Wan, and Suan Zao Ren Wan. He reports a complete disappearance of herpes lesions and deeper sleep, but some remaining genital itching and prodromal pain at times. Herbs are changed to Chai Hu Long Gu Mu Li Wan, Suan Zao Ren Wan, and Tian Wang Bu Xin Wan for a one-month course. At his next appointment he reports the disappearance of genital itching, prodromal symptoms, and calm sleep. He is talking more slowly, softly, and has a new part-time job at a local LGBT-owned store to help him meet people and build community.

CLIENT EXAMPLE

A married heterosexual female in her mid 50s has been coming in for headaches, hot flashes, and emotional upset (Grief, Sadness, Anger) for six months. These symptoms began when an intense, four-month-long affair (with a married male cheating on his own wife) suddenly ended. In the course of that relationship, she discovered BDSM, realized her Dominant and polyamorous nature, and amicably opened her own marriage to pursue these interests. She has not yet found another lover or play-partner for her newfound kinks. Treatments to unwind Repression and Craving have targeted clearing Liver Qi Stagnation-Heat or Liver Yang Rising, while nourishing Liver–Kidney Yin. Symptoms have been improving, with relapses whenever she has contact with the former lover, even though she has been advised against seeing him. Two weeks ago she had plastic surgery to relocate fat deposits for a 'better' body shape and she wants assistance with fast post-surgical healing. Because of extensive swelling and leg edema, Medical Qigong is used to clear Heat and Blood Stasis in the bruised areas instead of Acupuncture. There is extreme Heat objectively felt over GB 30 (especially on the right), and at Ren 17. She is sent home with press beads on ST 36, KI 3, SP 9, and LI 11, with Jin Gu Die Shang Wan (internal) and Zheng Gu Shui (external) Herbal Formulae. She returns three weeks later with a chestnut-sized lump in her right breast that is distinct, hard, objectively hot, with a slight shadow on the skin. She is referred to her Primary Care Physician for urgent evaluation, and is diagnosed with a quick-growing, metastatic cancer. Her breast is removed a week later. *Note: It is assumed that the plastic surgery released more Repressed Heat from latency than could be properly processed. When combined with post-surgical Blood Stasis, Damp obstruction, and Qi Deficiency, along with the already present Qi Stagnation-Heat, Yang Rising, and Yin Deficiency, it created the ideal conditions for cancer to arise.*

SUMMARY

» Desire is an attraction to an experience or thing stimulated by touch, sight, sound, or emotion. Desire or Craving can be oriented toward sex, material objects, achievement of status or relationship. Desire is healthy and natural when it is allowed to arise, be satisfied, and resolve.

» Pathological Desire or Craving are forms of 'clinging,' tightly holding on to something with persistence, stubbornness, or unhealthy dependence. Buddhism, Confucianism, and Daoism each consider this the root of human suffering.

» Chronic states of Desire or Craving can arise on their own through lack of mindful self-control, or they can be created by other chronic states that obstruct Qi movement and increase Heat in the Lower Jiao, including Extraordinary Vessel damage (abuse, etc.), Fear, Shame, Guilt, Secrecy, and Repression.

» Craving is a more intense – *and always pathological* – version of Desire. Craving is a chronically unresolved, unsatisfied Desire that an individual maintains well beyond any reasonable period of time.

» Each of the Five Elements supports healthy sexual Desire. Wood is the element of *action*, providing direction and courage to engage and initiate. Fire is the element of *stability* in maintaining focused Desire over a period of time. Metal is the element of *guidance*, helping align Desire with reason, self-knowledge, and *Li*. Water is the element of *engagement*, providing the foundation for Desire and sexual energy. Earth is the element of *integration*, including acceptance of one's Desires (physical, emotional, and spiritual). It is also the element in charge of creating Post-Natal Qi, which provides the day-to-day energy that dictates one's ability to form Desire or to participate in sex.

» In a healthy state of sexual, intellectual, or spiritual Desire, the *Ming Men* Fire stirs the Jing-Essence and Yang aspect of Kidney energy. When Desire is frustrated, *Ming Men* Fire continues to stir the Lower Jiao, affecting the Kidneys and genitals. Thwarted from proper movement, Heat only continues to build, congealing Lower Jiao fluids until some of the Heat 'escapes' through the *Bao Mai* to the Heart, Pericardium and Middle Jiao organs (Liver/Gallbladder, Stomach, etc.).

» When chronic Craving is allowed to 'run amok', the *Ming Men* Fire will no longer be contained in the Lower *Dan Tian*. As Heat is merely another form of Qi, *Ming Men* Fire will follow the mind's intention, increasing temperature in whatever system Desire is grasping at while stirring up Internal Wind.

» One of the greatest challenges in treating Desire or Craving is that Heat easily feeds itself. It does so by 'cooking' the Yin Substances, leading to Yin or Blood Deficiency, Blood Stasis, and Phlegm, all of which create Empty-Heat or Stagnation patterns that can promote the development of more Heat.

» Mental rest, Herbal Formulae, and Diet are the most critical components to repairing the Yin Substances injured by Desire and Craving.

Chapter 15

DESCENT INTO DARKNESS
Self-Loathing and Suicide

- A Ray of Light: Hope

- Darkest Before the Dawn

- The Journey Home

When man's five viscera are diseased, they might be compared to conditions of thorns, stains, knots, or obstructions. Thorns, although embedded for a long time, still can be pulled out. Stains, although filthy for a long time, still can be washed away. Knots, although tied for a long time, still can be untied. Obstructions, although blocked for a long time, still can be opened up. Some people say chronic disease cannot be cured. This is speaking incorrectly. The skilful acupuncturist can take hold of the disease in the same way he pulls out thorns, washes out stains, unties knots, or breaches obstructions. Disease, although chronic, still can be ended. Those who say diseases are incurable have not mastered the technique of acupuncture.

– Ling Shu[1]

Self-Loathing and Suicidal Ideation are the darkest and heaviest of emotional states. They are conditions of hopelessness and stagnation, in which a blend of difficult and chronic emotional states are already at play. Energetically tapping into these conditions manifests thick, sticky, heavy, dense, black 'clouds' at the core of the body (see Figures 15.4 and 15.5). To get to this point, all Five Elements are likely suffering, but it is the Earth and Metal Elements that play dominant roles.

---

1   As quoted in Jing-Nuan 1993, p.5.

Earth corresponds to both Post-Heaven Qi and the human existence level of the Three Treasures (i.e., the blend of Earth and Heaven energies). The Earth Element is in charge of self-acceptance, and must be severely obstructed or depleted in order for Self-Loathing to develop. This is common with chronic, enduring Shame, where Dampness and Phlegm contribute to depletion and obstruction of the Spleen and the Qi Mechanism. Disgust with one's physical form – such as can occur with body dysmorphic disorder (BDD), history of sexual abuse, or desperate Craving to match un-attainable ideals – are all common pathways to Shame and Self-Loathing. Anger or Frustration towards one's self (emotional forms of Wood invading Earth) are also commonplace with Self-Loathing, typically due to Guilt or Repression from strict cultural upbringing. As Disgust is an emotional state that pertains to the Stomach, any Wood–Earth patterns from Anger or Frustration may focus on the Stomach, not the Spleen, with primary symptoms of belching and nausea along with other digestive and systemic concerns.

Supported by the self-acceptance of Earth, Metal mitigates the balance between personal beliefs and cultural or familial expectations (*Li*). When Earth cannot nourish Metal, one's ability to navigate this terrain will suffer and impact their approach to the lessons of the Nine Palaces. If Metal then stagnates for any reason, such as with the Grief of unfulfilled Desire or the Qi Stagnation of Repression, Self-Loathing can set in more easily. This is especially true for DGS individuals that must constantly 'find their center' – i.e., re-anchor to Earth, self-acceptance, and their own personal beliefs – under the constant onslaught of cultural oppression.

The Metal Element also corresponds to the Po, the aspect of *Wu Shen* that relates to the physical body and both physical and spiritual 'inspiration.' When Metal and its Po are damaged, unprocessed Grief or Sadness can overwhelm the system, obstructing inspiration and dramatically dimming the promise of Hope. Common causes of damage to the Po include emotional Shock and Trauma, especially with events that involved physical sensation and harm. East–West Axial Trauma breaks from extreme emotional stress can also damage any aspect of the *Wu Shen* – including the Po – when a history of childhood Trauma gets re-triggered by a new event. Regardless of the cause, if profound Sadness disrupts inspiration and overwhelms the promise of change, it becomes easy for Suicidal Ideation – *the Po's allowance of death* – to set in.

All Five Elements require treatment to successfully navigate this dark and heavy terrain, but Earth and Metal are at the top of the priority list for Self-Loathing or Suicidality. The interaction of self-acceptance and contentment (Earth Element) with inspiration and the soul of the body (Metal Element) must be fully supported with compassion and grace to re-ignite the spirit of Hope and foster permanent emotional change. Only once this stage has begun can the joy of Fire, the motivation of Water, and the courage of Wood take hold to guide the individual back to a state of true emotional health.

The impact of cultural oppression and the threat of physical violence in the creation of Suicidality cannot be underestimated. A 2016 USCDC report on Sexual Identity and other behaviors of teenage youth in the United States demonstrated that lesbian, gay, bisexual, and questioning youth were experiencing acts of violence and contemplating suicide at twice or more the rate of their heterosexual-identified peers, along with increased incidence of bullying and substance use (Kann *et al.* 2016, p.77). Areas of serious concern for increased risk included:

- Physical and sexual assault

- Not attending school because of personal safety concerns

- Feeling extremely sad or hopeless

- Considering suicide, making plans or attempting suicide.

It must be noted that rates of suicide and suicide attempts among transgender individuals are even worse, at three to four times that of the United States general population.

The role of Hope in diminishing these risks must not be underestimated: research published in 2017 showed a dramatic decrease in rates of contemplating and attempting suicide among LGBT youth in the individual US states that legalized same-sex marriage between 1999 and 2015, when the US Supreme Court eventually ruled same-sex marriage to be legal throughout the nation (Raifman *et al.* 2017).

A RAY OF LIGHT: HOPE

There are two very different definitions for the word 'hope.' The Hope that is needed to combat Self-Loathing or Suicidality is a powerful feeling of *trust* or *belief* in being 'on the path,' which aligns with the principles of Daoism and the Heavenly Contract. In this sense, Hope is about knowing who you are, enabling the ability to make choices in alignment with self-knowledge, self-acceptance, and having faith in this combination to support the process of one's journey. When this Hope is consistently cultivated, it is a brilliant and blinding white light that supports and bolsters the *Zheng*/Upright Qi of the entire system (see Figure 15.3). In cultures where Shame, Fear, and Guilt force people to conform to *Li*, the inner light of Hope must be consistently cultivated. For it is only when up against the intensity of Hope's light that the blackness of Self-Loathing or Suicidal Ideation are simply unable to take hold.

Translating Hope

The Chinese language offers a variety of character combinations that all mean 'hope.' Hope that combats Self-Loathing or Suicidal Ideation is best represented by Xìn Xīn, which translates as trust, faith, and confidence. It depicts a confidence or trust in one's own Heart center, placing self-reliance and self-acceptance at the forefront of cure.

信心   Xìn Xīn   Hope: confidence, faith, trust

The brilliant light of Hope results from proper alignment of the Three Treasures (Earth, Humankind, and Heaven) and the activation of the Taiji pole. Proper positioning of the Three Treasures relies upon the actualization of the authentic self, which is a combination of accepting the human form (Jing-Earth), who you are supposed to become (Shen-Heaven), and how or what to do in order to get there, as manifested through one's day-to-day actions (Qi-Humankind). Unfortunately, these are major life lessons that many people shirk away from, and in doing so they neglect the cultivation of internal Hope.

Each of the Five Elements and their corresponding aspect of *Wu Shen* are involved in cultivating Hope. Generation of Hope starts and ends at the center, with the Earth Element and Yi-Intellect manifesting self-acceptance and contentment in the midst of change. Each of the other Elements support Hope through various activities. Figure 15.1 shows this through the axial orientation of the Five Elements, with Metal offering inspiration and the ability to navigate *Li,* Water motivating the Will to enact Destiny, Wood providing the courage to face what must change, and Fire providing a sense of joy in each moment. In other words, when *Li* is not allowed to interfere with one's natural state of self-cultivation, the correct path of Destiny will be enforced in one's life, bringing Joy to nourish contentment and firmly establish a sense of self-acceptance. All of these are natural, uncontrived, 'effortless actions' akin to *Wu Wei* principles of 'non-effort' that enable Hope to flow forth without struggle.

Unfortunately, Hope wavers in the face of consistent oppression, such as endured by DGS individuals. It can simply become too difficult for any person to muster up the courage to 'face the demons,' demand better for one's self, or feel inspired again and again. Anytime one of the Five Elements suffers or the Qi Mechanism is obstructed, the Upright Qi may falter and true Hope can dim. This is where the more inferior definition of hope enters, where it is only a dim dream or aspiration for future results or events. Someone might hope to be noticed, or to get a new job, or that a family dinner will go smoothly. A DGS individual might hope their conservative family will accept them, or that being seen at a public BDSM event won't negatively impact their career. When we look underneath this interpretation of hope, the etiological root is in Water, where it merely serves to neutralize Fear.

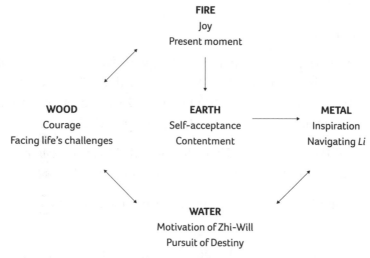

Figure 15.1: The Elements of Hope

In mild hopelessness, where there is lack of self-acceptance or an acute sense of extreme Grief, but no long-standing Self-Loathing or any form of Suicidal Ideation, the trust, belief, and intense light of true Hope can be easily kindled with Chinese Medicine.

Stabilizing Hope

Treatment to stabilize Hope is a form of 'Destiny Work,' where Heaven and Earth energies are realigned through the human form, using the Chong Mai and the Taiji pole that travel through the center. The following treatment suggestions are useful for those experiencing mild hopelessness, but are also a maintenance program for those that have been to the darkest place and are firmly on the way back. Care must be exercised to not overtreat and cause further damage to the Chong Mai or Taiji pole, which occurs more commonly with Acupuncture than other modalities. In a 2017 lecture on doing harm with Acupuncture, Jeffrey Yuen specified that injury to Kidney 6 (which is used to access both the Ren and Yin Qiao Mai) could lead to faltering self-esteem and potential for suicidality; *extreme caution should therefore be used if considering this acupoint.*

As 'Stabilizing Hope' is a purely Spirit-level treatment, needle technique must be gentle, or can be replaced by Essential Oils, Gemstones, Moxabustion, or Medical Qigong. 'Bach Flower Remedies' (internal or external application) are also appropriate to foster internal radiance.

- Treatment Principles: Rectify the Five Elements, Harmonize the Three Treasures and the Micro-cosmic Orbit (Taiji pole, Chong, Ren, and Du Channels).

- Acupuncture:

  - Three Treasures: *Jing*–Ren 3, 4, 6, with KI 14, also Du 3, 4, UB 23, 52 (with Moxa); *Qi*–Ren 11, 12, 13 with ST 21, also ST 36, UB 20, 21; *Shen*–Ren 15, 17, 19/20 with KI 23/24 (or anywhere along the sternum), also UB 14, 15, 43, 44, Yintang, Du 24

  - Taiji Pole activation: KI 1, Ren 8–with Moxa (or combine Ren 7, 9, Kidney 16), Du 20; *all points can be done with Moxa treatment*

  - Chong Mai (SP 4–LV 3–PC 6) or points along the channel (ST 30, SP 12, etc.)

  - Ren Mai (Lu 7–KI 6), Ren 2, 3, 4, 6, 10, 12, 15, 17, 22 (palpate for flaccidity) – *middle and lower Jiao points can be treated with Moxa if cold or flaccid*

  - Du Mai (SI 3–UB 62), Du 2, 3, 4, 5–12 (palpate for stickiness), Du 13, 14, 15, 20.

- Medical Qigong:

  - Stimulate each *Dan Tian* individually with touch, light, color, sound, and/or intention

  - 'Holding the Three *Dan Tian*' with vision of an internal column of bright white light connecting them (i.e., the Taiji pole).

- Gemstones : Dioptase, Opal (Pink Andean, Rainbow), Sodalite, Sunstone, Unakite.

- Qigong: Five Healing Sounds; Five Healing Colors; Microcosmic Orbit; Taiji Meditation.

- Bach Flower Remedies: Elm–Ren 8, Honeysuckle–LU 3, Larch–SJ 15, Mimulus–KI 24, 25, Olive–UB 42–44, Rock Rose–Ren 4, Sweet Chestnut–Du 1, Wild Rose–Du 10, 11 (Craydon and Bellows 2005).

- Affirmation: 'I belong.'

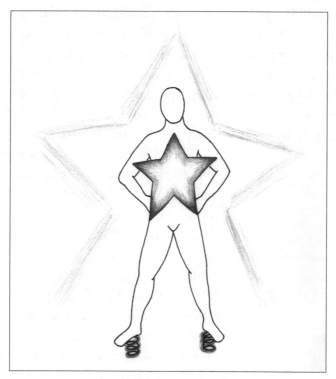

Figure 15.2: The Shape of Pride

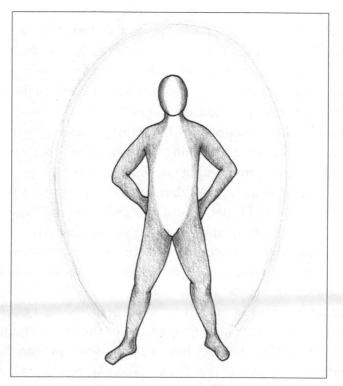

Figure 15.3: The Shape of Hope

DARKEST BEFORE THE DAWN

Self-Loathing and Suicidal Ideation both present as heavy blackness near the core of the body. In Self-Loathing, this darkness is located in the Middle and Upper Jiaos only, impacting the Earth, Metal, and Fire Elements (see Figure 15.4). The Earth Element is at the root of this condition, as it fosters self-acceptance. Self-acceptance is adversely impacted by any Earth deficiency or obstruction, such as Spleen Qi Deficiency, Qi Fall, or Damp-Phlegm in the Middle Jiao, but is not typically impacted by a pure excess Earth condition like Stomach Fire.

Metal is the child of Earth, so will surely suffer from any Earth pathology. The Grief and Sadness one experiences with loss of self-acceptance, or the chronic emotional pain of a restrictive culture that limits authenticity can both injure Metal. Metal can also deplete its 'mother' and foster the development of Shame when self-destructive behaviors that injure the Po are allowed to take root.

Regardless of initial etiology, the black cloud of Self-Loathing starts within Earth and Metal, but will quickly spread to Fire. Fire organs manage all emotions, but Fire is also Earth's 'mother' and Metal's Upper Jiao partner in the formation of *Zong*/Chest Qi, so there are multiple routes to Fire involvement. The depletion of Earth and Metal will put too much of a burden on Fire leading to decreased capacity to experience of Joy as well as limited ability to process all emotions. Eventually, the individual will feel emotionally numb with no sense of happiness, leading to reduction in physical sensation as well.

A wide array of conditions can manifest from the combination of inability to self-accept, self-destruction of the Po, and physical and emotional numbness. These include eating disorders and anorexia, body dysmorphic disorder, and alterations to one's flesh (i.e., cutting, flesh binding, genital stapling, etc.). As a practitioner, one must be acutely aware of the energetic difference between healthy kink practices such as branding, cutting, waist binding, or genital alteration and any form of self-infected physical damage caused by Self-Loathing. Those using kink for sexual arousal and exploration will still have an intact sense of self-acceptance, along with Pride and Hope radiating from within (see Figures 15.2 and 15.3).

In order to develop the depth of darkness associated with Suicidal Ideation (see Figure 15.5), all Five Elements must now be involved. First, self-acceptance (Earth), inspiration (Metal), and Joy (Fire) are consumed by Self-Loathing. Second, lack of self-confidence depletes the courage of Wood, leaving the individual unable to face life's challenges or pursue spiritual growth. Between lack of courage and loss of inspiration, the Will of Water will fail, and the individual will arrest their own pursuit of Destiny. Over time, the light of Hope (i.e., the radiance of the Taiji pole and the alignment of the Three Treasures) will be *extinguished*. The sufferer will not have a strong sense of who they are (Jing-Essence-Earth), who they are meant to be (Shen-Spirit-Heaven), or how to get there (Qi-Emotion-Humankind), creating a state of extreme hopelessness.

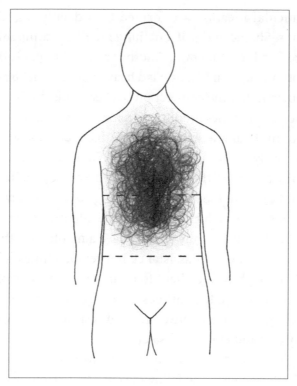

Figure 15.4: Blackening Clouds – The Shape of Self-Loathing

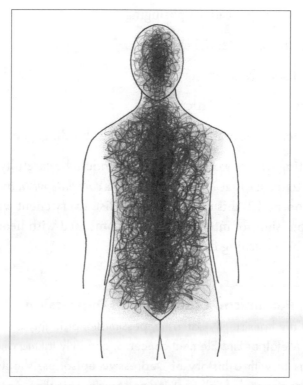

Figure 15.5: Descent into Darkness – The Shape of Suicidality

The roots of Suicidal Ideation are formed by a deeply ingrained medley of difficult emotions. Shame and Self-Loathing are likely companions as both are related to severe Earth dysfunction. Another reason Shame is likely involved is due its heavy nature; Suicidal Ideation is a heavier state than Self-Loathing alone. Giovanni Maciocia noted the connection between cultural Shame and Suicide, stating, 'Shame can sometimes produce extreme circumstances, as when Japanese businessmen commit suicide when they are disgraced socially' (2013, p.297). Other emotions likely at play include Guilt or Trauma, which contribute Blood Stasis to the dark nature of the condition, and Secrecy or Repression, which contribute Bound Qi from the inability to change or move forward.

As practitioners, we are lucky when clients identify their own issues with suicide. These clients will typically already have a mental health professional on their team, or have sought this assistance in previous times of crisis. If we are diving in deeply enough with a client to clear away the roots of suicidality, the risk of short-lived 'dips' into the darkness – lasting a few hours or days – is high. Requiring the client to see a licensed mental health professional is critical to ensure their physical and emotional safety.

Unfortunately, many clients do not realize that their emotions are putting them in a high-risk category. The following concerns strongly correlate with the presence of Self-Loathing or Suicidal Ideation:

- Repressive, conservative upbringing

- Hopelessness, existential crisis

- Eating disorders, anorexia

- Body dysmorphic disorder

- Flesh alterations: branding, cutting, waist binding, genital alteration.

Clients presenting with any of these concerns should be carefully monitored, but it is important to realize that 1) these conditions *correlate with, but do not indicate* Suicidal Ideation, and 2) this is an incomplete list. Every client will have a unique presentation, but signs of internal darkness combined with heavy self-criticism should always be a warning flag.

Sarcasm, Pessimism, Criticism, and Depression

Clients that are consistently sarcastic, pessimistic, or highly critical of others, with Earth, Metal, or Fire Element concerns, currently taking anti-depressant medications or with a history of Depressive episodes, should be closely monitored for potential of Self-Loathing and Suicidal Ideation. As Leon Hammer wrote, 'Negativity is a perfect cultural medium for *depression*... Underneath are feelings of worthlessness, self-depreciation, inadequacy, and low self-esteem' (2005, p.156).

THE JOURNEY HOME

The most important act of healing is meeting a client exactly 'where they are at,' without judgment or platitudes. This is especially important for clients suffering from Self-Loathing or Suicidality, as their family, friends, and community have likely already uttered every version of 'But you are so pretty – smart – kind... Your family loves you... I'll miss you... You are being so selfish.' Instead, we must provide objective and empathetic emotional support without question, criticism, or adding to the burden of *Li*.

As Leon Hammer wrote, clients come to us 'for our ability to recognize the positive quest for contact beneath the negative emotions and behavior; this need is especially great for those who have already come to disdain themselves' (2005, p.156). Considering this quest for connection, the following statements may prove more helpful:

- I am sorry this weighs on you like this.

- I am here to help.

- Please let my eyes offer another vision of the world.

Learning Self-Love

To combat Self-Loathing, treatment is always focused on strengthening Fire, Earth, and Metal, along with dispersing the darkness near the core and fostering a sense of Hope. Disease will be found in the corresponding organs and tissues, so various physical symptoms may present. Heavy and unforgiving self-criticism is also likely, which is often masked by laughter or sarcasm. Through the energetic exchange of the client–practitioner relationship, we can help clients change their mindset by consistently bringing positivity and Hope to the treatment room. Areas of pathology and their associated symptoms include the following:

- Fire: Heart, Pericardium, Blood Vessels, Tongue, Shen-Spirit – anxiety, insomnia, palpitations, difficulty finding words/stuttering.

- Earth: Spleen, Stomach, Pancreas, Muscles, Mouth, Yi-Intellect – eating disorders, digestive difficulties, diabetes Type II, heavy physical sensations, prolapse, gum and teeth concerns, difficulty concentrating.

- Metal: Lung, Large Intestine, Skin, Nose, Po-'Body' – respiratory/sinus concerns, frequent colds/immune system insufficiency, irregular bowel movements, eczema, cutting or other abuse of the flesh.

- Treatment Principles: Harmonize Fire–Earth–Metal Elements, Clear Obstructions, 'Lift' Qi (i.e., promote Joy, self-acceptance, and inspiration).

Primary Modalities

- Acupuncture:

  - Earth–Fire–Metal: UB 13, 14, 15, 20, 21, 22, 23, 25, 42, 43, 44, 49, 50, 51; ST 36, SP 3, 6, 9, HT 3, 5, 6, 7, PC 6, LU 1, 2, 3, 4, 5, 7–9

  - Clear Obstructions: this must be individually evaluated for channel or organ issues, underlying emotions causing obstructive patterns, etc.

  - Lift Qi: LI 10, Du 20, Sishencong (directed upward); Moxabustion on ST 36, Ren 4, 6, 8; needle from feet to head in general.

- Herbal Formulae: Si Jun Zi Wan, Nu Ke Ba Zhen Wan, Yu Ping Feng San Wan, Gui Pi Wan, Bu Zhong Yi Qi Wan.

- Medical Qigong:

  - 'Clearing Darkness from the Spirit' – counterclockwise rotations at the spirit level; 'sword finger' may be used for thick obstruction

  - 'Holding the Three *Dan Tian*' with vision of an internal column of bright white light connecting them (i.e., the Taiji pole).

- Affirmation: 'I am loveable, deserving, and special.'

Secondary Modalities

- Qigong: Wuji Pose–standing or moving; Hun Yuan Gong–Opening and Closing Heaven and Earth; Sheng Zhen Qigong: Heart Spirit as One/Jesus Sitting, Releasing the Heart/Mohammed Standing – Pure Heart Descends.

- Bach Flower Remedies: Agrimony–PC 6, Cerato–HT 7, Cherry Plum–Du 14, Crab Apple–LI 18, Gentian–KI 21–23, Gorse–LI 14, Hornbeam–UB 1, 67, Mustard–KI 20–21, Pine–LU 1, Rock Water–Ren 15, Wild Rose–Du 10, 11 (Craydon and Bellows 2005).

- Gemstones: Diamond, Green Aventurine, Hemimorphite, Meteorite, Moldavite, Rose Quartz, Ruby, Snowflake Obsidian, Tektite, Turquoise.

Letting Light Shine

Treatment for Suicidal Ideation is more complex, as all Five Elements are now involved, interrupting the Qi Mechanism, the San Jiao, the Three Treasures, and the Taiji Pole. The Chong Mai is worth mentioning again in this chapter, for in Medical Qigong theory it correlates to the Taiji pole and can be used to help clear the darkness from all three Jiaos, especially if there is underlying Guilt or Blood Stasis.

Multiple emotions are involved at the root of Suicidality, so one must look for the emotions and patterns involved to guide individual treatment. Shame, Guilt, and a history of Trauma are likely, with their accompanying Dampness/Phlegm, Blood Stasis, and axial breaks. Qi Stagnation is always present with Suicidality due to the disruption of the Generating Sequence and the Qi Mechanism, so Repression or Secrecy may be more difficult to discern. Suicidality is a chronic condition with a 'cloud of darkness' that hides the root condition, so it will take time to identify and treat each aspect of the etiology.

Individuals can live with Self-Loathing and mild forms of Suicidality for a long time, perhaps not even knowing how close they are to the edge. Regardless of the individual's level of awareness, the involvement of multiple emotions and patterns allow complex, 'knotty' diseases to form, including auto-immune conditions and severe organ damage. Once true Suicidality has entered the conscious level, it can take years to come back from, with multiple relapses – *even if for only a few seconds at a time* – into dark thought patterns. Deconstruction of inappropriate belief structures that lie at the root of emotional stressors, and the conscious choice to live an authentic life without Shame, Secrecy, or the denial of Desire holding an individual back, are all critical for full recovery. This may require drastic life changes, such as physically moving to another, more accepting location, or cutting off contact with one's family-of-origin. When attempting to rise fully out of the darkness, there are three ingredients that must also not be ignored: mental health counseling, exercise and/or meditation, and long-term maintenance of self-care.

- Typical Presentation: Multiple-system health concerns, auto-immune diseases, cancer.

- Treatment Principles: Support and nurture the Five Elements and the generating sequence, Harmonize the Qi Mechanism, the San Jiao, the Three Treasures, and the Taiji pole. *Note: Other Treatment Principles will be dictated by the accompanying emotions.*

- Primary Modalities: Acupuncture, Medical Qigong, Qigong, Gemstones, Bach Flower Remedies, Affirmations.

- Secondary Modalities: Herbal Formulae, Tuina or other bodywork.

- Lifestyle: Individualized and long-term self-care routines are critical for effective resolution, including mental health counseling and exercise or meditation.

- Affirmations: 'I am grateful for all that I have.'

CLIENT EXAMPLE

A female aged 16 presents with a recent diagnosis of Depression after she was found cutting her inner thighs. She was already referred to a psychiatrist and is being evaluated for medication. The client also experiences anxiety, insomnia, environmental allergies, and generalized physical fatigue. Her complexion is very pale, with thick, dark, shiny hair. She has a slight 'hump' on her upper back from slouching forward. Her menses is 30–32 days, deep red, clotted, with cramps. Her tongue is pale, thin, slightly dry, and curled under at the tip. Her pulse is thin and weak overall, extremely frail in both front positions. She is diagnosed with Spleen and Lung Qi Deficiency, Heart Blood Deficiency, and Blood Stasis due to Self-Loathing and Repression. She is treated with Acupuncture (ST 36, SP 6, Ren 6, 12 – all with Moxa; LV 3, GB 34, HT 6, PC 6, Yintang), and tumbled Gemstones (Bloodstone, Malachite, Rose Quartz, Tiger Eye – placed bilaterally on Lao Gong). After treatment, her pulses are much stronger, but now also wiry and slightly rapid. She is given a six-month course of Jia Wei Xiao Yao Wan and Nu Ke Ba Zhen Wan in conjunction with bi-weekly or monthly treatments. She is also instructed to wear Gemstone bracelets each day (selected from the list above). At three months of treatment the menstrual cycle has stabilized, her energy, sleep, and anxiety are markedly improved, pulses are stronger but still thin, and the tongue is no longer pale or dry, but still curled under. Herbal Formulae are continued, but reduced to 'as needed.' *Note: After one year of Chinese Medicine treatment, in conjunction with talk therapy and psychiatric medication, the client revealed they were pansexual, gender-queer/non-binary, and kink-oriented.*

CLIENT EXAMPLE

A queer, married female in her late 30s presents with post-partum PTSD and Suicidal Ideation after a medication allergy and hypovolemic shock almost killed both her and her child during delivery six months prior. The near-death experience PTSD re-triggered PTSD from childhood sexual abuse. She is experiencing multiple flashbacks daily, with extreme Fear, overwhelming Sadness and Guilt about lack of breast milk, and Shame regarding bonding difficulties. She also has extreme pain and numbness near the surgical scar. She is already working with her long-time mental health therapist, massage, craniosacral, and shiatsu practitioners. Her tongue is swollen, pale, peeled and orange on the sides, dry center, thin red tip. Pulse is slippery, wiry, forceful, and weak, with no rear pulses on either side. She is diagnosed with Blood, Yin and Qi Deficiency, Spleen and Kidney Deficiency, Damp-Phlegm, Blood Stasis, Metal Disharmony, and Restless Spirit. Treatment uses a blend of weekly Acupuncture and Medical Qigong treatment, with daily Herbal Formulae, Diet recommendations, and mild exercise/movement (stretching and short walks). Overall emphasis is on Herbal Formulae (Nu Ke Ba Zhen Wan with Tian Wang Bu Xin Wan) and Diet (Blood and Qi strengthening with Damp-Phlegm clearing) to stabilize the Shen as quickly as possible.

Blood, Qi, Earth, Metal, and Water stabilized within three to four months: she now experiences more positive mood, no nightmares, limited flashbacks, and 'moments of complete normality.' Her menses has also returned, bringing 'an overwhelming flood of emotion' with bleeding. As her body got stronger, a new emotion appeared: Anger, with outbursts of rage. The next phase of treatment focused on East–West Trauma (from the recent adult-onset near-death experience), and North–South Trauma (from the childhood abuse), while clearing Blood Stasis from both the Uterus and Heart. She continued with therapy, bodywork, weekly Acupuncture, and Qigong exercises at home (Gathering the Rice; Hun Yuan Gong–Grinding the Corn; Daoist Napping/ Shao Yin Circulation; Qi Circulation/Tai Yang Circulation), but the principal treatment modality remained Herbal Formulae, alternating a combination of Tian Wang Bu Xin Wan and Liu Jun Zi Wan for days 1–14 of the menstrual cycle, and Xue Fu Zhu Yu Wan with Chai Hu Long Gu Mu Li Wan for days 15–28. She also had other formulas to manage symptoms: Pe Min Kan Wan for seasonal allergies, Er Chen Wan for occasional respiratory and digestive Phlegm that only appeared with increased humidity, and Bi Xie Sheng Shi Wan for extreme bloating at ovulation. After another four months, Anger flared only when she spoke about the medical mistake, and 'mood drops' were now only with extreme fatigue and stress. Through therapy she uncovered 'pools of Self-Loathing and Shame' from the sex abuse, so Gemstones were added to the protocol (Amethyst, Carnelian, Coral, Hematite, Yellow Jade, Snowflake and Black Obsidian, Tiger Eye, Sunstone). Within two more months of treatment she found a physical therapist that specialized in pelvic floor damage, and dramatically reduced her work hours in order to focus on her family and prevent relapses. Due to cost issues, Acupuncture, massage, and shiatsu were reduced to bi-weekly or monthly, but therapy, Qigong, Gemstones and Herbal Formulae remained consistent, except for minor changes based on season or symptoms.

At three years' post-birth, she said it felt 'like a veil lifted.' Ruby and Unakite were added to support the ongoing cultivation of Hope, and treatment focus shifted to address prevention of relapse and occasional health concerns (seasonal changes, allergies, digestion, headaches, menstrual irregularities, etc.). *Note: Unlike post-partum Anxiety or Depression, post-partum (PP) PTSD's recovery time-frame averages three to five years. One explanation is the pre-existing Trauma and/or extreme life stressors that are statistically consistent in the PP-PTSD population. Making sure a client with PP-PTSD has strong emotional and community support throughout this entire recovery period is critical not only to the success of treatment, but also to their very survival.*

SUMMARY

» Self-Loathing and Suicidal Ideation are conditions of hopelessness and stagnation, where difficult and chronic emotional states are already at play, manifesting as thick, sticky, heavy, dense, black 'clouds' at the core of the body.

» Hope is a powerful feeling of *trust* or *belief* in knowing who you are, granting the ability to make choices in alignment with self-knowledge, self-acceptance, and faith in the process of one's own journey.

» Hope results from the activation of the Taiji pole, which is based in proper alignment of the Three Treasures (Earth, Humankind, and Heaven). Positioning the Three Treasures relies upon the actualization of the authentic self, through a combination of accepting the human form (Jing-Earth), who you are supposed to become (Shen-Heaven), and how or what to do in order to get there, as manifested through one's day-to-day actions (Qi-Humankind).

» In the face of consistent oppression, anytime one of the Five Elements suffers or the Qi Mechanism is obstructed, the Upright Qi may falter and Hope can dim. To cultivate Hope, Metal offers inspiration and the ability to navigate *Li*, Water motivates the Will to enact Destiny, Wood provides the courage to face what must change, Fire provides a sense of joy in each moment, and Earth manifests self-acceptance and contentment in the midst of change.

» In the development of Self-Loathing and Suicidal Ideation, it is the Earth and Metal Elements that play dominant roles.

» Earth must be severely obstructed or depleted for self-acceptance to wane, which is common with the Dampness and Phlegm associated with chronic, enduring Shame. The etiology of Earth dysfunction may also include Disgust with one's physical form, or Anger and Frustration towards one's self (Wood invading Earth) due to Guilt or Repression.

» When Earth cannot nourish Metal, the ability to navigate personal and cultural beliefs will suffer, especially for DGS individuals under the constant onslaught of cultural oppression. When Metal stagnates, Self-Loathing can set in more easily. If Sadness disrupts Metal's inspiration and overwhelms the promise of change, Suicidal Ideation – *the Po's allowance of death* – can set in.

» The darkness of Self-Loathing is located in the Middle and Upper Jiao. It starts within Earth and Metal, but will quickly spread to Fire. Due to the impact on Fire and Metal, the individual suffering from Self-Loathing will eventually feel emotionally numb, with no sense of happiness and a reduction in physical sensation. To combat Self-Loathing, treatment is always focused on strengthening Fire, Earth, and Metal, along with dispersing the darkness near the core and fostering a sense of Hope.

» There are distinct energetic differences between healthy kink practices of branding, cutting, waist binding, and genital alteration, versus those due to Self-Loathing. Those using kink for sexual arousal and exploration will still have self-acceptance, Pride, and Hope radiating from within (also see Chapter 9).

» In the depth of darkness that precedes Suicidal Ideation, the sufferer will have lost the sense of who they are (Jing-Essence-Earth), who they are meant to be (Shen-Spirit-Heaven), or how to get there (Qi-Emotion-Humankind). If chronic, the alignment of the Three Treasures and radiance of the Taiji pole will eventually be extinguished, creating a state of extreme hopelessness where all Five Elements are suffering.

» Suicidal Ideation is formed by a deeply ingrained medley of emotion. Shame and Self-Loathing are likely companions as both are related to severe Earth dysfunction. Other emotions likely at play include Guilt or Trauma, which contribute Blood Stasis, and Secrecy or Repression, which contribute Bound Qi.

» Signs of internal darkness – heavy self criticism or criticism of others, sarcasm, and pessimism – combined with Earth, Metal, or Fire Element concerns, anti-depressant medications or a history of Depressive episodes, should be closely monitored for potential of Self-Loathing and Suicidal Ideation.

» The most important act of healing for Self-Loathing and Suicidal Ideation is meeting a client exactly 'where they are at,' without judgment or platitudes. Deconstruction of inappropriate belief structures that lie at the root of emotional stressors, and the conscious choice to live an authentic life without holding back are both critical for full recovery. The importance of long-term self-care and periods of mental health counseling cannot be overemphasized.

Five Element Chart

	Wood	Fire	Earth	Metal	Water
Yin organ(s)	Liver	Heart Pericardium	Spleen (Pancreas)	Lung	Kidney
Yang organ(s)	Gallbladder	Small Intestine San Jiao	Stomach	Large Intestine	Urinary Bladder
Color	Green	Red	Yellow	White	Blue-Black
Sound	Shouting	Laughing	Singing	Crying	Groaning
Emotion(s)	Anger	Joy	Pensiveness	Sadness and Worry	Fear
Taste	Sour	Bitter	Sweet	Pungent	Salty
Sense organ	Eyes	Tongue	Mouth	Nose	Ears
Body tissue	Sinews	(Blood) Vessels	Muscles	Skin	Bones
Climate/EPF	Wind	Heat	Damp	Dry	Cold
Season	Spring	Summer	Late Summer	Fall	Winter
Compass direction	East	South	Center	West	North
Development	Birth	Growth	Transformation	Harvest	Storage
Spirit *Wu Shen*	Hun	Shen	Yi	Po	Zhi
	Wood	**Fire**	**Earth**	**Metal**	**Water**

Emotion Chart

This chart is included for quick reference of the material only, and is not meant to serve as a 'one size fits all' diagnostic tool.

Emotion	Primary Pathology	Location	Associated Emotions
Fear	Channel Stagnation Reduced Movement	Above Diaphragm Liver, Heart, Kidneys	Trauma, Shame, Guilt, Craving, Self-Loathing
Trauma			
Indirect	Blood Deficiency	Heart	Emotional stress
Complex	Blood Stasis and/or Phlegm	Heart	More severe stress
North–South Axis	*Varied*	Heart, Kidney	Anxiety, Fear
		Spleen/Stomach	Worry, Shame
East–West Axis	*Varied*	Liver/Gallbladder, Lungs/Large Intestine	Anger, Sadness
		Spleen/Stomach	Worry, Guilt
San Jiao and Wei Qi	Fluid Stasis (Dampness, Phlegm) Poor 'boundaries'	*Systemic & Varied*	Emotional immaturity Elevated environmental sensitivity
Guilt	Blood Stasis	Middle and Lower Jiao	Secrecy, Repression
Shame	Phlegm	Lower Jiao	Self-Loathing, Fear
Secrecy and Lying	Qi Stagnation and Heat	Kidneys, Throat Liver, Heart, San Jiao Spleen/Stomach	Primary: Fear Secondary: Guilt, Shame, Desire, Craving
Repression	Qi Stagnation and 'Bound' Heat	Bone level, Deep 'necks,' *systemic*	Passive-Aggression, Self-Loathing

cont.

Emotion	Primary Pathology	Location	Associated Emotions
Desire	Heat	Heart, Liver	Anxiety, Irritability
Craving	Heat/Fire Wind Yin Substances	Heart, Liver, Stomach (Kidneys)	Fear, Trauma, Shame, Guilt, Secrecy, Repression
Self-Loathing	Dark, Heavy Earth, Metal, Fire	Middle and Upper Jiao	Shame, Disgust, Anger, Frustration
Suicidal Ideation	Darker, Heavier All Five Elements	San Jiao Three Treasures Taiji pole	Shame, Self-Loathing, Sadness, Guilt, Trauma, Secrecy, Repression

Qigong Exercises

This list is provided as a guide to those unfamiliar with the Qigong Exercises recommended in this book, but it is not meant to teach the practice of Qigong. Learning Qigong takes time, patience, and personal growth, and is best done with the guidance of an experienced instructor. As noted in Chapter 2, I have personally abandoned all sex-based rules (hand positioning, directional flow, etc.) in my practice and teaching of Qigong. I have consistently found that personal comfort while practicing is always more important for an individual's physical, emotional, and spiritual health than 'following the rules.'

Many of these exercises are available via internet sites or detailed in other source materials. The primary published sources used in this book are Ken Cohen's *The Way of Qigong,* Jerry Alan Johnson's *Chinese Medical Qigong Theory: A Comprehensive Classical Text,* and Jun Feng Li's *Sheng Zhen Wuji Yuan Gong,* as noted in the list of forms below. Qigong exercises without any written or internet source material come from my original Qigong teachers, Master 'Luke' Chang-Shin Jih, Donna Price, or Nate Summers, to whom I am indebted for their compassion and expertise. There are also a few movements I have personally developed, practiced, and taught for many years. After twenty years of practicing, I can only hope I have honored my teachers and the tradition of Qigong by translating these movements well.

- Abdominal Round-Rubbing: Johnson, 'Circling the Abdomen,' pp.706–707.

- Buddhist Greeting – *seated form*: Johnson, pp.319–320; similar to Cohen's 'The Meditating Buddha,' p.195.

- Butterfly Form: From a wide stance, inhaling as arms slowly lift at the sides of the body over the head until the back of the palms almost touch. Exhaling, arms slowly fall at the sides of the body as the knees bend deeply. Arms cross (one slightly on top of the other) in front of the lower abdomen at the end of the exhale. Repeat 6–24 times, with arms alternating the cross each time. End by exhaling without bending the knees, allowing arms to settle at the sides of the body into Wuji posture. *Caution: When done quickly, this is an intense cardiovascular exercise.*

- Combing the Hair: From Wuji posture, inhaling as one arm crosses in front of the body bringing the palm toward the opposite ear. Without touching the head, bring the palm over that side of the head, then as far back as one can comfortably reach. At the maximum point of circle and breath, the palm turns away from the body before the arm sinks back to the side of the body on the exhale. This is all done in one fluid circular movement. Repeat 6–18 times for each arm, either one at a time, or alternating back-and-forth. *Note: Can also be performed in 'bow' stance.*

- Daoist Napping/Shao Yin Circulation: Lying on one's back, with small pillows for head and knee propping to support the spine as needed. The left palm rests on Ren 4–6. The right palm rests on Ren 17, the Front Mu of the Pericardium. Pillows are used to prop the arms into place. Breathing deeply into the lower abdomen, one can rest quietly in this pose for 10 or more minutes. *Caution: This posture will raise the Qi, so it is best done in the morning or afternoon, not at night.*

- Eight Brocades–Archer: An old form of Qigong, with many variations. Cohen's 'Open the Bow as Though Shooting the Buzzard' is found on pp.186–188.

- Five Dragons Beat the Drum: Using the tips of all ten fingers, gently tapping over the entire chest area to break up stagnations.

- Five Breaths to Dawn: In a wide stance facing eastward in the early morning, the right hand forms a gentle fist in front of Ren 4–6, cupped from below by the left hand. Five deep inhalations bring the energy of dawn's light into the Lower *Dan Tian*. When finished, palms turn to lie flat for a moment at Ren 8 – one crossed over the other – before they slowly separate to settle at the sides of the body.

- Five Healing Sounds: An old form of Qigong, with many variations. Cohen's 'The Six Qi Method' can be found on pp.165–166; Johnson's 'Six Healing Sound Prescriptions' is found on pp.660–665.

- Five Healing Colors: An old form of Qigong, with many variations. Cohen's 'Colored Light Meditation' can be found on pp.167–168.

- Five Animal Frolics–Bear, Crane: An old form of Qigong, with many variations. Cohen's can be found on pp.199–209.

- Gathering the Rice: From a wide stance, inhaling as elbows bend, allowing palms to face upward, fingertips toward each other, rising in front of the body from lower abdomen to shoulder height. Exhaling, palms turn to face outward, expanding/pushing Qi out and away from the sides of the body at shoulder height. *(Repeat from here.)* Inhaling, palms turn to face the body, drawing Qi inward to the width of the shoulder joints. Exhaling, palms turn to face forward as the waist bends and the arms open wide and go down as far as possible with palms turning to face each other. Inhaling, arms move toward each other to 'scoop' Qi from the Earth. Still inhaling, palms turn to face upward, fingertips toward each other, rising in front of the body from the ground to the navel. As the breath shifts, palms turn to face the body. Exhaling, palms turn away from the body as they rotate upward to face Heaven, fingertips point toward each other as palms push toward the sky. Inhaling, palms separate and arms open wide to the sides of the body at shoulder height, with palms facing out and fingertips up toward Heaven. Continuing to inhale, elbows bend and palms soften, allowing hands to return to shoulder width. Exhaling, palms turn to face outward, expanding/pushing Qi out and away from the sides of the body at shoulder height again. Repeat 6–18 times. End by inhaling as palms turn to face forward and then down; exhale as elbows relax and arms settle to the sides of the body.

- Golden Rooster Shakes his Feathers: A four-step movement from either shoulder-width or wide stance. Breath is natural throughout all movements. 1) Elbows are bent at shoulder height with fingertips toward Heaven. Hands quickly rotate side to side, shaking the wrists and arms. Continue for 30–90 seconds, then slowly stop. 2) Arms are down at the sides of the body with elbows bent and hands forward. Use the combined force of the arms and waist to twist the pelvis and hips back and forth quickly, shaking the buttocks, thighs, and back. Continue for 30–90 seconds, then slowly stop. 3) Arms are loose at the sides of the body. Quickly lift one heel at a time, bending the knees, shaking the entirety of both legs. Continue for 30–90 seconds, then slowly stop. 4) Starting with movement 1, add in each movement together, without stopping. Once all three movements are being performed simultaneously, continue for 30–90 seconds, and then slowly stop. *Note: This is very dispersive to the Qi. Resettle Qi back to the Lower* Dan Tian *before continuing one's practice.*

- *Hun Yuan Gong:* Although not an old form, there are still many variations:

  - Descending the Yang, Ascending the Yin: Johnson, pp.691–693.

  - Grinding the Corn: *Beginner:* From a wide stance with relaxed arms at the sides, shift the weight side to side and back to front while drawing a horizontal figure 8 with the perineal floor. Specifically, start with weight on the right leg, rotating the pelvis and weight forward on the right foot, before crossing the weight over to the back side of the left leg. Rotate the pelvis and weight forward on the left leg, before crossing the weight over to the back side of the right leg. Repeat 6–18 times. *Intermediate:* Same leg movements, but with palms facing the ground, fingertips toward each other at the level of Ren 4–8. The palms will remain facing down at all times. As the weight rotates on the right foot, the hands circle outward from the body, palms still facing down. As the weight crosses to the opposite leg, the palms are at their furthest circular point from the body, but centered to the midline/navel. As the weight shifts fully to the left leg, palms continue their wide circle to the left, then come in toward the lower abdomen. As the weight shifts to the right leg, the palms pass close in front of the body. Repeat this counterclockwise circling 6–18 times before changing direction to a clockwise circle. *Note: The leg movements do not change. One always starts with weight placed on the back of a leg before moving to the front of that same side. (Similar to Johnson, 'Turning and Winding the Belt Vessel', pp.693–695.)*

  - Holding the three *Dan Tian:* Shoulder-width stance. Breathing is natural and deep into the Lower Jiao for 6–18 breaths per position. Palms face each other, slightly turned toward the body, approximately 6–8 inches apart in five different positions: in front of Ren 4–6; in front of Ren 12–14; in front of Yintang; again in front of Ren 12–14; ending in front of Ren 4–6. *Note: Always end in the Lower* Dan Tian.

  - Opening and Closing Heaven and Earth: From a wide stance, body weight and central pole are shifted to the right leg. Palms face each other, slightly turned toward the body, approximately 6–8 inches apart in front of Ren 4–6. *(Repeat from here.)* Inhaling, palms continue to face each other as body weight shifts to the left leg and extended arms rise in front of the midline of the body all the way over the head above Du 20. As the breath shifts from inhale to exhale, palms turn away from each other over Du 20. Exhaling, the arms open and fall to the sides of the body as the body weight shifts back to the right leg. As the breath shifts from exhale to inhale, the palms turn to face each other again at Ren 4–6. Repeat 6–12 times, and then *reverse*: Palms face each other, slightly turned toward the body, approximately 6–8 inches apart in front of Ren 4–6. Inhaling, body weight shifts to the left leg as the arms open and palms face up, rising at the sides of the body all the way over the head until the palms face each other, approximately 6–8 inches apart over Du 20. Exhaling, body weight shifts to the right leg as the palms retain their position while the extended arms fall in front of the midline to the level of Ren 4–6. Repeat 6–12 times. End by bringing palms down to Ren 4–6, then slowly separating them to the sides as weight shifts to balance on both legs equally. (Similar to Johnson, pp.695–696.)

- Opening and Closing the Lower *Dan Tian*: From a wide stance, body weight and central pole are shifted to the right leg. Palms face each other, slightly turned toward the body, approximately 6–8 inches apart in front of Ren 4–6. Inhaling, palms continue to face each other as body weight shifts to the left leg and arms open at the sides to hip height. Exhaling, weight shifts back to the right leg as arms and palms return to the original position. Repeat 6–18 times. *Optional: As hands come toward each other on inhalation lift the perineum; relax again on exhalation. (Similar to Johnson, pp.687–689.)*

- Opening and Closing the Three *Dan Tian*: Starting with 'Opening and Closing the Lower *Dan Tian*,' perform this same side-to-side movement with hands at the five positions mentioned in 'Holding the three *Dan Tian*.' in front of Ren 4–6; in front of Ren 12–14; in front of Yintang; again in front of Ren 12–14; ending in front of Ren 4–6. (Similar to Johnson, 'Opening and Closing the Upper, Middle, and Lower Burners,' pp.687–689.)

- Microcosmic Orbit: Johnson, pp.678–681.

- Passing Clouds: From a shoulder-width Wuji stance with arms at the sides. *Beginner:* Inhaling, palm facing the body, the right arm crosses in front of the body to the height of the left shoulder joint while weight subtly shifts to the left leg. At the shift of the breath, the right palm crosses in front of the throat as body weight shifts to center. Exhaling, the right arm extends fully out to the right side at shoulder height while weight shifts to the right leg, then the arm slowly drops, palm facing down, to the side of the body. Repeat 6–18 times, then do the same for the left arm. *Intermediate:* Alternate the arms back-and forth so that as one arm is extending out to the side, the other is crossing the body. *Note: Beginner form can also be performed in 'bow' stance.*

- Pounding and Scrubbing: An old form of Qigong self-massage, with many variations. The basics are to hold a loose fist and gently tap on Acupuncture points and channels to disperse stagnations. Johnson outlines this clearly in 'Massage Tapping,' pp.702–706:

  - Gallbladder Channel: Fingertip tapping or scrubbing along the temporal region of the head, followed by vigorous rubbing of GB 20, and individual pounding of GB 21. Then simultaneous pounding on GB 30 before bending the waist to pound downward along both iliotibial bands and outer sides of the calf region, following the Gallbladder Channel. End by sweeping off the tops of the feet from ankles (GB 40) to the toes

  - Yang Channels (upper body): Fingertip tapping or scrubbing along the temporal, occipital, vertex, and forehead, followed by tapping/pounding on GB 20, SJ 15, LI 16, LI 11–9, and LI 4. Follow by scrubbing or 'wiping' both outer arms.

- Qi Circulation/Tai Yang Circulation: Lying on one's back, with pillows under the knees to lengthen the spine and soften the lumbar area. Palms face down near the sides, with armpits open, elbows softly bent, and scapula gently pulled apart. Breathing deeply into the lower abdomen, one can rest quietly in this pose for 10 or more minutes. *Caution: This posture is cooling, so use a blanket!*

- Qi Pouring/Pouring Qi: From a wide stance with knees bent, start with weight and center of the body in one leg. The 'weight-side' arm is elbow bent with palm face up at hip-to-waist height. The other palm rests over the first, facing each other with 4–8 inches between. Inhale as legs lift the body, weight shifts to the center, and the top palm rises to a level just above the head, but still in front of the body. Exhaling, weight continues to shift to the opposite side and knees soften as the top palm comes to rest face up at waist-to-hip height position. Simultaneously, the former bottom palm rises over the head to settle with palms facing each other again (4–8 inches between). Repeat side-to-side, 6–18 times per side.

- Rotating the Sun and Moon: Johnson, pp.689–691.

- Sheng Zhen Qigong: A modern form of Qigong[1]:

---

1   See www.shengzhen.org.

- Heart Spirit as One/Jesus Sitting: Li, pp.76–85

- Heaven Nature/Kuan Yin Standing–Boat Rowing in the Stream of Air, Traveling Eastward Across the Ocean (movement 1 and 2): Li, pp.53–57

- Releasing the Heart/Mohammed Standing–Pure Heart Descends (movement 9): Li, pp.158–159.

- Sinking the Turbid and Washing the Organs: Johnson, 'Descend the Qi and Cleanse the Organs,' pp.682–684.

- Silk-Reeling Qigong: An old form of Qigong that focuses on clockwise and counterclockwise rotations of all the joints (neck, shoulders, elbows, wrists, hips, knees, ankles, etc.) to clear the 'spaces' and allow Qi to flow freely. Both 'Combing the Hair' and 'Winding the Silken Thread' are variations of Silk-Reeling.

- Taiji Meditation: Typically done in a seated position, but can also be done lying or standing. While breathing deeply and slowly into the Lower *Dan Tian,* focus is placed on visualizing an internal column of bright white light inter-connecting the three *Dan Tian* from the pelvic floor (Ren 1– Du 1) to Du 20. *Note: It may be easier to focus on one area at a time (i.e., lower, middle, then upper* Dan Tian*) before attempting the entire pole.*

- Warrior Attendant – *seated form*: Johnson, pp.319–320.

- Winding the Silken Thread: From a 'bow' stance (where weight can shift back-and-forth between the legs on a slight angle), breathing is natural into the lower *Dan Tian.* The same arm as the forward leg rises up to shoulder height. The hand begins to rotate on the wrist in one direction. This movement gets larger until the three arm joints (wrist, elbow, shoulder) are all in rotation, allowing the body weight to gently shift back and forth with the motion. Repeat 6–18 times, then reverse direction, starting again just from the wrist. Change legs in the bow stance, and repeat both directions for the opposite arm.

- Wuji Pose – *standing*: The most basic standing pose of Qigong, described in Cohen, 'The Posture of Power,' pp.86–96, and 'Standing Like a Tree,' pp.133–143, as well as in Johnson 'The Eighteen Rules of Proper Medical Qigong Structure,' pp.321–330.

- Wuji Pose – *moving*: Starting from Wuji posture, inhale as the wrists gently glide forward, allowing the weight to shift subtly forward on the feet and the fingers drag behind the hands as though creating trails in the air. Exhale as the wrists move gently backward, slightly behind the buttocks, allowing the weight to shift subtly to the heels (without lifting the toes). Always lead the arm movements by the wrists, not the fingers. Repeat, back-and-forth for 12–36 passes. To end, decrease the degree of forward and back movement on each pass until the physical body reaches stillness. *Note: This is a good alternative to Wuji standing for those with too much stagnation to be still for even short periods of time.*

Bibliography

Abbate, S. (2001) 'A Simplified Approach to the Treatment of Scars with Oriental Medicine.' *Acupuncture Today 2*, 11. Accessed on October 19, 2018 at www.acupuncturetoday.com/mpacms/at/article.php?id=27842.

Aaron, M. (2016) 'Analysis: How the AASECT Sex Addiction Statement Was Created: An insider's perspective of AASECT's sex addiction statement.' *Psychology Today*, Nov 30. Accessed on September 25, 2018 at www.psychologytoday.com/us/blog/standard-deviations/201611/analysis-how-the-aasect-sex-addiction-statement-was-created.

American Association of Sexuality Educators, Counselors and Therapists (AASECT) (n.d.) 'AASECT Position on Sex Addiction.' Accessed on September 25, 2018 at www.aasect.org/position-sex-addiction.

Baum, I. (2018) 'Sexual Fantasies You Might Have That Are Totally Normal.' *Popsugar*. Accessed on October 19, 2018 at www.popsugar.com/love/Common-Sexual-Fantasies-44150552.

Blackless, M., Charuvastra, A., Derryck, A., Fausto-Sterling, A., Lauzanne, K., and Lee, E. (2000) 'How Sexually Dimorphic Are We? Review and Synthesis.' *American Journal of Human Biology 12*, 151–166. Accessed on October 16, 2018 at https://pdfs.semanticscholar.org/f7c9/37560ae809fd8046adaac73827a9f5f8968a.pdf.

Bornstein, K. (1994) *Gender Outlaw: On Men, Women, and the Rest of Us*. New York: Vintage Books.

Borresen, K. (2018) 'Six Of The Most Common Sexual Fantasies, According To Sex Therapists.' *Huffington Post*. Accessed on October 19, 2018 at www.huffpost.com/entry/common-sexual-fantasies_n_5ae20d7ee4b02baed1b80971.

Brennet, N. (2017) *We Belong*. Flaming Dame Records.

Brown, B. (2010) *The Gift of Imperfection: Let Go of Who You Think You're Supposed to Be and Embrace Who You Are*. Center City, MN: Hazelden.

Brown, B. (2012a) *Daring Greatly: How the Courage to Be Vulnerable Transforms the Way We Live, Love, Parent, and Lead*. New York: Gotham Books.

Brown, B. (2012b) 'TED2012 lecture: Listening to Shame.' Accessed on February 19, 2019 at www.youtube.com/watch?v=psN1DORYYV0.

Cecil-Sterman, A. (2012) *Advanced Acupuncture: A Clinic Manual*. New York: Classical Wellness Press.

Chengnan, S. (ed.) and Qiliang, W. (trans.) (2000) *Chinese Bodywork: A Complete Manual of Chinese Therapeutic Massage*. Berkeley, CA: Pacific View Press.

Ching, N.T. (2016) 'Chinese Medicine from a Queer Perspective.' May 5, 2016. 47th International TCM Kongress in Rothenburg, May 3–7, 2016.

Cohen, K.S. (1997) *The Way of Qigong: The Art and Science of Chinese Energy Healing*. New York: Ballantine Books.

Colapinto, J. (2000) *As Nature Made Him: The Boy Who Was Raised as a Girl*. New York: HarperCollins Publishers.

CPS, TASHRA, and NCSF (2017) 'Addiction to Sex and/or Pornography: A Position Statement from the Center for Positive Sexuality (CPS), The Alternative Sexualities Health Research Alliance (TASHRA), and the National Coalition for Sexual Freedom (NCSF).' *Journal of Positive Sexuality 3*, 40–44.

Craydon, D. and Bellows, W. (2005) *Floral Acupuncture: Applying the Flower Essences of Dr. Bach to Acupuncture Sites.* Berkeley, CA: The Crossing Press.

Davidson, M.R. (2012) *A Nurse's Guide to Women's Mental Health.* New York: Springer Publishing Company.

Diemer, E., Grant, J., Munn-Chernoff, M., Patterson, D., and Duncan, A. (2015) 'Gender Identity, Sexual Orientation, and Eating Related Pathology in a National Sample of College Students.' *Journal of Adolescent Health 57*, 2, 144–149.

Doyle, K. (2015) 'Sexual Orientation, Gender Identity Tied to Eating Disorder Risk.' Accessed on October 19, 2018 at www.reuters.com/article/us-eating-disorder-gender-idUSKBN0NT2E020150508.

Easton, D. and Hardy, J.W. (2009) *The Ethical Slut: A Practical Guide to Polyamory, Open Relationships, and Other Adventures* (Second Edition). Berkeley, CA: Celestial Arts.

Eno, R. (2018) 'The Analects of Confucius: An Online Teaching Translation. Version 2.21.' Accessed on October 26, 2018 at www.indiana.edu/%7Ep374/Analects_of_Confucius_(Eno-2015).pdf.

Feng, G-F. and English, J. (1972) *Lao Tsu: Tao Te Ching.* New York: Random House.

Fernando, G. (2018) 'Sydney dominatrix Mistress Tokyo opens up about things she'll never do.' Accessed on October 19, 2018 at www.news.com.au/lifestyle/relationships/sex/sydney-dominatrix-mistress-tokyo-opens-up-about-things-shell-never-do/news-story/ae1bfb871a6cbb0fb7e37d2bd5ebeddf.

Flaws, B. and Sionneau, P. (2001) *The Treatment of Modern Western Medical Diseases with Chinese Medicine: A Textbook and Clinical Manual.* Boulder, CO: Blue Poppy Press.

Franks, L.J. (2016) *Stone Medicine: A Chinese Medical Guide to Healing with Gems and Minerals.* Rochester, VT: Healing Arts Press.

Furth, C. (1999) *A Flourishing Yin: Gender in China's Medical History 960–1665.* Berkeley, CA: University of California Press.

Gerson, M.N. (2015) 'BDSM Versus the DSM: A history of the fight that got kink de-classified as mental illness.' *The Atlantic.* Accessed on October 19, 2018 at www.theatlantic.com/health/archive/2015/01/bdsm-versus-the-dsm/384138.

Hammer, L. (2005) *Dragon Rises, Red Bird Flies: Psychology and Chinese Medicine* (Revised Edition). Seattle, WA: Eastland Press, Inc.

Hicks, A., Hicks, J., and Mole, P. (2011) *Five Element Constitutional Acupuncture* (Second Edition). Edinburgh: Churchill Livingston.

Holman, CT (2018) *Treating Emotional Trauma with Chinese Medicine: Integrated Diagnostic and Treatment Strategies.* London: Singing Dragon.

hooks, b., Salzberg, S., and Mcleod, M. (2017) *The Power of Real Love: A Conversation with Sharon Salzberg and bell hooks.* New York: Jewish Community Centre. Accessed on September 6, 2018 at www.lionsroar.com/the-power-of-real-love.

Jarrett, L.S. (2001) *Nourishing Destiny: The Inner Tradition of Chinese Medicine.* Stockbridge, MA: Spirit Path Press.

Jing-Nuan, W. (trans.) (1993) *Ling Shu or The Spiritual Pivot.* Honolulu, HI: University of Hawai'i Press.

Johnson, J.A. (2000) *Chinese Medical Qigong Therapy: A Comprehensive Clinical Text.* Pacific Grove, CA: The International Institute of Medical Qigong.

Kann, L., Olsen, E.O., McManus, T., *et al.* (2016) 'Sexual Identity, Sex of Sexual Contacts, and Health-Related Behaviors Among Students in Grades 9–12 – United States and Selected Sites, 2015.' *Center of Disease Control: Morbidity and Mortality Weekly Report (MMWR), Surveillance Summaries 65,* 9.

Kaptchuk, T. (1983) *The Web That Has No Weaver.* New York: Contemporary Books.

Killerman, S. (2013) 'Understanding the Complexities of Gender: Sam Killerman at TEDxUofIChicago.' Accessed on July 26, 2018 at www.youtube.com/watch?v=NRcPXtqdKjE.

Kinkly (n.d.) 'Cutting Fetish.' Accessed on October 19, 2018 at www.kinkly.com/definition/10737/cutting-fetish.

Leggett, D. (1994) *Helping Ourselves: A Guide to Traditional Chinese Food Energetics.* Totnes: Meridian Press.

Li, J.F. (2004) *Sheng Zhen Wuji Yuan Gong – A Return to Oneness: Qigong of Unconditional Love.* Twin Lakes, WI: Lotus Press.

Maciocia, G. (2005) *The Foundations of Chinese Medicine: A Comprehensive Text for Acupuncturists and Herbalists* (Second Edition). Edinburgh: Churchill Livingston.

Maciocia, G. (2013) *The Practice of Chinese Medicine: The Treatment of Disease with Acupuncture and Chinese Herbs* (Second Edition). Edinburgh: Churchill Livingston.

MacEowen, F. (2002) *The Mist-Filled Path: Celtic Wisdom for Exiles, Wanderers, and Seekers.* Novato, CA: New World Library.

Maclean, W. (2017) 'The Primary Pathological Triad.' *Mayway Mailer,* August. Accessed on February 19, 2018 at www.mayway.com/pdfs/maywaymailers/Mailers_2017/Mayway_Mailer_August_2017/Maclean-Pathological-Triad-Article-2017.pdf.

Maclean, W. and Taylor, K. (2016) *Clinical Manual of Chinese Herbal Patent Medicines* (Third Edition). Sydney: Pangolin Press.

Matsumoto, K. and Birch, S. (1986) *Extraordinary Vessels.* Brookline, MA: Paradigm Publications.

Moses, G. (2009) 'Queer Poetics: How to Make Love to a Trans Person.' Accessed on February 19, 2019 at http://wildgender.com/queer-poetics-how-to-make-love-to-a-trans-person/2401.

Myss, C. (n.d.) 'Three Popular Ways of Avoiding Powerful Guidance.' Carolyn's Blog. Accessed on June 9, 2018 at www.myss.com/three-popular-ways-avoiding-powerful-guidance.

Nhat Hanh, Thich (2014) *No Mud, No Lotus.* Berkeley, CA: Parallax Press.

Newell, J. (2011) 'Translation & Commentary by Gu Shen Yu.' *Old Oak Taiji School,* October. Accessed on July 11, 2019 at http://oldoakdao.org/yahoo_site_admin/assets/docs/Dao_De_Jing_Chapter_42.1230151.pdf.

Parkin, J.C. (2014) *fuck it: the ultimate spiritual way* (Revised Edition). Carlsbad, CA: Hay House, Inc.

Raifman, J., Moscoe, E., Austin, B., and McConnell, M. (2017) 'Difference-in-Differences Analysis of the Association Between State Same-Sex Marriage Policies and Adolescent Suicide Attempts.' *JAMA Pediatrics 171,* 4, 350–356.

Rekink (2018) 'List Of Fetishes And List Of Kinks And Terminology.' Accessed on October 19, 2018 at https://rekink.com/guides/kinks.

Rosen, R. (2018) *Heart Shock: Diagnosis and Treatment of Trauma with Shen-Hammer and Classical Chinese Medicine.* London: Singing Dragon.

Sommers, E. and Porter, K.E. (2003a) 'The Dance of Yin and Yang: Transgender Health, Part One.' *Acupuncture Today 4,* 5.

Sommers, E. and Porter, K.E. (2003b) 'The Dance of Yin and Yang: Transgender Health, Part Two.' *Acupuncture Today 4,* 8.

Sumedho, A. (2011) *The Four Noble Truths*. Hemel Hempstead: Amaravati Publications.

Taormino, T. (2008) *Opening Up: A Guide to Creating and Sustaining Open Relationships*. San Francisco, CA: Cleis Press.

Taormino, T. (ed.) (2012) *The Ultimate Guide to Kink: BDSM, Role Play, and the Erotic Edge*. Berkeley, CA: Cleis Press.

Twain, M. (1984) *The Innocents Abroad, Roughing It*. New York: Literary Classics of the United States.

United Nations (n.d.) 'Intersex Factsheet.' Free and Equal United Nations for LGBT Equality. Accessed on October 16, 2018 at https://unfe.org/system/unfe-65-Intersex_Factsheet_ENGLISH.pdf.

Yuen, J.C. (2002) *Materia Medica of Essential Oils: Based on a Chinese Medical Perspective*. Los Angeles, CA: Lotus Center for Integrative Medicine.

Yuen, J. (2017a) 'Essential Oils for Common Pediatric Conditions.' American University of Complementary Medicine, Los Angeles, CA, Presented September 22, 2017.

Yuen, J. (2017b) 'When Acupuncture Can Be Harmful,' Lecture at the American University of Complementary Medicine, Los Angeles, CA, Presented May 7, 2017.

Wilms, S. (2018) *Humming with Elephants: The Great Treatise on the Resonant Manifestations of Yin and Yang – A Translation and Discussion of Chapter Five of the Yellow Emperor's Inner Classic Plain Questions*. Whidbey Island, WA: Happy Goat Productions.

Index